Maturation Phenomenon in Cerebral Ischemia III

Springer

Berlin
Heidelberg
New York
Barcelona
Budapest
Hong Kong
London
Milan
Paris
Singapore
Tokyo

U. Ito · C. Fieschi · F. Orzi · T. Kuroiwa
I. Klatzo (Eds.)

Maturation Phenomenon in Cerebral Ischemia III

Defensive Mechanisms Versus Apoptosis

Neuronal Recovery and Protection in Cerebral Infarction

Third International Workshop, April 20–22, 1998, Pozzili, Italy
Istituto Neurologico Mediterraneo „Neuromed",
Pozzilli (Isernia), Italy

With 67 Figures, some in Color, and 20 Tables

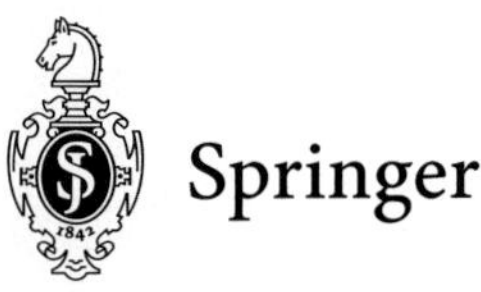 Springer

UMEO ITO
Musashino Red Cross Hospital
Department of Neurosurgery
1-26-1 Kyonan-cho, Musashino-shi
Tokyo 180, Japan

CESARE FIESCHI
Università di Roma "La Sapienza"
Dipartimenti di Scienze Neurologiche
Viale dell'University 30
00185 Roma, Italy

FRANCESCO ORZI
Istituto Neurologico Mediterraneo
NEUROMED Research Laboratories
Via Atinense 18
86077 Pozzilli (Isernia), Italy

TOSHIHIKO KUROIWA
Tokyo Medical and Dental University
Department of Neuropathology
Medical Research Institute
1-5-45 Yushima, Bunkyo-ku
113 Tokyo, Japan

IGOR KLATZO
National Institutes of Health
Laboratory of Neuropathology
and Neuroanatomical Sciences, NINDS
Bethesda, MD 20892-4128, USA

Third International Workshop, April 20–22, 1998
Istituto Neurologico Mediterraneo "Neuromed", Pozzilli (Isernia), Italy
Chairmen: C. Fieschi and U. Ito. **Cochairmen:** F. Orzi and T. Kuroiwa
Secretaries: U. Ito (general), F. Otzi (local)
International Advisory Board: A. Baethmann, N. G. Bazan, D. W. Choi, K.-A. Hossmann, T. Kirino, I. Klatzo, K. Kogure, J. Krieglstein, F. Plum, F. R. Sharp, M. Tomita and T. Wieloch
Local Organizers: F. Orzi, V. Colangelo, R. Di Grezia, G. Sette
Secretariats: I) General: Department of Neurosurgery, Musashino Red Cross Hospital, 1-26-1 Kyonan-cho, Musashino-shi. Tokyo 180, Japan, Tel: +81-422-32-3111, Fax: +81-422-32-9551, e-mail: umeo-ito@po.iijnet.or.jp 2) Local: INM Neuromed, Via Atinense 18, 86077 Pozzilli (IS), Ital. Tel: +39-865-915266/91521, Fax: +39-865-927575, e-mail: forzi@tin.it

ISBN 3-540-65023-7 Springer-Verlag Berlin Heidelberg New York

Library of Congress Cataloging-in-Publication Data.
Maturation phenomenon in cerebral ischema III: defensive mechanisms versus apoptosis neuronal recovery and protection in cerebral infarction / U. Ito ... [et al.] (eds.) New York : Springer, 1999. p. cm. RC388.5.M3632 1999 616.8/1 21. 3540650237 (softcover). Proceedings of the 3rd International Symposium on Matuation Phenomenon in Cerebral Ischemia, held in Pozilly Italy in April 1998. Includes bibliographical references and index. Cerebral ischemia – Pathophysiology – Congresses. Cerebral ischemia – Molecular aspects – Congresses. Apoptosis – Congresses. Neuroplasticity – Congresses. Nervous system – Regeneration – Congresses. Ito, U. (Umeo) International Symposium on Maturation Phenomenon in Cerebral Ischemia (3rd : 1998 : Pozilly, Italy). 98044835

Production: PRO EDIT GmbH, Heidelberg
Cover design: Design & Production GmbH, Heidelberg
Typesetting: Mitterweger Werksatz GmbH, Plankstadt
SPIN: 10663915   19/3133 – 5 4 3 2 1 0 – Printed on acid-free paper

Preface

The Maturation Phenomenon, described by Ito et al. in 1975 [3] on the basis of histological observations in the hippocampus as well as other portions of the cerebral hemisphere, refers to the hours or days of delay in the development of pathological changes in various parameters of ischemic injury following the restoration of blood flow to the ischemic brain. There is a direct relationship between the intensity of ischemic insult and the speed and rate of maturation of ischemic injury, a lesser intensity being associated with slower and less severe development of the lesions. The delayed neuronal death of CA1 pyramidal cells of the hippocampus [8] is a classic example. In the cerebral cortex, with increasing intensity of the ischemic insult, the maturation phenomenon of ischemic injuries intensifies, seamlessly, from less extensive to more extensive disseminated selective neuronal necrosis (DSNN), and then further to cerebral infarction upon reaching a critical threshold [1, 2, 4, 6, 7]. We also have found that following ischemic insults just under the threshold level required to induce infarction, only disseminated selective neuronal necrosis (DSNN) progresses, while following ischemic insults at the threshold level, initially only DSNN develops, followed by the evolution of a gradually enlarging infarcted focus [5, 7].

The reporting of this phenomenon boosted research in the field, as it became evident that ischemic damage is not a sudden event, but a process potentially susceptible to therapeutic intervention. Since then a growing number of studies have improved our knowledge regarding the mechanisms of cell death and recovery following this event. In September 1990, at the first international symposium on "Maturation Phenomenon in Cerebral Ischemia" in Tokyo, the nature and mechanisms of the phenomenon were discussed. The second symposium was organized in Tokyo in March-April 1996, with the subtitle "Neuronal Recovery and Plasticity". New development, particularly in the field of molecular biology, have been rapidly yielding information on the molecular nature and the dynamics of mechanisms of cell death and recovery.

It can be assumed that the Maturation Phenomenon represents a continuing struggle between the acceleration of tissue or neuronal death and the activation of defensive mechanisms leading to neuronal recovery. The elucidation of these mechanisms is important for developing the ability to manipulate them during a long-lasting "therapeutic window". This volume presents the third international symposium held in Pozzilli, Italy in April 1998, with the subtile. "Defensive Mechanisms Versus Apoptosis and/or Necrosis, Neuronal Recovery and Protection in Cerebral Infarction." The book outlines the present status of investigations and provides further stimulation for research in this field.

The focus is on the elucidation of (1) genetic expression and neuronal apoptosis and/or necrosis in cerebral ischemia, (2) factors and mechanisms enhancing susceptibility or tolerance (growth factors, etc.) in cerebral ischemia, (3) factors modulating neuronal plasticity and the course of maturation phenomenon (metabolic and inflammatory factors) in cerebral ischemia, and (4) ischemic infarction: threshold, experimental and clinical dynamics, and therapeutic designs for the prevention or reduction of its intensity.

December, 1998   Umeo Ito and coeditors

References

1. Hanyu, S, Ito U, Hakamata Y, Yoshida M (1995) Transition from ischemic neuronal necrosis to infarction in repeated ischemia. Brain Res 686:44–48
2. Hanyu S, Ito U, Hakamata Y, Nakano I (1997) Topographical analysis of cortical neuronal loss associated with dissemenated selective neuronal necrosis and infarction after repeated ischemia. Brain Res 767:154–157
3. Ito U, Spatz M, Walker J Jr, Klatzo I (1975) Experimental cerebral ischemia in mongolian gerbils. I. Light microscopic observations. Acta Neuropathol (Berl) 32:209–223
4. Ito U, Yamaguchi T, Tomita H, Tone O, Shishido T, Hayashi H, Yoshida M (1992) Maturation phenomenon of ischemic injuries observed in Mongolian gerbils: introductory remarks. In: Ito U, Kirino T, Kuroiwa T, Klatzo I (eds) Maturation phenomenon in cerebral ischemia I. Springer, Berlin Heidelberg New York, pp 1–13
5. Ito U, Hanyu S, Hakamata Y, Nakamura, M, Arima K (1996) Ultrastructure of astrocytes associates with progressing selective neuronal death or impending infarction after repeated ischemia. In: Krieglstein J (ed) Pharmacology of cerebral ischemia. Medpharm, Stuttgart, pp 385–392
6. Ito U, Hanyu S, Hakamata Y, Kuroiwa T, Yoshida M (1997) Features and threshold of infarct development in ischemic maturation phenomenon. In: Ito U, Kirino T, Kuroiwa T, Klatzo I (eds) Maturation phenomenon in cerebral ischemia II. Springer, Berlin Heidelberg New York, pp 115–121
7. Ito U, Hanyu S, Hakamata Y, Arima K, Oyanagi K, Kuroiwa T, Nakano I (1999) Temporal profile of cortical injury following ischemic insult just below and at the threshold level for induction of infarction–light and electron microscopic study. In: Ito U, Fieschi C, Orzi F, Kuroiwa T, Klatzo I (eds) Maturation phenomenon in cerebral ischemia III. Springer, Berlin, Heidelberg New York (this volume)
8. Kirino T (1982) Delayed neuronal death in the gerbil hippocampus following ischemia. Brain Res 239:57–69

Contents

I Role of Genetic Expression and Neuronal Apoptosis and/or Necrosis

II Factors and Mechanisms Enhancing Susceptibility or Tolerance (Growth Factors)

III Factors Modulating Neuronal Plasticity and the Course of Maturation Phenomenon in Cerebral Ischemia (Metabolic and Inflammatory Factors)

IV Ischemic Infarction: Threshold, Experimental and Clinical Dynamics and Therapeutic Design for Prevention or Reduction of Intensity

V Special Lecture

VI Poster Presentations (Abstracts)

VII Round Table Discussion

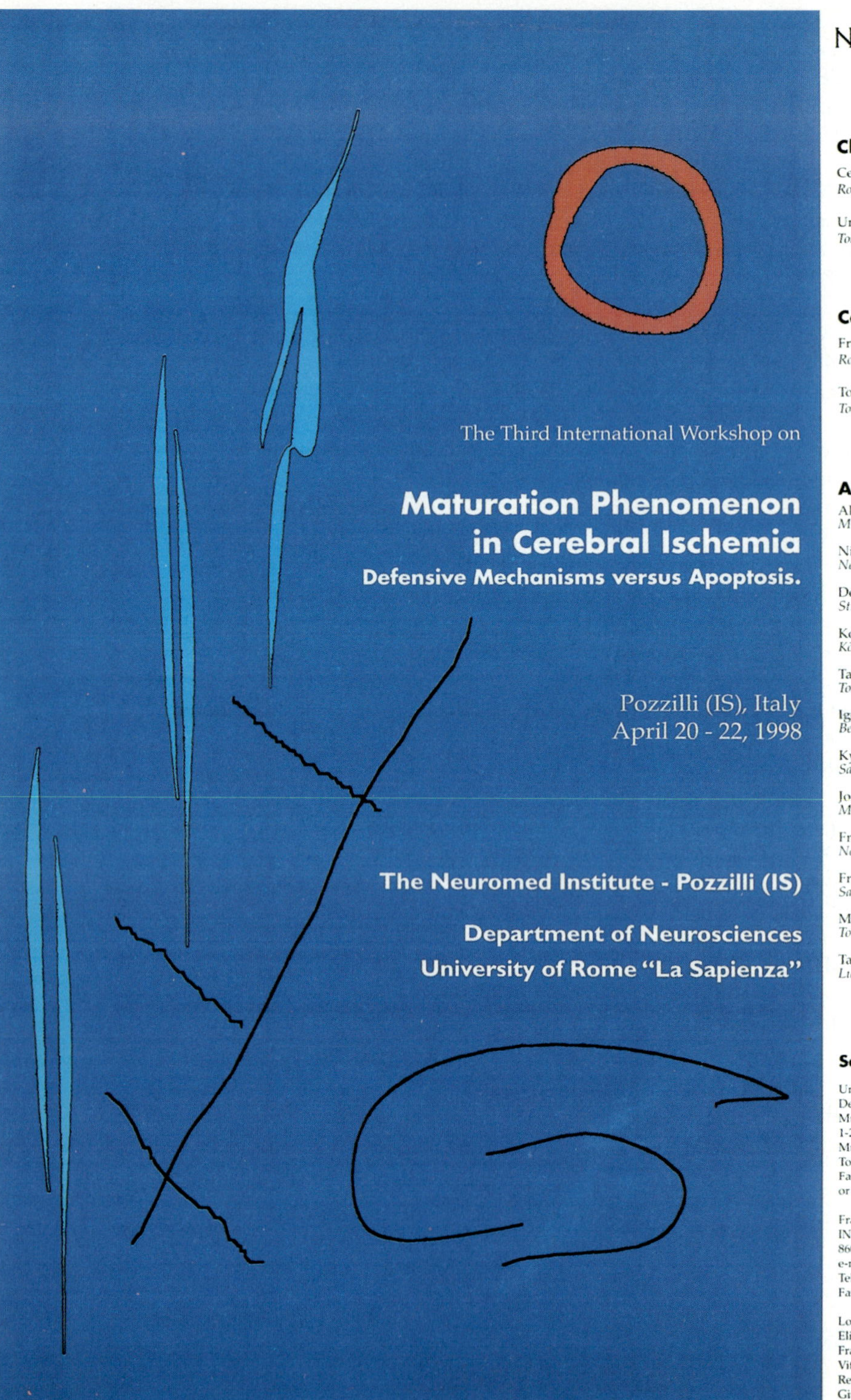

NEUR✛MED

Chairmen
Cesare Fieschi
Rome, Italy

Umeo Ito
Tokyo, Japan

Co-Chairmen
Francesco Orzi
Rome, Italy

Toshihiko Kuroiwa
Tokyo, Japan

Advisory Board
Alexander Baethmann
München, FRG

Nicolas G. Bazan
New Orleans, USA.

Dennis Choi
St. Louis, USA

Konstantin A. Hossman
Köln, FRG

Takaaki Kirino
Tokyo, Japan

Igor Klatzo
Bethesda, USA

Kyuuya Kogure
Saitama - Ken, Japan

Joseph Krieglstein
Marburg, FRG

Fred Plum
New York, USA

Frank R. Sharp
San Francisco, USA

Minoru Tomita
Tokyo, Japan

Tadeusz Wieloch
Lund, Sweden

Secretaries
Umeo Ito (General Affairs)
Department of Neurosurgery
Musashino Red Cross Hospital
1-26-1, Kyonan-cho
Musashino-shi
Tokyo 180, Japan
Fax +81 3 3301 5600
or +81 422 32 9551

Francesco Orzi (Local Affairs)
INM Neuromed, Via Atinense 18
86077 Pozzilli (IS), Italy
e-mail: forzi@tin.it
Tel. + 39 865 915245
Fax + 39 865 927575

Local Organizers:
Elisa Lombardozzi
Francesco Orzi
Vittorio Colangelo
Renato Di Grezia
Giuliano Sette
Tel. + 39 865 929600 - 915225 -
929322
Fax + 39 865 927575

The Third International Workshop on

Maturation Phenomenon
in Cerebral Ischemia
Defensive Mechanisms versus Apoptosis.

Pozzilli (IS), Italy
April 20 - 22, 1998

The Neuromed Institute - Pozzilli (IS)

Department of Neurosciences

University of Rome "La Sapienza"

List of First-Named Authors

ASANO, T.
Department of Neurosurgery, Saitama Medical Center/School, Kamoda, Kawagoe, Saitama 350, Japan

BOLDYREV, A.
Institute of Neurology, Russian Academy of Medical Sciences, 123367 Moscow, Russia

CHEN, J.
Department of Neurology, University of Pittsburgh, 3550 Terrace Street, Pittsburgh, PA 15217, USA

CHOPP, M.
Henry Ford Health Science Center, Henry Ford Hospital, Neurology Department, 2799 West Grand Boulevard, Detroit, MI 48202, USA

COLANGELO, V.
LSUMC Neuroscience Center of Excellence, 2020 Gravier St., Suite D, New Orleans, LA 70112, USA

COLBOURNE, F.
Alberta Stroke Program, Department of Pathology, Faculty of Medicine, Health Sciences Center, University of Calgary, 3330 Hospital Dr. NW, Calgary, AB, Canada T2N 4N1

DAWSON, D.
Stroke Branch, National Institute of Neurological Disorders and Stroke, National Institutes of Health, Bldg. 36, Rm. 4A03, 36 Convent Drive MSC 4128, Bethesda, MD 20982 – 4128, USA

DEGRACIA, D.J.
Department of Emergency Medicine, Wayne State University, Detroit, MI 48202, USA

DEMBO, T.
Department of Neurology, School of Medicine, Keio University, 35 Shinanomachi, Shinjuku-ku, 160-8582 Tokyo, Japan

FIESCHI, C.
Department of Neurological Sciences, University "La Sapienza",
Viale dell' Universita 30, 00185, Rome, Italy

GARCIA, J.H.
Department of Pathology, Henry Ford Hospital, K-6 2799W Grand Boulevard,
Detroit, MI 48202-2689, USA

GILLARDON, F.
Max Planck Institute for Neurological Research, Department of Experimental
Neurology, Gleueler Straße 50, 50931 Cologne, Germany

GORDON, W.C.
LSUMC Neuroscience Center of Excellence, 2020 Gravier St., Suite D, New Orleans,
LA 70112, USA

GORTER, J.A.
Department of Experimental Dierkunde, University of Amsterdam, Kruislaan 320,
1098 SM Amsterdam, The Netherlands

HANYU, S.
Department of Neurology, Jichi Medical School, 3311-1 Yakushiji, Minamikawachi-
machi, Kawachi, Tochigi, 329-04 Japan

HERMANN, D.M.
Max Planck Institute for Neurological Research, Department of
Experimental Neurology, Gleueler Straße 50, 50931 Cologne, Germany

HOSSMANN, K.-A.
Max Planck Institute for Neurological Research, Department of
Experimental Neurology, Gleueler Straße 50, 50931 Cologne, Germany

HUNGERHUBER, E.
Institute for Surgical Research, Klinikum Grosshadern, Ludwig-Maximilians-
Universität, Marchioninistraße 15, 81377 Munich, Germany

IADECOLA, C.
Laboratory of Cerebrovascular Biology and Stroke, Department of Neurology,
University of Minnesota Medical School, Box 295 UMHC, 420 Delaware St. S.E.,
Minneapolis, MN 55455, USA

ITO, U.
Department of Neurosurgery, Musashino Red Cross Hospital, 1-26-1 Kyonan-cho,
Musashino-shi, Tokyo 180, Japan

JOHANSSON, B.B.
Section for Experimental Neurology, Wallenberg Neuroscience Center,
Lund University, University Hospital, 221 85 Lund, Sweden

KATO, H.
Department of Neurology, Tohoku University School of Medicine, 1-1 Seiryomachi, Aoba-ku, Sendai 980-8574, Japan

KAWASE, M.
Department of Neurosurgery, Neurology & Neurological & Sciences, Stanford University School of Medicine, Palo Alto, CA 94304, USA

KRIEGLSTEIN, J.
Institut für Pharmakologie und Toxikologie, Fachbereich Pharmazie und Lebensmittelchemie, Philipps-Universität, Ketzerbach 63, 35032 Marburg, Germany

KUROIWA, T.
Deparment of Neuropathology, Medical Research Institute, Tokyo Medical and Dental University, 1-5-45 Yushima, Bunkyo-ku, Tokyo 113, Japan

MATSUMOTO, M.
Division of Strokology, First Department of Medicine, Osaka University School of Medicine, 2 – 2 Yamada-oka, Suita, Osaka 565-0871, Japan

MIMA, T.
Deparment of Neurosurgery, Kochi Medical School, Kohasu, Okatoyo-cho, Nanngoku City, Kochi, 738 Japan

MIYAZAWA, T.
Deparment of Neurosurgery, National Defense Medical College, Namiki 3-2, Tokorozawa, Saitama 359, Japan

OHARA, Y.
Naval Medical Research Institute, Bethesda, Maryland, USA

PICHIULE, P.
Department of Anatomy, Case Western Reserve University, School of Medicine, Cleveland, OH 44106 – 4938, USA

REISER, G.
Institut für Neurobiochemie, Medizinische Fakultät der Universität Magdeburg, Leipziger Straße 44, 39120 Magdeburg, Germany

SAGER, T.N.
Dept. of Pharmacology, 26B Smedeland, 2600 Glostrup, Denmark

SCHMID-ELSAESSER, R.
Department of Neurosurgery, Klinikum Grosshadern, Ludwig-Maximilians-Universität, Marchioninistraße 15, 81377 Munich, Germany

SCHUMANN, P.
Division of Experimental Neurology, Department of Neurology, Charité Hospital,
10098 Berlin, Germany

SEIWERT, T.
Institute for Neurosurgical Pathophysiology, Johannes Gutenberg University,
Langenbeckstraße 1, 55101 Mainz, Germany

SHARP, F.R.
Department of Neurology, University of California at San Francisco,
and Department of Veterans Affairs Medical Center, 4150 Clement Street,
San Francisco, CA 94121, USA

SIESJÖ, B.K.
Center for the Study of Neurological Disease, The Neuroscience Institute,
Queen's Medical Center, 1356 Lusitana Street, 8th Floor, Honolulu, HI 96813, USA

SNIDER, B.J.
Center for the Study of Nervous System Injury, and Department of Neurology,
Washington University Medical School, St. Louis, MO 63110, USA

SOKOLOFF, L.
Laboratory of Cerebral Metabolism, National Institute of Mental Health,
Building No. 36, Room 1A-05, Bethesda, MD 20892, USA

TAKAGI, K.
Department of Neurosurgery, Teikyo University School of Medicine, 2-11-1, Kaga,
Itabashi-ku, Tokyo, 173 – 8605, Japan

TAMURA, A.
Department of Neurosurgery, Teikyo University School of Medicine, 2-11-1, Kaga,
Itabashi-ku, Tokyo, 173 – 8605, Japan

TANAKA, K.
Department of Neurology, School of Medicine, Keio University, 35 Shinanomachi,
Shinjuku-ku, Tokyo 160 – 8582, Japan

TATEISHI, N.
Minase Research Institute, Ono Pharmaceutical Co., Ltd., Osaka 618, Japan

TOMITA, M.
Department of Neurology, School of Medicine, Keio University, 35 Shinanomachi,
Shinjuku-ku, Tokyo 160 – 8582 Tokyo, Japan

YAMADA, K.
Department of Neurosurgery, Nagoya City University Medical School,
1 Kawasumi, Mizuho-ku, Nagoya 467-0001, Japan

I Role of Genetic Expression an Neuronal Apoptosis and/or Necrosis

Multiple Molecular Penumbras Associated with Focal Ischemia in Brain

F. R. Sharp, M. Bergeron, J. Honkaniemi, A. Mancuso, S. Massa, and P. R. Weinstein

Introduction: Penumbra

The concept of a penumbra around an area of focal infarction in the brain has undergone constant revision [6, 38, 46, 58, 119, 120]. It has been defined as an area outside of the infarction that is electrophysiologically silent [119], is depolarized, demonstrates decreased perfusion [38], increased oxygen extraction [30], decreased protein metabolism [46] and decreased glucose metabolism [35] as well as other parameters [7, 28, 40]. The application of molecular methods to the study of cerebral ischemia has provided support for all of these definitions of the penumbra related to molecular markers [58]. Recent data from many laboratories demonstrate that there are several penumbras around an area of infarction that can be defined in molecular terms, and that correlate with the more classical "penumbra" defined on the basis of blood flow, metabolic, biochemical and physiological parameters.

Immediately surrounding areas of infarction is a narrow zone, in which selective neuronal cell death occurs. This selective neuronal cell death can be detected using conventional hematoxylin and eosin staining [89], as well as with more recently described TUNEL staining of brain [15, 26, 68, 74, 118]. Outside this zone is a region in which heat-shock protein 70 (HSP70) messenger RNA (mRNA) and HSP70-protein expression occurs in neurons [51, 52, 90, 94, 114, 131]. It is proposed that the HSP70-protein expression is an index of the zone of protein denaturation [81, 113]. This region would also represent a region of decreased blood flow that was not severe enough to produce infarction. Outside this zone is another, in which blood flow is chronically reduced, resulting in the induction of hypoxia inducible factor (HIF). The zone of HIF induction would delineate the zone of chronic hypoxia [11, 108]. Finally, the most distant zone from the core of infarction is defined by the induction of immediate early genes, such as c-fos and NGFIA [2, 32, 47, 53, 54]. This distant induction is related to ischemia-induced spreading depression and depolarization, which may spread throughout the rodent hemisphere and cross the corpus callosum.

Ischemic Core of Infarction

The core of an ischemic region appears to undergo rapid ionic changes, which are associated with changes in the diffusion of water and can be detected within minutes of ischemia by diffusion magnetic resonance imaging (D-MRI) [8, 86, 128]. One of the earliest molecular changes is decreased protein synthesis in the area of ischemia [46]. A number of factors that regulate protein translation, including elongation initi-

Maturation Phenomenon in Cerebral Ischemia III
U. Ito et al. (Eds.)
© Springer-Verlag Berlin Heidelberg 1999

ation factor 2 (eIF2), appear to trigger this decrease of translation [13, 14, 22, 64, 80]. The biochemistry of this response is discussed in this volume (pp. 47–52). In addition to decreased translation, transcription for many genes is decreased or blocked in regions where blood flow is quite low and where ATP levels fall dramatically [62].

Within areas of infarction, the HSP70 protein is generally not expressed in neurons or glial cells [57, 58, 67, 69]. HSP70 mRNA may be expressed in the core of the infarction if the ischemia is not too severe [54, 57, 58]. However, areas of severe middle cerebral artery (MCA) ischemia demonstrate no induction of either HSP70 mRNA or c-fos mRNA, presumably because of a block of transcription, related either to energy failure [62] or another effect of ischemia that blocks transcription. It is notable that HSP70 protein can be expressed in endothelial cells in areas of MCA infarction [31, 37, 57, 115]. Whether these endothelial cells survive the infarction, due in part to the presence of HSP70, is unknown; it is possible that they do. Therefore, some areas of infarction may have vascular elements survive even though the neurons and glia die.

Selective Neuronal Cell Death: TUNEL/Apoptotic Cell Death?

Selective neuronal cell death has been described following global ischemia, with the death of CA 1 pyramidal neurons being particularly well studied [59–61, 92, 135]. Only recently, has it been clear that selective neuronal cell death occurs following focal ischemia. Hematoxylin and eosin staining shows eosinophilic neurons within a few millimeters of focal infarction [89]. More recently, TUNEL staining has demonstrated that isolated neurons at the edges of focal infarction can demonstrate DNA fragmentation [15, 16, 19, 26, 68, 70, 74]. In some instances, the nuclei appear to have apoptotic bodies, typical of cells that die via apoptosis. In other cases, there is a uniform degradation of DNA in neuronal nuclei, which might occur in necrotic cells where the DNA is secondarily degraded [70, 76–78]. In either case, the TUNEL staining clearly demonstrates that there is selective neuronal cell death in a small rim surrounding a focal infarction. These TUNEL-positive cells generally do not express HSP70 protein [118]. This suggests that either HSP70 protein expression protects cells from dying, or cells with DNA fragmentation cannot or do not express HSP70 protein [18, 26, 44, 73, 78, 118].

Not only does focal MCA ischemia cause selective neuronal cell death around areas of infarction, but MCA occlusions in rodents and, perhaps, in man lead to selective cell death in the hippocampus, thalamus and other structures [118]. Approximately one-third of rodents that sustain MCA occlusions demonstrate selective neuronal cell death in the hippocampus [118].

These results suggest that following MCA occlusions, there is a zone of selective neuronal cell death around the area of infarction. In addition, there is selective neuronal cell death in other regions, including the hippocampus, thalamus and substantia nigra, which may relate to moderate ischemia in those regions [118], excitotoxic injury [118] or to loss of trophic support following cortical and basal-ganglia infarction [39, 88, 102–104, 121, 134].

Zone of Protein Denaturation: HSP70

Following both temporary and permanent MCA occlusions, HSP70 mRNA is expressed throughout the MCA distribution, both within the areas of infarction and in regions adjacent to the infarction [1, 17, 43, 51, 52, 57, 58, 90, 91, 93, 97, 105, 114, 125, 131]. The HSP70 mRNA is induced by the presence of denatured proteins within cells [21, 85, 96]. Injections of denatured proteins into cells induces HSP70 [3]. Plant amino acids, when incorporated into mammalian proteins, cause abnormalities of tertiary structure that are tantamount to denaturation and also induce HSP70 in cells [4, 71]. Hence, the region of HSP70-mRNA induction can be viewed as the zone within and around an infarction where denatured proteins are found within cells [81, 114].

A schematic diagram of the possible mechanisms of HSP70 induction following focal ischemia is shown in Fig. 1. HSP70 mRNA is induced in neurons in the core of the infarct, as well as in the penumbra, where denatured proteins within these cells stimulate heat-shock factors (HSFs), which then form a trimer and bind to the heat-shock element on the HSP70 gene [81, 85]. This initiates transcription of HSP70 mRNA in these neurons.

In the infarct core, which will go on to infarct, the HSP70 mRNA cannot be translated into protein. The inability of the cells to make HSP70 protein may contribute to their death [81]. Outside areas of infarction, cells that made HSP70 mRNA are able to

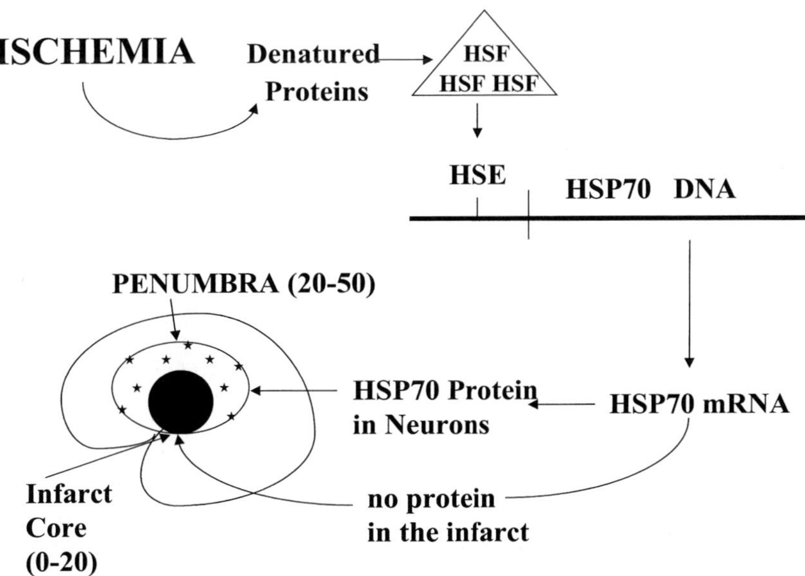

Fig. 1. Diagram showing the mechanism of HSP70 mRNA and HSP70 protein induction in brain following focal ischemia. Ischemia produces denatured proteins within neurons, glia and endothelial cells. Denatured proteins activate heat-shock factors that form a trimer and bind to heat-shock elements on the HSP70 gene. This triggers transcription of HSP70 mRNA. In the core of the infarction HSP70 mRNA cannot be translated. In the penumbra the HSP70 mRNA is translated into HSP70 protein in neurons that generally survive the ischemic injury

translate this into HSP70 protein [54, 57, 58, 81, 114]. Astrocytes and microglia at the periphery of infarcts express high levels of HSP70 protein [31, 97, 115]. Neurons also express HSP70 protein outside the areas of infarction. If the MCA occlusion is brief, without producing infarction, HSP70 protein can be expressed in neurons throughout the MCA distribution. If the MCA occlusion is permanent, with infarction throughout the MCA distribution, then HSP70 protein may be expressed in a limited number of neurons at the border zones between the middle, anterior and posterior cerebral arteries [58, 81].

HSP70 expression in the neurons outside areas of infarction is presumed to protect these cells from further protein denaturation [9, 10]. Moreover, the HSP70 expression may promote protein renaturation and promote cell survival [5, 34, 84, 106, 107, 122–124]. Overexpression of HSP70 protein in transgenic mice markedly protects the brain against focal ischemic infarction and moderately protects against global ischemic injury [98, 99].

The results suggest that the zone of HSP70 protein expression outside of an area of infarction represents the zone in which protein denaturation occurred within cells (Fig. 3). This zone can be quite narrow and coincide with other zones, or it can be quite widespread and involve the entire MCA distribution.

Zone of Persistent Hypoxia: HIF

HIF has been found to play a key role in regulating transcriptional responses to hypoxia [100, 108, 109, 127]. Hypoxia upregulates erythropoetin, which in turn increases the proliferation of red blood precursors [112]. HIF appears to be a key intermediary, which induces erythropoetin and other hypoxia-inducible genes [110].

Hypoxia may be sensed by a heme protein or a similar oxygen sensor [12]. This sensor then activates HIFα transcription and may stabilize HIFα protein [49, 100]. HIFα then binds to HIFβ, the aromatic hydrocarbon-receptor nuclear translocator (Arnt), which is constitutively expressed in a cell [132]. The HIFα and HIFβ dimer then bind to hypoxia response elements on the promoters of target genes to stimulate their transcription [108, 126]. A number of genes have been identified that have hypoxia response elements in their promoters. These include the glycolytic enzymes such as lactate dehydrogenase [27, 66, 110, 111]. The HIF target genes also include erythropoetin [108], vascular endothelial growth factor (VEGF) [29, 75], glucose transporter [36], heme oxygenase-1 [65], inducible nitric-oxide synthase (NOS) [83] and transferrin [101]. Therefore, the induction/activation of HIF could play a key role in the response of hypoxic/ischemic brain to decrease the effects of hypoxia (Fig. 2). Induction of HIF would promote increased ATP production during hypoxia, with increases of glycolytic enzymes and the glucose transporter. HIF induction would promote increased blood flow by induction of NOS and production of new blood vessels via VEGF.

Examination of HIF expression following MCA occlusion has shown that HIF mRNA is expressed in the distribution of the MCA and anterior cerebral arteries (ACA), which are in the parietal neocortex and cingulate cortex [11]. The HIFα mRNA was markedly induced in the ACA distribution, whereas there was little induction of HIFβ [11]. Recent MR studies in our laboratory demonstrate that perfusion in

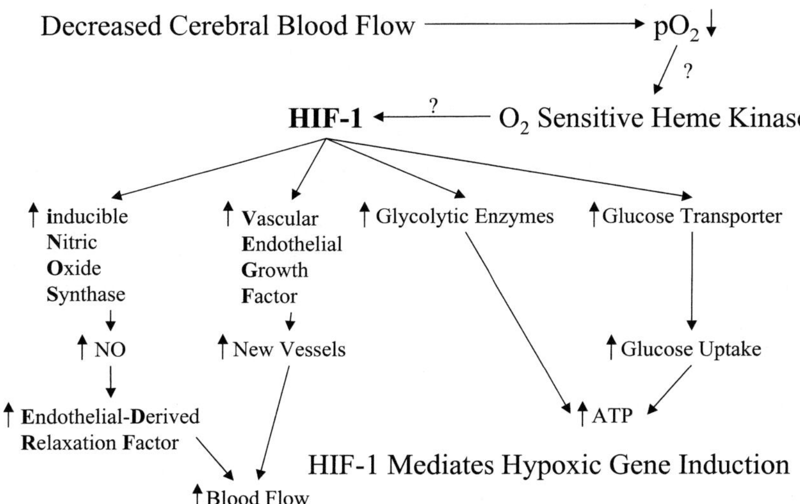

Fig. 2. Diagram showing the possible role of hypoxia inducible factor (HIF) in cerebral ischemia. Hypoxia is sensed by an unknown protein. This activates HIFα transcription. HIFα binds to HIFβ to form a dimer that then binds to hypoxia-inducible elements on target genes. This triggers transcription of the target genes such as those for glycolytic enzymes, inducible nitric oxide synthase (iNOS), the glucose transporter, and vascular endothelial growth factor (VEGF). These target genes then lead to increased ATP, increased blood flow, and increased glucose transport into hypoxic cells

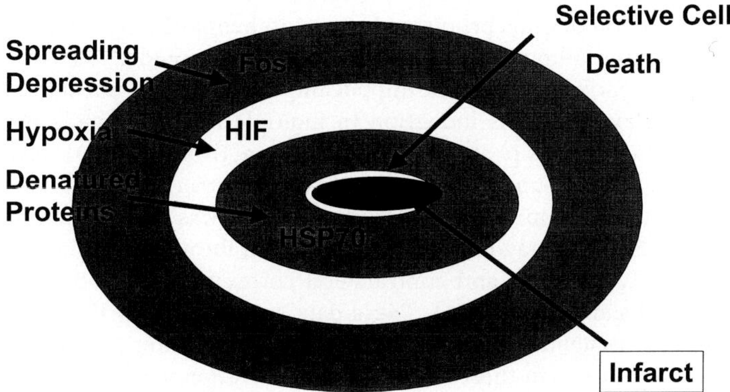

Fig. 3. Proposed molecular penumbras in brain based on the genes that are induced and the factors that likely induce these genes. Around the infarct core is a zone of selective neuronal cell death that may represent apoptotic cell death, at least to some degree. In this zone, pro-apoptotic gene expression is presumed to overcome anti-apoptotic gene expression in the cells that die. Around this is a zone of HSP70 heat-shock protein expression in neurons that represents a zone of protein denaturation. Blood flow must have been impaired in this zone sometime during or after the focal ischemia. Surrounding or adjacent to this is a zone of HIF expression that represents a region of persistent hypoxia – that probably represents a region of decreased blood flow. The zone most distant from the ischemic core is the area where immediate early genes, such as c-fos, are induced. This region likely represents all areas that have been transiently depolarized by the focal ischemia and could include contralateral cortex, hippocampus, thalamus and other subcortical and cortical structures that are directly or indirectly connected to cortex

the distribution of the ACA is decreased with the suture-occlusion model used in these studies, though the decreased perfusion in the ACA distribution is quite modest compared with the marked decrease of perfusion in the MCA distribution [79].

The data suggest that HIFα is induced in the cingulate cortex in a distribution consistent with decreased blood flow in the ACA distribution. We postulate that the decreased blood flow in the ACA distribution leads to moderate hypoxia, which induces HIFα, which in turn should lead to induction of HIFα target genes, such as the glycolytic enzymes and VEGF. Hence, the region of HIFα expression would demonstrate the region of sustained hypoxia outside of the area of infarction and show the region of persistently decreased blood flow and hypoxia around the infarct (Fig. 3).

Zone of Spreading Depression: Fos

A consistent finding in all focal-ischemia studies has been the induction of c-fos, NGFIA and other selected transcription factors throughout an ischemic hemisphere [2, 20, 25, 33, 45, 47, 48, 50, 53, 72, 87, 105, 116, 131]. c-fos is induced in the entire MCA territory as well as in cingulate cortex, frontal cortex and occipital cortex [54, 55]. Because of the widespread induction of the gene, it was assumed that it was due to spreading depression. In addition, application of potassium chloride to cortex and focal cortical injuries similarly induced c-fos throughout the hemisphere [41, 42, 117, 133], further supporting spreading depression as the mechanism of c-fos induction. Finally, prior administration of N-methyl-D-aspartate (NMDA) antagonists, such as MK801, were shown to block ischemia-induced spreading depression; they blocked the whole hemisphere induction of c-fos produced by focal ischemia [20, 33, 32, 56].

Of equal importance, we and others showed that focal ischemia could also induce c-fos and other immediate early genes in the hippocampus, thalamus, substantia nigra and contralateral cortex [56]. This induction in multiple regions outside the areas of middle cerebral ischemia was postulated to be due to activation of pathways in and around the ischemic cortex, and this, in turn, activated structures anatomically connected to the ischemic region via NMDA receptors. This was again tested by the prior administration of NMDA antagonists, which prevented the distant induction of c-fos in the hippocampus, thalamus and contralateral cortex [56]. They did not block c-fos induction in substantia nigra [56]. These data suggest that cortical outputs from ischemic and peri-ischemic cortex activated neurons in distant regions via NMDA receptors and induced c-fos in these regions. Such activation was blocked by NMDA receptor antagonists.

The data suggest that there are zones well outside the zone of focal MCA ischemia that express c-fos and other transcription factors in response to depolarization produced by the focal ischemia. This penumbra of depolarization can extend well outside the region of decreased blood flow as well as to subcortical brain structures and the cortex in the contralateral hemisphere.

This distant induction of transcription factors could form the basis for plasticity observed around focal ischemic regions in primate and human cortex [95]. This could also form a molecular basis for altered patterns of blood-flow activation in ipsilateral and contralateral cortex following focal subcortical infarctions [129, 130].

Spreading depression does occur in human cortex, though it is not likely that spreading depression progresses throughout a hemisphere, because of the presence of cortical gyri [23, 24, 82]. However, it is possible that spreading depression could progress down a gyrus, and activation of corticofugal pathways to adjacent gyri, the opposite cortex and subcortical structures could mediate long-term changes of gene expression in those structures and promote the plasticity noted following ischemic brain injury [63, 95].

References

1. Abe K, Kawagoe J, Araki T, Aoki M, Kogure K (1992) Differential expression of heat shock protein 70 gene between the cortex and caudate after transient focal cerebral ischaemia in rats. Neurol Res 14: 381–385
2. An G, Lin TN, Liu JS, Xue JJ, He YY, Hsu CY (1993) Expression of c-fos and c-jun family genes after focal cerebral ischemia [see comments]. Ann Neurol 33: 457–464
3. Ananthan J, Goldberg AL, Voellmy R (1986) Abnormal proteins serve as eukaryotic stress signals and trigger the activation of heat shock genes. Science 232: 522–524
4. Andersson H, Lindqvist E, Olson L (1997) Plant-derived amino acids increase hippocampal BDNF, NGF, c-fos and hsp70 mRNAs. Neuroreport 8: 1813–1817
5. Artigues A, Iriarte A, Martinez-Carrion M (1997) Refolding intermediates of acid-unfolded mitochondrial aspartate aminotransferase bind to hsp70. J Biol Chem 272: 16852–16861
6. Astrup J, Siesjo BK, Symon L (1981) Thresholds in cerebral ischemia – the ischemic penumbra. Stroke 12: 723–725
7. Back T, Zhao W, Ginsberg MD (1995) Three-dimensional image analysis of brain glucose metabolism-blood flow uncoupling and its electrophysiological correlates in the acute ischemic penumbra following middle cerebral artery occlusion. J Cereb Blood Flow Metab 15: 566–577
8. Baird A, Benfield A, Schlaug G, Siewert B, Lovblad KO, Edelman RR, Warach S (1997) Enlargement of human cerebral ischemic lesion volumes measured by diffusion-weighted magnetic resonance imaging [see comments]. Ann Neurol 41: 581–589
9. Beckmann RP, Lovett M, Welch WJ (1992) Examining the function and regulation of hsp 70 in cells subjected to metabolic stress. J Cell Biol 117: 1137–1150
10. Beckmann RP, Mizzen LE, Welch WJ (1990) Interaction of Hsp 70 with newly synthesized proteins: implications for protein folding and assembly. Science 248: 850–854
11. Bergeron M, Solway KE, Ferriero DM, Sharp FR (1997) Induction of hypoxia inducible factor-1 in rat brain after middle cerebral artery occlusion. Soc Neuroscience Abstracts 27: 229.229
12. Bunn HF, Poyton RO (1996) Oxygen sensing and molecular adaptation to hypoxia. Physiol Rev 76: 839–885
13. Burda J, Martin ME, Garcia A, Alcazar A, Fando JL, Salinas M (1994) Phosphorylation of the alpha subunit of initiation factor 2 correlates with the inhibition of translation following transient cerebral ischaemia in the rat. Biochem J 302: 335–338
14. Burda J, Martin ME, Gottlieb M, Chavko M, Marsala J, Alcazar A, Pavon M, Fando JL, Salinas M (1998) The intraischemic and early reperfusion changes of protein synthesis in the rat brain. eIF-2 alpha kinase activity and role of initiation factors eIF-2 alpha and eIF-4E, J Cereb Blood Flow Metab 18: 59–66
15. Charriaut-Marlangue C, Margaill I, Represa A, Popovici T, Plotkine M, Ben-Ari Y (1996) Apoptosis and necrosis after reversible focal ischemia: an in situ DNA fragmentation analysis. J Cereb Blood Flow Metab 16: 186–194
16. Chen J, Graham SH, Chan PH, Lan J, Zhou RL, Simon RP (1995) bcl-2 is expressed in neurons that survive focal ischemia in the rat. Neuroreport 6: 394–398
17. Chen J, Graham SH, Zhu RL, Simon RP (1996) Stress proteins and tolerance to focal cerebral ischemia. J Cereb Blood Flow Metab 16: 566–577
18. Chen J, Simon R (1997) Ischemic tolerance in the brain. Neurology 48: 306–311
19. Chopp M, Li Y, Jiang N, Zhang RL, Prostak J (1996) Antibodies against adhesion molecules reduce apoptosis after transient middle cerebral artery occlusion in rat brain. J Cereb Blood Flow Metab 16: 578–584
20. Collaco-Moraes Y, Aspey BS, de Belleroche JS, Harrison MJ (1994) Focal ischemia causes an extensive induction of immediate early genes that are sensitive to MK-801. Stroke 25: 1855–1861

21. Craig EA, Gambill BD, Nelson RJ (1993) Heat shock proteins: molecular chaperones of protein biogenesis. Microbiol Rev 57402–414
22. de Haro C, Mendez R, Santoyo J (1996) The eIF-2alpha kinases and the control of protein synthesis. Faseb J 10: 1378–1387
23. Diener HC (1997) Positron emission tomography studies in headache. Headache 37: 622–625
24. do Carmo RJ, Somjen GG (1994) Spreading depression of Leao: 50 years since a seminal discovery. J Neurophysiol 72: 1–2
25. Dragunow M, Beilharz E, Sirimanne E, Lawlor P, Williams C, Bravo R, Gluckman P (1994) Immediate-early gene protein expression in neurons undergoing delayed death, but not necrosis, following hypoxic-ischaemic injury to the young rat brain. Brain Res Mol Brain Res 25: 19–33
26. Du C, Hu R, Csernansky CA, Hsu CY, Choi DW (1996) Very delayed infarction after mild focal cerebral ischemia: a role for apoptosis? J Cereb Blood Flow Metab 16: 195–201
27. Firth JD, Ebert BL, Ratcliffe PJ (1995) Hypoxic regulation of lactate dehydrogenase A. Interaction between hypoxia-inducible factor 1 and cAMP response elements. J Biol Chem 270: 21021–21027
28. Folbergrova J, Memezawa H, Smith ML, Siesjo BK (1992) Focal and perifocal changes in tissue energy state during middle cerebral artery occlusion in normo- and hyperglycemic rats. J Cereb Blood Flow Metab 12: 25–33
29. Forsythe JA, Jiang BH, Iyer NV, Agani F, Leung SW, Koos RD, Semenza GL (1996) Activation of vascular endothelial growth factor gene transcription by hypoxia-inducible factor 1. Mol Cell Biol 16: 4604–4613
30. Furlan M, Marchal G, Viader F, Derlon JM, Baron JC (1996) Spontaneous neurological recovery after stroke and the fate of the ischemic penumbra [see comments]. Ann Neurol 40: 216–226
31. Gaspary H, Graham SH, Sagar SM, Sharp FR (1995) HSP70 heat shock protein induction following global ischemia in the rat. Brain Res Mol Brain Res 34: 327–332
32. Gass P, Herdegen T, Bravo R, Kiessling M (1993) Induction and suppression of immediate early genes in specific rat brain regions by the non-competitive N-methyl-D-aspartate receptor antagonist MK-801. Neuroscience 53: 749–758
33. Gass P, Spranger M, Herdegen T, Bravo R, Kock P, Hacke W, Kiessling M (1992) Induction of FOS and JUN proteins after focal ischemia in the rat: differential effect of the N-methyl-D-aspartate receptor antagonist MK-801. Acta Neuropathol (Berl) 84: 545–553
34. Gebauer M, Zeiner M, Gehring U (1997) Proteins interacting with the molecular chaperone hsp70/hsc70: physical associations and effects on refolding activity FEBS. Lett 417: 109–113
35. Ginsberg MD (1990) Local metabolic responses to cerebral ischemia. Cerebrovasc Brain Metab Rev 2: 58–93
36. Gleadle JM, Ratcliffe PJ (1997) Induction of hypoxia-inducible factor-1, erythropoietin, vascular endothelial growth factor, and glucose transporter-1 by hypoxia: evidence against a regulatory role for Src kinase. Blood 89: 503–509
37. Gonzalez MF, Lowenstein D, Fernyak S, Hisanaga K, Simon R, Sharp FR (1991) Induction of heat shock protein 72-like immunoreactivity in the hippocampal formation following transient global ischemia. Brain Res Bull 26: 241–250
38. Hakim AM (1987) The cerebral ischemic penumbra. Can J Neurol Sci 14: 557–559
39. Hara H, Harada K, Sukamoto T (1993) Chronological atrophy after transient middle cerebral artery occlusion in rats. Brain Res 618: 251–260
40. Heiss WD, Graf R (1994) The ischemic penumbra. Curr Opin Neurol 7: 11–19
41. Herrera DG, Robertson HA (1990) Application of potassium chloride to the brain surface induces the c- fos proto-oncogene: reversal by MK-801. Brain Res 510: 166–170
42. Herrera DG, Robertson HA (1996) Activation of c-fos in the brain. Prog Neurobiol 50: 83–107
43. Higashi T, Takechi H, Uemura Y, Kikuchi H, Nagata K (1994) Differential induction of mRNA species encoding several classes of stress proteins following focal cerebral ischemia in rats. Brain Res 650: 239–248
44. Honkaniemi J, Massa SM, Sharp FR (1996) Global ischemia induces apoptosis associated genes in gerbil hippocampus. Mol Brain Res (in press)
45. Honkaniemi J, Sagar SM, Pyykonen I, Hicks KJ, Sharp FR (1995) Focal brain injury induces multiple immediate early genes encoding zinc finger transcription factors. Brain Res Mol Brain Res 28: 157–163
46. Hossmann KA (1994) Viability thresholds and the penumbra of focal ischemia [see comments]. Ann Neurol 36: 557–565
47. Hsu CY, An G, Liu JS, Xue JJ, He YY, Lin TN (1993) Expression of immediate early gene and growth factor mRNAs in a focal cerebral ischemia model in the rat. Stroke 24:178
48. Ikeda J, Nakajima T, Osborne OC, Mies G, Nowak TS, Jr (1994) Coexpression of c-fos and hsp70 mRNAs in gerbil brain after ischemia: induction threshold, distribution and time course evaluated by in situ hybridization. Brain Res Mol Brain Res 26: 249–258

49. Kallio PJ, Pongratz I, Gradin K, McGuire J, Poellinger L (1997) Activation of hypoxia-inducible factor 1alpha: posttranscriptional regulation and conformational change by recruitment of the Arnt transcription factor. Proc Natl Acad Sci U S A 94: 5667–5672

50. Kamii H, Kinouchi H, Sharp FR, Epstein CJ, Sagar SM, Chan H (1994) Expression of c-fos mRNA after a mild focal cerebral ischemia in SOD-1 transgenic mice. Brain Res 662: 240–244

51. Kamii H, Kinouchi H, Sharp FR, Koistinaho J, Epstein CJ, Chan PH (1994) Prolonged expression of hsp70 mRNA following transient focal cerebral ischemia in transgenic mice overexpressing CuZn-superoxide dismutase. J Cereb Blood Flow Metab 14: 478–486

52. Kawagoe J, Abe K, Sato S, Nagano I, Nakamura S, Kogure K (1992) Distributions of heat shock protein (HSP) 70 and heat shock cognate protein (HSC) 70 mRNAs after transient focal ischemia in rat brain. Brain Res 587: 195–202

53. Kiessling M, Gass P (1994) Stimulus-transcription coupling in focal cerebral ischemia. Brain Pathol 4: 77–83

54. Kinouchi H, Sharp FR, Chan PH, Koistinaho J, Sagar SM, Yoshimoto T (1994) Induction of c-fos, junB, c-jun, and hsp70 mRNA in cortex, thalamus, basal ganglia, and hippocampus following middle cerebral artery occlusion. J Cereb Blood Flow Metab 14: 808–817

55. Kinouchi H, Sharp FR, Chan PH, Koistinaho J, Sagar SM, Yoshimoto T (1994) Induction of NGFI-A mRNA following middle cerebral artery occlusion in rats: in situ hybridization study. Neurosci Lett 171: 163–166

56. Kinouchi H, Sharp FR, Chan PH, Mikawa S, Kamii H, Arai S, Yoshimoto T (1994) MK-801 inhibits the induction of immediate early genes in cerebral cortex, thalamus, and hippocampus, but not in substantia nigra following middle cerebral artery occlusion. Neurosci Lett 179: 111–114

57. Kinouchi H, Sharp FR, Hill MP, Koistinaho J, Sagar SM, Chan PH (1993) Induction of 70-kDa heat shock protein and hsp70 mRNA following transient focal cerebral ischemia in the rat. J Cereb Blood Flow Metab 13: 105–115

58. Kinouchi H, Sharp FR, Koistinaho J, Hicks K, Kamii H, Chan PH (1993) Induction of heat shock hsp70 mRNA and HSP70kDa protein in neurons in the 'penumbra' following focal cerebral ischemia in the rat. Brain Res 619: 334–338

59. Kirino T (1982) Delayed neuronal death in the gerbil hippocampus following ischemia, Brain Res 239: 57–69

60. Kirino T, Tamura A, Sano K (1985) Selective vulnerability of the hippocampus to ischemia – reversible and irreversible types of ischemic cell damage. Prog Brain Res 63: 39–58

61. Kirino T, Tamura A, Sano K (1986) A reversible type of neuronal injury following ischemia in the gerbil hippocampus. Stroke 17: 455–459

62. Kobayashi S, Welsh FA (1995) Regional alterations of ATP and heat-shock protein-72 mRNA following hypoxia-ischemia in neonatal rat brain. J Cereb Blood Flow Metab 15: 1047–1056

63. Kogure K, Kato H (1993) Altered gene expression in cerebral ischemia. Stroke 24: 2121–2127

64. Krause GS, Tiffany BR (1993) Suppression of protein synthesis in the reperfused brain. Stroke 24: 747–756

65. Lee PJ, Jiang BH, Chin BY, Iyer NV, Alam J, Semenza GL, Choi AM (1997) Hypoxia-inducible factor-1 mediates transcriptional activation of the heme oxygenase-1 gene in response to hypoxia. J Biol Chem 272: 5375–5381

66. Li H, Ko HP, Whitlock JP (1996) Induction of phosphoglycerate kinase 1 gene expression by hypoxia. Roles of Arnt and HIF1alpha. J Biol Chem 271: 21262–21267

67. Li Y, Chopp M, Garcia JH, Yoshida Y, Zhang ZG, Levine SR (1992) Distribution of the 72-kd heat-shock protein as a function of transient focal cerebral ischemia in rats. Stroke 23: 1292–1298

68. Li Y, Chopp M, Jiang N, Zaloga C (1995) In situ detection of DNA fragmentation after focal cerebral ischemia in mice. Brain Res Mol Brain Res 28: 164–168

69. Li Y, Chopp M, Zhang ZG, Zhang RL, Garcia JH (1993) Neuronal survival is associated with 72-kDa heat shock protein expression after transient middle cerebral artery occlusion in the rat. J Neurol Sci 120: 187–194

70. Li Y, Sharov VG, Jiang N, Zaloga C, Sabbah HN, Chopp M (1995) Ultrastructural and light microscopic evidence of apoptosis after middle cerebral artery occlusion in the rat. Am J Pathol 146: 1045–1051

71. Lindquist S (1992) Heat-shock proteins and stress tolerance in microorganisms. Curr Opin Genet Dev 2: 748–755

72. Lindsberg PJ, Frerichs KU, Siren AL, Hallenbeck JM, Nowak TS, Jr (1996) Heat-shock protein and c-fos expression in focal microvascular brain damage. J Cereb Blood Flow Metab 16: 82–91

73. Linnik MD, Miller JA, Sprinkle-Cavallo J, Mason PJ, Thompson FY, Montgomery LR, Schroeder KK (1995) Apoptotic DNA fragmentation in the rat cerebral cortex induced by permanent middle cerebral artery occlusion. Brain Res Mol Brain Res 32: 116–124

74. Linnik MD, Zobrist RH, Hatfield MD (1993) Evidence supporting a role for programmed cell death in focal cerebral ischemia in rats. Stroke 24: 2002–2009
75. Liu Y, Cox SR, Morita T, Kourembanas S (1995) Hypoxia regulates vascular endothelial growth factor gene expression in endothelial cells. Identification of a 5' enhancer. Circ Res 77: 638–643
76. MacManus JP, Hill IE, Huang ZG, Rasquinha I, Xue D, Buchan AM (1994) DNA damage consistent with apoptosis in transient focal ischaemic neocortex. Neuroreport 5: 493–496
77. MacManus JP, Hill IE, Preston E, Rasquinha I, Walker T, Buchan AM (1995) Differences in DNA fragmentation following transient cerebral or decapitation ischemia in rats. J Cereb Blood Flow Metab 15: 728–737
78. MacManus JP, Linnik MD (1997) Gene expression induced by cerebral ischemia: an apoptotic perspective. J Cereb Blood Flow Metab 17: 815–832
79. Mancuso A, Derugin N, Ono Y, Hara K, Chen SF, Sharp FR, Weinstein PR (1997) Correlation of HSP:70 and c-fos mRNA expression with regional depolarization determined by diffusion MRI following MCA occlusion in rats. Soc Neurosci Abstracts 27: 558.510
80. Marin P, Nastiuk KL, Daniel N, Girault JA, Czernik AJ, Glowinski J, Nairn AC, Premont J (1997) Glutamate-dependent phosphorylation of elongation factor-2 and inhibition of protein synthesis in neurons. J Neurosci 17: 3445–3454
81. Massa SM, Swanson RA, Sharp FR (1996) The stress gene response in brain. Cerebrovascular Brain Metab Rev 8: 95–158
82. Mayevsky A, Doron A, Manor T, Meilin S, Zarchin N, Ouaknine GE (1996) Cortical spreading depression recorded from the human brain using a multiparametric monitoring system. Brain Res 740: 268–274
83. Melillo G, Taylor LS, Brooks A, MxKP>usso T, Cox GW, Varesio L (1997) Functional requirement of the hypoxia-responsive element in the activation of the inducible nitric oxide synthase promoter by the iron chelator desferrioxamine. J Biol Chem 272: 12236–12243
84. Michels AA, Kanon B, Konings AW, Ohtsuka K, Bensaude O, Kampinga HH (1997) Hsp70 and Hsp40 chaperone activities in the cytoplasm and the nucleus of mammalian cells. J Biol Chem 272: 33283–33289
85. Morimoto RI (1993) Cells in stress: transcriptional activation of heat shock genes. Science 259: 1409–1410
86. Moseley ME, Butts K, Yenari MA, Marks M, de Crespigny A (1995) Clinical aspects of DWI. NMR Biomed 8: 387–396
87. Munell F, Burke RE, Bandele A, Gubits RM (1994) Localization of c-fos, c-jun, and hsp70 mRNA expression in brain after neonatal hypoxia-ischemia. Brain Res Dev Brain Res 77: 111–121
88. Nakane M, Teraoka A, Asato R, Tamura A (1992) Degeneration of the ipsilateral substantia nigra following cerebral infarction in the striatum. Stroke 23: 328–332
89. Nedergaard M, Diemer NH (1987) Focal ischemia of the rat brain, with special reference to the influence of plasma glucose concentration. Acta Neuropathol (Berl) 73: 131–137
90. Nimura T, Weinstein PR, Massa SM, Panter S, Sharp FR (1996) Heme oxygenase-1 (HO-1) protein induction in rat brain following focal ischemia. Brain Res Mol Brain Res 37: 201–208
91. Noga M, Hayashi T, Tanaka J (1997) Gene expressions of ubiquitin and hsp70 following focal ischaemia in rat brain. Neuroreport 8: 1239–1241
92. Nowak TS Jr (1993) Synthesis of heat shock/stress proteins during cellular injury. Ann N Y Acad Sci 679: 142–156
93. Nowak TS Jr, Jacewicz M (1994) The heat shock/stress response in focal cerebral ischemia. Brain Pathol 4: 67–76
94. Nowak TS Jr, Osborne OC, Suga S (1993) Stress protein and proto-oncogene expression as indicators of neuronal pathophysiology after ischemia. Prog Brain Res 96: 195–208
95. Nudo RJ, Wise BM, SiFuentes F, Milliken GW (1996) Neural substrates for the effects of rehabilitative training on motor recovery after ischemic infarct (comments). Science 272: 1791–1794
96. Pelham HR (1986) Speculations on the functions of the major heat shock and glucose-regulated proteins. Cell 46: 959–961
97. Planas AM, Soriano MA, Estrada A, Sanz O, Martin F, Ferrer I (1997) The heat shock stress response after brain lesions: induction of 72 kDa heat shock protein (cell types involved, axonal transport, transcriptional regulation) and protein synthesis inhibition. Prog Neurobiol 51: 607–636
98. Plumier JC, Krueger AM, Currie RW, Kontoyiannis D, Kollias G, Pagoulatos GN (1997) Transgenic mice expressing the human inducible Hsp70 have hippocampal neurons resistant to ischemic injury. Cell Stress Chaperones 2: 162–167
99. Rajdev S, Solway KE, Mestril R, Dillmann WH, Sharp FR (1997) Heat shock protein 70 expression in brains of transgenic mice overexpressing the rat inducible heat shock protein 70 protection against global ischemia. Soc Neurosci Abstracts 27: 848.815

100. Ratcliffe P, Rourke J, Maxwell P (1998) Oxygen sensing, hypoxia-inducible factor-1 and the regulation of mammalian gene expression. J Exp Biol 201: 1153–1162
101. Rolfs A, Kvietikova I, Gassmann M, Wenger RH (1997) Oxygen-regulated transferrin expression is mediated by hypoxia-inducible factor-1. J Biol Chem 272: 20055–20062
102. Saji M, Cohen M, Blau AD, Wessel TC, Volpe BT (1994) Transient forebrain ischemia induces delayed injury in the substantia nigra reticulata: degeneration of GABA neurons, compensatory expression of GAD mRNA. Brain Res 643: 234–244
103. Saji M, Reis DJ (1987) Delayed transneuronal death of substantia nigra neurons prevented by gamma-aminobutyric acid agonist. Science 235: 66–69
104. Saji M, Volpe BT (1993) Delayed histologic damage and neuron death in the substantia nigra reticulata following transient forebrain ischemia depends on the extent of initial striatal injury. Neurosci Lett 155: 47–50
105. Sanz O, Estrada A, Ferrer I, Planas AM (1997) Differential cellular distribution and dynamics of HSP70, cyclooxygenase-2, and c-Fos in the rat brain after transient focal ischemia or kainic acid. Neuroscience 80: 221–232
106. Saris N, Holkeri H, Craven RA, Stirling CJ, Makarow M (1997) The Hsp70 homologue Lhs1p is involved in a novel function of the yeast endoplasmic reticulum, refolding and stabilization of heat-denatured protein aggregates. J Cell Biol 137: 813–824
107. Schumacher RJ, Hansen WJ, Freeman BC, Alnemri E, Litwack G, Toft DO (1996) Cooperative action of Hsp70, Hsp90, and DnaJ proteins in protein renaturation. Biochemistry 35: 14889–14898
108. Semenza GL (1994) Regulation of erythropoietin production. New insights into molecular mechanisms of oxygen homeostasis, Hematol Oncol Clin North Am 8: 863–884
109. Semenza GL (1998) Hypoxia-inducible factor 1 and the molecular physiology of oxygen homeostasis. J Lab Clin Med 131: 207–214
110. Semenza GL, Jiang BH, Leung SW, Passantino R, Concordet JP, Maire P, Giallongo A (1996) Hypoxia response elements in the aldolase A, enolase 1, and lactate dehydrogenase A gene promoters contain essential binding sites for hypoxia-inducible factor 1. J Biol Chem 271: 32529–32537
111. Semenza GL, Roth PH, Fang HM, Wang GL (1994) Transcriptional regulation of genes encoding glycolytic enzymes by hypoxia-inducible factor 1. J Biol Chem 269: 23757–23763
112. Semenza GL, Wang GL (1992) A nuclear factor induced by hypoxia via de novo protein synthesis binds to the human erythropoietin gene enhancer at a site required for transcriptional activation. Mol Cell Biol 12: 5447–5454
113. Sharp FR (1995) Stress proteins are sensitive indicators of injury in the brain produced by ischemia and toxins. J Toxicol Sci 20: 450–453
114. Sharp FR, Kinouchi H, Koistinaho J, Chan PH, Sagar SM (1993) HSP70 heat shock gene regulation during ischemia. Stroke 24:I72–75
115. Sharp FR, Lowenstein D, Simon R, Hisanaga K (1991) Heat shock protein hsp72 induction in cortical and striatal astrocytes and neurons following infarction. J Cereb Blood Flow Metab 11: 621–627
116. Sharp FR, Sagar SM (1994) Alterations in gene expression as an index of neuronal injury: heat shock and the immediate early gene response. Neurotoxicology 15: 51–59
117. Sharp JW, Sagar SM, Hisanaga K, Jasper P, Sharp FR (1990) The NMDA receptor mediates cortical induction of fos and fos-related antigens following cortical injury. Exp Neurol 109: 323–332
118. States BA, Honkaniemi J, Weinstein PR, Sharp FR (1996) DNA fragmentation and HSP70 protein induction in hippocampus and cortex occurs in separate neurons following permanent middle cerebral artery occlusions. J Cereb Blood Flow Metab 16: 1165–1175
119. Symon L (1980) The relationship between CBF, evoked potentials and the clinical features in cerebral ischaemia. Acta Neurol Scand Suppl 78: 175–190
120. Symon L, Lassen NA, Astrup J, Branston NM (1977) Thresholds of ischaemia in brain cortex. Adv Exp Med Biol 94: 775–782
121. Tamura A, Tahira Y, Nagashima H, Kirino T, Gotoh O, Hojo S, Sano K (1991) Thalamic atrophy following cerebral infarction in the territory of the middle cerebral artery. Stroke 22: 615–618
122. Terada K, Kanazawa M, Bukau B, Mori M (1997) The human DnaJ homologue dj2 facilitates mitochondrial protein import and luciferase refolding. J Cell Biol 139: 1089–1095
123. Torella C, Mattingly JR Jr, Artigues A, Iriarte A, Martinez-Carrion M (1998) Insight into the conformation of protein folding intermediate(s) trapped by GroEL. J Biol Chem 273: 3915–3925
124. Vandenbroeck K, Martens E, Billiau A (1998) GroEL/ES chaperonins protect interferon-gamma against physicochemical stress – study of tertiary structure formation by alpha-casein quenching and ELISA. Eur J Biochem 251: 181–188
125. Wagstaff MJ, Collaco-Moraes Y, Aspey BS, Coffin RS, Harrison MJ, Latchman DS, de Belleroche JS (1996) Focal cerebral ischaemia increases the levels of several classes of heat shock proteins and their corresponding mRNAs. Brain Res Mol Brain Res 42: 236–244

126. Wang GL, Semenza GL (1993) Characterization of hypoxia-inducible factor 1 and regulation of DNA binding activity by hypoxia. J Biol Chem 268: 21513–21518
127. Wang GL, Semenza GL (1996) Molecular basis of hypoxia-induced erythropoietin expression. Curr Opin Hematol 3: 156–162
128. Warach S, Boska M, Welch KM (1997) Pitfalls and potential of clinical diffusion-weighted MR imaging in acute stroke (editorial; comment). Stroke 28: 481–482
129. Weiller C, Chollet F, Friston KJ, Wise RJ, Frackowiak RS (1992) Functional reorganization of the brain in recovery from striatocapsular infarction in man. Ann Neurol 31: 463–472
130. Weiller C, Ramsay SC, Wise RJ, Friston KJ, Frackowiak RS (1993) Individual patterns of functional reorganization in the human cerebral cortex after capsular infarction. Ann Neurol 33: 181–189
131. Welsh FA, Moyer DJ, Harris VA (1992) Regional expression of heat shock protein-70 mRNA and c-fos mRNA following focal ischemia in rat brain. J Cereb Blood Flow Metab 12: 204–212
132. Wood SM, Gleadle JM, Pugh CW, Hankinson O, Ratcliffe PJ (1996) The role of the aryl hydrocarbon receptor nuclear translocator (ARNT) in hypoxic induction of gene expression. Studies in ARNT-deficient cells. J Biol Chem 271: 15117–15123
133. Woodburn VL, Hayward NJ, Poat JA, Woodruff GN, Hughes J (1993) The effect of dizocilpine and enadoline on immediate early gene expression in the gerbil global ischaemia model. Neuropharmacology 32: 1047–1059
134. Yamada K, Kinoshita A, Kohmura E, Sakaguchi T, Taguchi J, Kataoka K, Hayakawa T (1991) Basic fibroblast growth factor prevents thalamic degeneration after cortical infarction. J Cereb Blood Flow Metab 11: 472–478
135. Zola-Morgan S, Squire LR, Rempel NL, Clower RP, Amaral DG (1992) Enduring memory impairment in monkeys after ischemic damage to the hippocampus. J Neurosci 12: 2582–2596

Aspects of the Maturation Phenomenon Observed by the TUNEL Method

W. C. Gordon, V. Colangelo, N. G. Bazan, and I. Klatzo

Summary. Comparative studies, using adjacent sections stained with cresyl violet and the TUNEL FITC-dUTP method, provided several observations relevant to the significance of the TUNEL reaction and the dynamics of maturation phenomenon in cerebral ischemia. Our investigations were performed in gerbils subjected to single ischemic exposures and to repeated exposures separated by various time intervals. Using the TUNEL method, our observations of animals sacrificed following a single 6 min ischemia produced by bilateral common carotid artery occlusion (BCAO), suggest that neurons for which TUNEL-positive staining is limited to nuclei are capable of recovery. This is evident in the subiculum, CA 2 and CA 3, indicating survival of many neurons that revealed, at certain post-ischemic times, transient TUNEL-positivity confined to their nuclei. Nissl-stained sections obtained from gerbils sacrificed on day 7 demonstrated slight neuronal loss in the subiculum, which was more pronounced in CA 2. In contrast, there was full preservation of CA 3 neurons, with centrally-located nuclei and distinct Nissl bodies. These observations indicate that TUNEL staining, associated with preservation of the nuclear membrane, does not invariably signify impending cellular death; the fragmented deoxyribonucleic acid (DNA) can still be repaired and neurons may recover fully. With regard to maturation phenomenon, our observations indicate that the selective vulnerability and sensitivity of the response to ischemic injury in various neuronal types are different and can be modified by changing the time interval between sublethal and lethal ischemic exposures. TUNEL labeling appears in the more resistant subiculum and CA 2 earlier than in CA 1, whereas for animals given a 1-h interval between exposures, the high vulnerability of CA 1 becomes overshadowed by some of the thalamic nuclei and cerebral cortex.

Introduction

It has become increasingly apparent that the dynamics of maturation phenomenon reflect, to a great extent, a fluctuating balance of genomic expression, leading either to recovery and neuroprotection or to accelerated apoptotic death. That sublethal hyperthermia is associated with the induction of stress proteins (heat shock proteins) and enhanced tolerance to a subsequent lethal thermal exposure [1, 4, 13] has been confirmed by the demonstration that a sublethal ischemic exposure may also induce neuronal tolerance to a lethal ischemic injury [11, 12]. Subsequent studies in this area have revealed the transient nature of induced tolerance and the relevance of the interval between various ischemic exposures [7, 9, 16]. Although it is well established that

Maturation Phenomenon in Cerebral Ischemia III
U. Ito et al. (Eds.)
© Springer-Verlag Berlin Heidelberg 1999

tolerance is developed when initial sublethal ischemia is followed within a few days by lethal insult, we have been interested in observing how shorter intervals may be reflected in apoptotic changes, as visualized by TUNEL staining. We have been particularly interested in investigating the enhanced, cumulative effect on ischemic injury when there is a 1-h interval between repeated exposures [6, 7].

The assumption that apoptosis plays an important role in the maturation of ischemic injury has prompted us to focus on various aspects of these processes. We have applied the sensitive, fluorescent, fluorescein isothiocyanate (FITC)-dUTP TUNEL method to outline the dynamic features of the development of ischemic injury in various topistic regions. Also, we are interested in ascertaining whether, as is generally assumed, positive TUNEL staining invariably denotes oncoming neuronal death, or whether it is possible that such cells are still capable of survival and eventual recovery. Finally, we have attempted to determine how induction of neuronal tolerance may be reflected in apoptotic changes as visualized by TUNEL staining.

Material and Methods

Experiments were carried out on female gerbils (60–80 g) subjected to bilateral complete arterial occlusion (BCAO) under 1.5 % halothane in 70 % N_2O, 30 % O_2 anesthesia. During and after the operation, rectal temperature was monitored and maintained at 37.5 °C. Groups of 4–6 gerbils were subjected either to a single 6-min BCAO and sacrificed by perfusion with buffered 4 % paraformaldehyde after 1, 2, 3, 4 or 7 days, or to an initial 2-min BCAO followed by a second 6-min BCAO after 15 min, 1 h, and 3 days of recirculation. Animals in the double-ischemic exposure groups were sacrificed 3 days after a 6-min exposure. In one additional group, gerbils undergoing the second (6-min) occlusion were terminated 7 days later. Brains were embedded in paraffin and sectioned (10-μm thick). Adjacent sections were stained with cresyl violet or labeled by the TUNEL FITC-dUTP method.

For imaging and analysis, sections were viewed with a Nikon Optiphot-2 with bright field or fluorescence optics. Identical regions in the hippocampus, thalamus and cortex were selected for comparison from each preparation. Images were detected with a SONY 3CCD color DXC-960MD camera and viewed on a SONY Trinitron color monitor at an initial magnification of 400×. Each neuronal cell body within the monitor field was counted to give regional densities, and these values were averaged for each treatment. Final results are presented as a percentage of control values ± SD.

Results

Gerbils sacrificed 1 day after a single 6-min episode of ischemia showed no abnormal changes that could be recognized in the cresyl violet preparations. On the other hand, TUNEL staining revealed, in the most mesial part of the hippocampal hilus, TUNEL-positive reactions within the nuclei of a few neurons. In gerbils sacrificed after 2 days, Nissl sections showed occasional accentuated staining of apical dendrites in CA 1. TUNEL-positive labeling was evident in scattered neurons in the subicular (Fig. 1B)

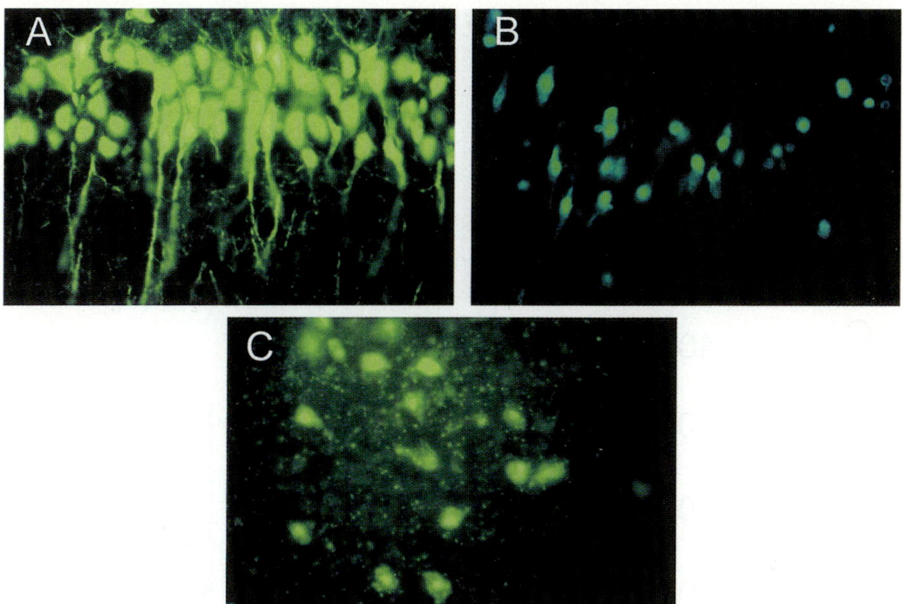

Fig. 1. A TUNEL labeling of CA 1 pyramidal neurons on day 3 after bilateral common carotid artery occlusion (BCAO), showing intense staining of the entire cell body, including processes (40×10). **B** Day 2 after 6-min BCAO. The subiculum reveals TUNEL labeling which is predominantly confined to neuronal nuclei (40×10). **C** TUNEL labeling in the area of the ventral thalamus, demonstrating an intense staining of neuronal bodies and numerous green fluorescent inclusions along the processes and in the neuropil. Gerbils subjected to 2 min ischemia, followed 1 h later by 6-min BCAO were sacrificed 3 days after the second insult (40×10)

and CA 2 regions, whereas the CA 1 and CA 3 segments remained completely TUNEL-negative.

Animals sacrificed after 3 days showed, in Nissl preparations, the expected severe injury in the CA 1 sector and occasional ischemic neuronal injury in the subicular and CA 2 regions. In corresponding TUNEL sections, the most conspicuous finding was staining of the CA 1 pyramidal neurons (Fig 1A). In addition to staining of their nuclei, these neurons also displayed a bright green fluorescence of their cytoplasm and, particularly, of their apical dendrites, which terminate in the stratum lacunosum-moleculare.

When the intensity of ischemic injury was not symmetric in both hemispheres, TUNEL staining in the less-affected hemisphere was confined to the neuronal cell bodies, without extension into processes. Also, in such asymmetrical cases, TUNEL staining of CA 1 neurons was correlated with the intensity of staining in the entorhinal cortex. It was observed that, on the side of more severe injury, intense TUNEL staining of CA 1 neurons and their processes was associated, on the ipsilateral side, with the staining of numerous neurons in the third layer of the entorhinal cortex. In contrast, in the less-affected hemisphere, in which the green fluorescence of CA 1 neurons did not extend into their processes, few or no TUNEL-positive neurons were found. Otherwise, in several gerbils with severe CA 1 injury, in addition to the ento-

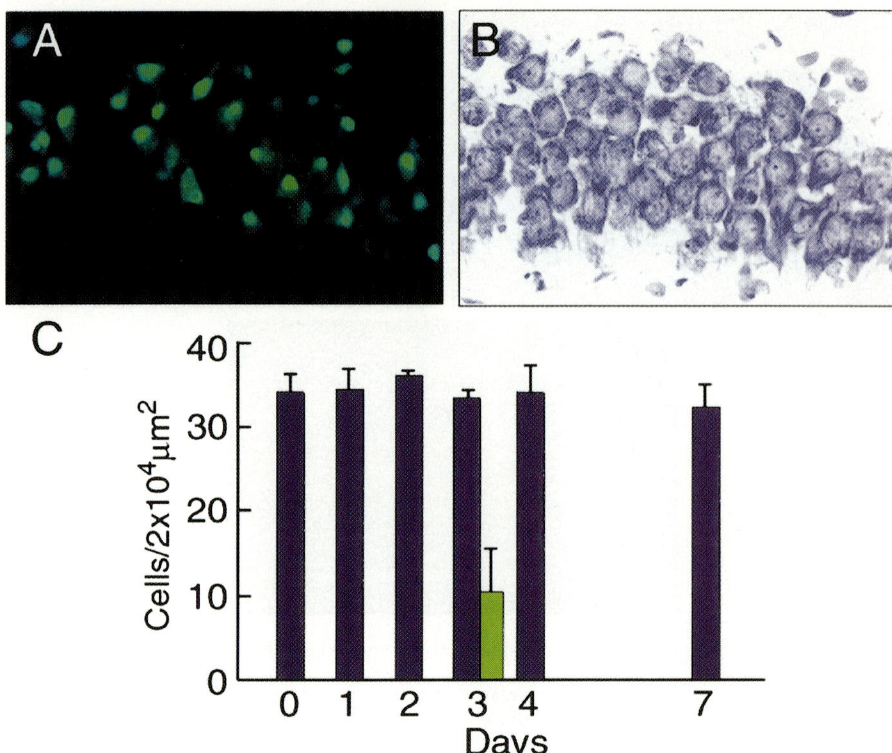

Fig. 2. A CA 3 sector on day 3 after bilateral common carotid artery occlusion (BCAO), showing TUNEL labeling of mostly eccentrically positioned nuclei (40×10). **B** Nissl stain. CA 3 on day 7, following 6-min BCAO. The neurons appear to be well preserved, with distinct Nissl bodies and mostly centrally located nuclei (40×10). **C** Graph showing the number of cells within a $2 \times 10^4\ \mu m^2$ area on the bend of the CA 3 region of the hippocampus. Gerbils were exposed to 6 min ischemia and allowed to recover for up to 7 days. Tissue was then prepared for Nissl stain (purple), which demonstrates no cell loss at any time, and for TUNEL-FITC dUTP labeling (green), which shows positive nuclear labeling on day 3

rhinal cortex, TUNEL staining was also positive in pyramidal neurons of the third layer of parietal cortex. In the subiculum, the mesial part showed TUNEL-positive staining in some neuronal nuclei, whereas more laterally, where the subiculum merged into CA 1, some neurons demonstrated TUNEL staining of the entire neuronal cell body, including proximal processes. In CA 2, in a number of neurons, TUNEL-positive labeling included their cytoplasm but no processes. Also, numerous TUNEL-positive neurons were observed most prominently where the CA 3 region curved in the direction of the hilus. TUNEL staining in CA 3 was almost always confined to neuronal nuclei, which were visibly translocated toward the periphery of the cell (Fig. 2A). Occasionally, some scattered TUNEL-positive neurons could also be seen in the hippocampal hilus.

In gerbils sacrificed after 4 days, Nissl-stained sections revealed an intensified microglial reaction in the severely-injured CA 1. The TUNEL reaction was similar to that of day 3, but was somewhat reduced in CA 1 and CA 2. Occasional TUNEL-positive neurons could be observed in the subiculum, but CA 3 was completely TUNEL-negative.

Nissl-stained sections of gerbils sacrificed after 7 days revealed severe destruction within CA 1, with the remaining pyramidal neurons appearing shrunken and pyknotic. In TUNEL-stained sections, shrunken pyramidal cells frequently showed, in the nuclei and sometimes in the cytoplasm, green fluorescent, bleb-like inclusions. Small, fluorescent inclusions were also occasionally observed in apical dendrites or lying free in the neuropil. The subiculum and CA 2 region demonstrated occasional TUNEL-positive neurons, whereas no TUNEL staining was seen in the CA 3 sector. Throughout this 7-day period, nerve cells were counted over equal areas ($2 \cdot 10^4$ μm^2) at the bend of the CA 3 region in both Nissl and TUNEL-labeled sections. Nissl stain (Fig. 2B) revealed no significant neuronal loss at any time (34.0 cell bodies±1.3 SD), even after transient TUNEL-positive staining on day 3 (10.3 cell bodies±5.3 SD) (Fig. 2C).

Groups of gerbils subjected to two (sublethal and lethal) ischemic exposures provided the following observations. Nissl sections from animals sacrificed 3 days after an initial 2-min period of ischemia, followed after 15 min by 6-min BCAO, revealed a slightly less intense injury in CA 1 and CA 2 than sections from animals sacrificed 3 days after a single 6-min period of ischemia. However, the cerebral cortex and thalamus demonstrated a number of scattered, dark neurons with distorted proximal neuronal processes. TUNEL staining in this double-exposure group displayed frequent positivity of CA 1 pyramidal cells, confined to the neuronal cell body; for cases in which the staining included apical dendrites, there was a clear association with conspicuous TUNEL positivity of neurons in the third layer of the entorhinal cortex on the ipsilateral side. Otherwise, there was frequent TUNEL positivity in CA 2 and CA 3, and in scattered neurons of the hilus. In contrast to animals sacrificed 3 days after a single 6-min occlusion, each animal in the double-exposure group displayed frequent TUNEL staining of scattered neurons in the parietal cortex, for which the intense green fluorescence was sometimes found to extend for a distance into the neuronal processes. One animal in this group revealed, in one hemisphere, TUNEL staining of neurons in the ventral region of the thalamus.

Animals sacrificed 3 days following exposure to a 1-h separation of 2-min and 6-min occlusions showed a marked enhancement of ischemic injury in the thalamus and parietal cortex. In some of the ventral thalamic nuclei, Nissl sections revealed severe ischemic injury, with chromatolytic or hyperchromatic neurons, some of which displayed cresyl violet-stained, twisted processes. Similar evidence of injury was also present in the parietal cortex. The TUNEL assay in this group revealed conspicuous staining in the thalamus, involving predominantly the ventral nuclei. In some neurons, only the nuclei were TUNEL positive, whereas, in others, the green fluorescence was also present in the cytoplasm and short processes. Also apparent in such areas was the frequent presence of brightly green fluorescent small inclusions, seen along neuronal processes or scattered in the neuropil (Fig. 1C). The parietal cortex in this group revealed frequent, intense TUNEL staining of the pyramidal neurons in the third layer. The CA 1 pyramidal cells were TUNEL stained with similar intensity and with similar synchronization in the asymmetrically-injured hemispheres (with staining in the entorhinal cortex) as described for the 15-min double-exposure group. TUNEL-positive staining, confined to the nuclei, was visible also in neurons of CA 2, and occasionally in a few neurons of CA 3.

For the group sacrificed 3 days following a 6-min ischemic exposure that was carried out 3 days after a 2-min period of ischemia, Nissl sections revealed complete preservation of CA 1 pyramidal neurons, with the exception of one gerbil that showed only moderate injury in the CA 1 sector. TUNEL staining in this group of animals was confined to the subiculum and CA 2, revealing nuclear staining in neurons very similar to that observed in the single 6-min period of ischemia in gerbils sacrificed 2 days later.

Discussion

Apoptosis, a process associated with DNA fragmentation and programmed cell death, remains a controversial subject, although its paramount role in cerebral ischemia maturation phenomenon has been generally accepted. One of the important, unresolved questions has been whether, in every case, apoptosis terminates with cellular death, thereby signifying from the time of its induction the point of no return, or whether this process may be reversed. This could be extremely important for potential therapeutic considerations. Although molecular studies in brain tissue subjected to ischemia clearly have associated fragmentation of DNA with the appearance of apoptotic oligonucleosomes, the meeting of morphological criteria for apoptosis frequently has been unsatisfactory, raising many suggestions that neurons in cerebral ischemia die mainly by necrosis. Relevant to this controversy, our observations appear to mollify some of these divergent points. First, they support the notion that apoptosis is not always associated with cell death; the induction of the apoptotic process may, when injury is severe enough, lead to death. This suggests that, when the injury is not too severe, some cells with nuclear TUNEL staining are capable of recovery, and this appears to be unequivocally demonstrated in our observations of the CA 3 neurons. In this hippocampal sector, following a single 6-min period of ischemia, numerous neurons revealed conspicuous TUNEL staining of nuclei (Fig. 2A) on day 3 and lasting for 1 day. However, neuronal cell counts in this group failed to reveal any significant neuronal loss (Fig. 2B) when gerbils were sacrificed 1 week later.

Reversibility of ischemic injury in CA 3 neurons has been previously reported by Ito et al. [8], who described a reactive change resembling that seen in central chromatolysis and similarly characterized by an eccentric translocation of neuronal nuclei facing a cytoplasm devoid of Nissl bodies. Hyden's [5] early ultraviolet (UV) spectrographic studies of central chromatolysis produced by peripheral nerve transection demonstrated that it is a very active and reversible process, requiring the intense production of RNA and basic proteins for the restoration of Nissl substance. Thus, it is conceivable that, in our study, the mildly-injured CA 3 neurons, showing the transitional appearance of TUNEL staining in eccentrically located nuclei, might be undergoing a similar restorative process towards recovery. The possibility of DNA restoration as it relates to the repair of DNA by endo-exonucleases has been reported by Fraser [3].

It would then appear that when ischemic injury is severe and acute, leaving insufficient time for the induction of apoptosis, neurons die by necrosis. In the case of less acute and less overwhelming cellular injury or irritation, induction of the apoptotic cascade occurs (with other genomic expressions), leading to DNA fragmentation and then, depending upon the severity of the injury, apoptosis may retreat and the neurons recover or, when the ischemic injury is more intense, apoptosis is joined or superseded by necrotic changes, terminating the life of the cell. It is conceivable that the loss of functional integrity of the nuclear membrane marks the point of no return and, based on our observations, we propose that the extension of TUNEL staining into the cytoplasm and processes may constitute a signpost for the irreversibility of ischemic cell injury.

In the pathophysiology of cerebral ischemia, two separate features should be recognized in affected brain tissue. One is the selective sensitivity of various specific neuronal populations in responding to sublethal noxae or irritations; the other is the well-recognized selective vulnerability, which relates to differences in the degree of injury in various neuronal units produced by ischemic episodes of the same intensity. The presented observations seem to demonstrate the distinction between these two features. Thus, the more resistant subiculum and CA 2 regions appear to be more sensitive in their response to a 6-min period of ischemia, revealing TUNEL labeling 1 day earlier than in the CA 1 sector. However, in spite of the simultaneous appearance of TUNEL staining in CA 1 and CA 3 areas on the third day after a 6-min period of ischemia, there is an obvious difference in the vulnerability of these sectors. This is clearly evident from neuronal survival rates, and is also reflected in the appearance of TUNEL staining in these two areas. Thus, whereas the CA 1 sector reveals intense TUNEL-positive staining of nuclei, cytoplasm and neuronal processes that persists for a number of days, CA 3 staining is confined to neuronal nuclei and lasts for only 1 day. This is consistent with the assumption that necrosis, but not apoptosis, plays the primary role in the abrupt demise of CA 1 pyramidal neurons on the third post-ischemic day.

Concerning the selective sensitivity of various neuronal populations to ischemia, it appears that transneuronal signaling may play a significant role. Transneuronal induction of tolerance has been demonstrated bilaterally in CA 1 of both hemispheres following unilaterally induced spreading depression and there is an early c-fos expression in both hippocampi [10]. Otherwise, bilateral tolerance in the CA 1 sector has been observed following ischemic infarction in one of the hemispheres [11]. A plausible explanation for these findings is that tolerance in both CA 1 sectors is induced by transneuronal signaling via the entorhinal cortex, which provides bilateral innervation for both hippocampi. In support of the assumption that apoptosis might be transneuronally induced, Charriaut-Marlangue et al. [2] observed TUNEL-labeling of some septal cells in the hemisphere contralateral to the side of infarction. Our own findings on the interrelationship of TUNEL-positivity between CA 1 and the entorhinal cortex may also be relevant to the transneuronal induction of apoptosis. The participation of neuroexcitotoxic mechanisms in CA 1 injury has been repeatedly demonstrated as an interference with the glutamatergic circuitry that extends through the entorhinal cortex, dentate gyrus, and Schaeffer's collaterals to the CA 1 pyramidal neurons [15]. In our studies, it appears plausible that neuroexcitation of an intensity resulting in necrosis of the CA 1 neurons could correlate with less neurotoxic excitation within the entorhinal cortex, expressing mainly reversible apoptotic changes.

 W. C. Gordon et al.

The elucidation of mechanisms responsible for altering selective vulnerability of various neuronal populations, by manipulating the time interval between ischemic exposures, could contribute considerably to an understanding of the maturation phenomenon. In the present study, the 1-h interval between ischemic insults was associated with greatly increased vulnerability of the cerebral cortex and thalamus, which was apparent in Nissl and in TUNEL preparations, but no enhancement and even a slight reduction in injury to CA 1. However, the day-3 interval was associated with marked preservation of the CA 1 sector and no thalamic injury was observed. This seems to emphasize the complexity of tolerance and of vulnerability phenomena and reminds us of the pathoclisis teachings of Vogt and Vogt [17], who recognized the selective vulnerability (pathoclisis) associated with each element of brain tissue, including its vasculature. Thus, in 1-h interval animals, damage of the thalamus, associated with previously described disturbances of the blood–brain barrier [14], could represent a cumulative effect of the vulnerability of both neurons and blood vessels.

Acknowledgements. The authors thank Thomas Harris, Jr. for excellent technical assistance and Josephine Wolfe for expert editorial assistance. This work was supported by NIH NS23002 and NIH EY02377.

References

1. Barbe MF, Tytell M, Gower DJ, Welch WJ (1988) Hyperthermia protects against light damage in the rat retina. Science 241: 1817–1820
2. Charriaut-Marlangue C, Margaill I, Plotkine M, Ben-Ari Y (1995) Early endonuclease activation following reversible focal ischemia. J Cereb Blood Flow Metab 15: 385–388
3. Fraser M (1994) Endo-exonucleases: enzymes involved in DNA repair and cell death? Bioessays 16: 761–766
4. Hahn GM, Li GC (1982) Thermotolerance and heat shock proteins in mammalian cells. Radiat Res 92: 452–457
5. Hyden H (1943) Protein metabolism in the nerve cell during growth and function. Acta Physiol Scand 6: 88–97
6. Ikeda J, Nagashima G, Nowak TS Jr, Mies G, Joo F, Xu S, Lohr J, Ruetzler CA, Wagner HG, Klatzo I (1989) Observations on accumulation of calcium in gerbils subjected to cerebral ischemia. In: Krieglstein J (ed) Pharmacology of cerebral ischemia. Wissenschaftliche Verlaggesellschaft, CRC Press, Stuttgart, pp 37–44
7. Ikeda J, Nagashima G, Saito N, Nowak TS Jr, Joo F, Mies G, Lohr JM, Ruetzler CA, Klatzo I (1990) Putative neuroexcitation in cerebral ischemia and brain injury. Stroke 21: 65–70
8. Ito U, Spatz M, Walker JT Jr, Klatzo I (1975) Experimental cerebral ischemia in mongolian gerbils. I. Light microscopic observations. Acta Neuropath 32: 209–223
9. Kawahara N, Ruetzler CA, Klatzo I (1995) Protective effect of spreading depression against neuronal damage following cardiac arrest cerebral ischemia. Neurol Res 17: 9–16
10. Kawahara N, Belayev L, Orzi F, Colangelo V, Klatzo I (1997) Transneuronal induction of tolerance in cerebral ischemia. In: Maturation phenomenon in cerebral ishemia II. U Ito, T Kirino, T Kuroiwa, I Klatzo (eds) Springer Verlag, Berlin, Heidelberg, New York, pp. 105–111
11. Kirino T, Tsujita Y, Tamura A (1991) Induced tolerance to ischemia in gerbil hippocampal neurons. J Cereb Blood Flow Metab 11: 299–307
12. Kitagawa K, Matsumoto M, Tagaya M et al. (1990) "Ischemic tolerance" found in the brain. Brain Res 528: 21–24
13. Li GC, Werb Z (1982) Correlation between the synthesis of heat-shock proteins and the development of thermotolerance in Chinese hamster fibroblasts. Proc Natl Acad Sci U S A 79: 3219–3222
14. Nagashima G, Nowak TS Jr., Joo F, Ikeda J, Ruetzler CA, Lohr J, Klatzo I (1990) The role of the blood–brain barrier in ischemic brain lesions. In: Johansson BB, Owman CH, Widner H (eds) Pathophysiology of the blood–brain barrier. Elsevier, New York, pp 311–321

15. Onodera H, Sato G, Kogure K (1986) Lesions of Schaeffer's collaterals prevent ischemic death of CA1 pyramidal cells. Neurosci Lett 68: 169–174
16. Tomida S, Nowak TS Jr., Vass K, Lohr JM, Klatzo I (1987) Experimental model for repetitive ischemic attacks in the gerbil: the cumulative effect of repeated ischemic insults. J Cereb Blood Flow Metab 7: 773–782
17. Vogt C, Vogt O (1922) Erkrankungen der Grosshirnrinde im Lichte der Topistic, Pathoklise und Pathoarchitektonik. J Psychiatr U Neurol 28: 9–68

Delayed Gene Expression and Ischemic Brain Injury

C. Iadecola, M. E. Ross, F. Zhang, S. Nogawa, M. Nagayama,
and T. Nagayama

Summary. There is increasing evidence that cerebral ischemic injury occurs at a slower pace than previously believed. Although in areas of severe ischemia tissue damage occurs relatively rapidly, in regions of less-severe ischemia, damage develops over the course of many hours or even days. In this chapter, we review data indicating that inducible nitric oxide synthase (iNOS) and cyclooxygenase-2 (COX-2) are upregulated following focal cerebral ischemia and that the products of their reaction contribute to the delayed progression of ischemic brain damage. Administration of iNOS and COX-2 inhibitors may be a useful therapeutic strategy to selectively target the progression of the brain damage that takes place during the post-ischemic period.

Introduction

There is a growing body of evidence indicating that cerebral ischemic damage develops at a slower pace than previously believed. Although in areas of severe ischemia irretrievable injury occurs relatively rapidly, in regions of less-severe ischemia, tissue damage develops over the course of many hours or even days. Several lines of evidence support this view. First, neuropathological studies following occlusion of the rat middle cerebral artery have shown that in the peripheral regions of the infarct, neuronal injury progresses over the course of 24–36 h [3, 8]. Second, studies using magnetic resonance imaging in stroke patients have found that signal abnormalities within the infarct evolve over days, suggesting delayed evolution of the damage [1, 34, 35]. Third, measurements of cerebral blood flow and cerebral oxygen utilization have suggested that viable brain tissue is present more than 12 h after ischemia [5, 13, 23]. The factors responsible for the delayed progression of damage have not been identified. In this chapter, evidence will be provided that two genes expressed in the post-ischemic period contribute to progression of the damage. These genes encode for the inducible or immunological isoform of nitric oxide synthase (iNOS) and for cyclooxygenase-2 (COX-2).

iNOS Produces Toxic Levels of NO

NOS comprises a family of enzymes that synthesize NO from oxidation of L-arginine [11]. Three main isoforms of NOS have been described (Table 1). Neuronal NOS (nNOS) is present in selected central and peripheral neurons and is activated by elevations in intracellular calcium through binding of calmodulin to the enzyme [9].

Maturation Phenomenon in Cerebral Ischemia III
U. Ito et al. (Eds.)
© Springer-Verlag Berlin Heidelberg 1999

Table 1. Isoforms of nitric oxide synthase (NOS)

Characteristics	nNOS	iNOS	eNOS
Molecular weight	≈ 160 kDa	≈ 133 kDa	≈ 130 kDa
Typical cell	Neuron	Macrophage	Endothelium
Subcellular localization	Cytosolic, membrane bound (PSD)	Cytosolic	Membrane bound (caveolae)
Expression	Constitutive, inducible (?)	Inducible	Constitutive
Regulation	Ca-CaM	Transcription	Ca–CaM
NO output	Pulse (pmol)	Continuous (μmol)	Pulse (pmol)

Ca-CaM calcium-calmodulin; *PSD* post-synaptic density. See text for references

Endothelial NOS (eNOS) is present mainly in endothelial cells and is also activated by calcium and calmodulin [31]. iNOS is not normally present in most cells, but its expression is induced in most cell types by endotoxins, cytokines and hypoxia [22]. Unlike nNOS and eNOS, iNOS produces micromolar amounts of NO continuously [22, 33]. High concentrations of NO are cytotoxic, an effect mediated by several mechanisms including deoxyribonucleic acid (DNA) damage, oxidative stress, and energy failure [12]. iNOS is induced in activated inflammatory cells, and NO produced by iNOS is responsible for the toxicity of activated macrophages and for the neurotoxicity of microglia and astrocytes [2, 14, 15, 22, 26].

iNOS is Expressed Following Focal Cerebral Ischemia in Rodents and Humans

Focal cerebral ischemia is associated with an inflammatory reaction involving the post-ischemic brain [4]. Ischemia induces expression of inflammatory mediators, including cytokines and adhesion molecules in the brain [4]. Blood-borne neutrophils invade the ischemic brain and astrocyte and microglia become activated [7, 8, 10]. Because inflammation induces iNOS expression in many organs, we tested the hypothesis that iNOS is also expressed in the brain following cerebral ischemia. In these studies, the rat middle cerebral artery (MCA) was either permanently ligated or transiently occluded with an intraluminal filament [37] for 2 h.

Permanent or transient MCA occlusion results in expression of iNOS messenger ribonucleic acid (mRNA) in the post-ischemic brain. In transient MCA occlusion, iNOS mRNA peaks 12 h after MCA occlusion and subsides at 96 h [18] (Fig. 1). In permanent MCA occlusion, iNOS expression was more delayed, starting at 12 h and reaching a peak at 48 h [17]. iNOS enzymatic activity, determined by the calcium-independent conversion of L-arginine to L-citrulline, increases with a time course similar to that of iNOS mRNA, suggesting that iNOS mRNA is translated into a functional protein [17, 18]. iNOS protein, assessed by immunocytochemistry, is observed in neutrophils infiltrating the post-ischemic brain and in blood vessels in the ischemic territory [17, 18]. iNOS immunoreactivity is also observed in acute human

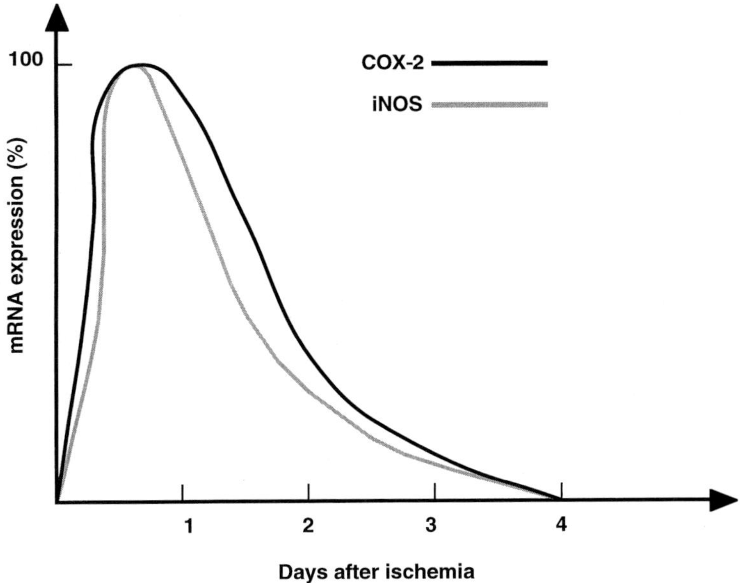

Fig. 1. Time course of messenger ribonucleic acid (mRNA) expression of nitric oxide synthase (iNOS) and cyclooxygenase-2 (COX-2) following focal cerebral ischemia produced by transient occlusion of the rat middle cerebral artery. See text for references

infarct. As in rodents, iNOS immunoreactivity is present in neutrophils and in the wall of cerebral blood vessels (C. Forster, H. B. Clark, M. E. Ross and C. Iadecola, unpublished observations). These observations suggest that, in rodents as well as in humans, cerebral ischemia is associated with expression of iNOS in the injured brain.

NO Produced by iNOS is Deleterious to the Post-Ischemic Brain

We then sought to explore the role of NO produced by iNOS in the mechanisms of cerebral ischemia. As a first approach, we studied the effect of the relatively selective iNOS inhibitor aminoguanidine on the size of the infarct produced by MCA occlusion in rats [16]. Aminoguanidine (100 mg/kg) was administered twice per day, beginning 24 h after permanent MCA occlusion. Rats were sacrificed 4 days after cerebral ischemia and infarct volume was assessed in thionine-stained brain sections, using an image analyzer [16]. Volumetric data were corrected for ischemic brain swelling. Aminoguanidine did not affect arterial pressure, rectal temperature or plasma glucose, but it did reduce infarct volume by 33 % – an effect associated with attenuation of iNOS, but not nNOS, enzymatic activity in the post-ischemic brain. Aminoguanidine treatment improved the recovery of motor deficits produced by MCA occlusion, suggesting that the reduction in infarct volume corresponds to a better functional outcome [24]. Aminoguanidine produced a comparable reduction in infarct volume following transient cerebral ischemia [18].

The data presented above suggest that pharmacological inhibition of iNOS reduces ischemic brain injury. To provide additional evidence for a role of iNOS in cerebral ischemia, we studied mice with deletion of the iNOS gene [21]. These knockout mice do not express iNOS and are relatively protected from the deleterious effects of inflammation [21]. As anticipated, iNOS-null mice did not express iNOS mRNA or protein following cerebral ischemia [19]. The extent of post-ischemic inflammation, as assessed by neutrophilic infiltration and astroglial activation, were comparable in iNOS-nulls and wild-type mice [19]. However, the infarct produced by MCA occlusion was ≈30 % smaller in iNOS-nulls than in wild-type controls (C57BL/6 or SV129) [19]. The reduction in infarct volume was observed 96 h, but not 24 h, after MCA occlusion [19]. Similarly, neurological deficits were reduced in iNOS-null mice, an effect observed 96 h, but not 24 h, after MCA occlusion [19]. Therefore, pharmacological iNOS inhibition or iNOS gene deletion attenuates focal cerebral ischemic damage.

The data provide evidence that iNOS expression and NO production are deleterious to the post-ischemic brain. In particular, the finding that the beneficial effects of iNOS inhibition or gene deletion are observed between 24 h and 96 h after ischemia suggests that NO produced by iNOS is one of the factors contributing to the progression of brain injury that occurs in the post-ischemic period.

COX-2

COX is a rate-limiting enzyme for prostanoid biosynthesis [32]. Two isoforms of COX have thus far been isolated and cloned (Table 2). COX-1 is constitutively expressed in most cells and produces prostanoids involved in normal cellular function [32]. COX-2 is normally not present in most cells, but its expression is upregulated in models of inflammation [32]. COX-2 is thought to contribute to the toxic effects of inflammation by producing reactive oxygen species and by synthesizing toxic prostanoids [30]. In brain, COX-2 is normally expressed at low levels in neurons and is upregulated following seizures or cerebral ischemia [36].

Table 2. Isoforms of cyclooxygenase (COX)

Characteristics	COX-1	COX-2
Other name	Prostaglandin H synthase 1	Prostaglandin H synthase 2
Molecular weight	≈65 kDa	≈70 kDa
Quaternary structure	Homodimer	Homodimer
Substrate	Arachidonic acid	Arachidonic acid
Reaction products	Prostaglandin H2, superoxide	Prostaglandin H2, superoxide
Typical cell	Most cell types	Inflammatory cells
Subcellular localization	Endoplasmic reticulum	Endoplasmic reticulum nuclear membrane
Expression	Constitutive	Constitutive in some cells, inducible in most cells

COX-2 and Ischemic Brain Injury

COX-2, but not COX-1, mRNA is upregulated following transient and permanent focal cerebral ischemia in rats [25]. The upregulation begins 6 h after transient MCA occlusion, peaks at 12 h and subsides at 48 h (Fig. 1). COX-2 protein is also upregulated with a time course similar to that of the corresponding mRNA [25]. After focal cerebral ischemia, COX-2 immunoreactivity is present in cells that have morphological characteristics of ischemic neurons in the region surrounding the ischemic core [25]. The COX-2 reaction product, prostaglandin E2 (PGE2), is increased in the post-ischemic brain, indicating increased COX catalytic activity. Considering that COX-1 is not upregulated in this model, the increased PGE2 production likely reflects COX-2 upregulation. We then investigated whether COX-2 is also expressed in the human brain after acute stroke. COX-2 immunoreactivity was observed in neurons at the periphery of the ischemic region (C. Forster, H. B. Clark, M. E. Ross and C. Iadecola, unpublished observations). In addition, COX-2 immunoreactivity was observed in neutrophils and in vascular cells. Therefore, COX-2 is also expressed in the human brain following cerebral ischemia.

To study the role of COX-2 reaction products in focal cerebral ischemia, we used the highly-selective COX-2 inhibitor NS398 [6]. NS398 (20 mg/kg; i.p.) was administered twice per day, starting 6 h after transient MCA occlusion [25]. Infarct volume was determined in thionine-stained brain sections 4 days after ischemia [25]. NS398 did not affect arterial pressure, rectal temperature or plasma glucose during the treatment period. However, NS398 blocked the post-ischemic increase in PGE2 and reduced infarct volume by 29 % compared with vehicle-treated controls [25].

The observation that NS398, administered 6 h after MCA occlusion, reduces ischemic damage suggests that products of COX-2 reaction contribute to the late stages of ischemic brain injury. Therefore, COX-2 may be another factor mediating progression of ischemic brain damage in the post-ischemic period.

Interactions between iNOS and COX-2

The fact that iNOS and COX-2 are expressed with a similar time course following focal cerebral ischemia raises the possibility of an interaction between NO produced by iNOS and COX-2. In models of inflammation, NO produced by iNOS activates COX-2 [27–29]. Preliminary results from our laboratory suggest that such interaction may also exist following cerebral ischemia. COX-2-positive neurons are located near iNOS-positive neutrophils, suggesting that NO produced by iNOS could influence COX-2. Furthermore, inhibition of iNOS by aminoguanidine attenuates post-ischemic production of PGE2 only in the ischemic region, where both iNOS and COX-2 are expressed, but not in the olfactory bulb, where only COX-2 is upregulated. Similarly, post-ischemic PGE2 accumulation is reduced in iNOS-null mice, which do not express iNOS. These observations raise the possibility that NO produced by iNOS activates COX-2 in the post-ischemic brain. COX-2 reaction products, therefore, might be an additional factor by which NO exerts its deleterious effects in the late stages of cerebral ischemia.

Conclusions

We have reviewed evidence suggesting that delayed expression of iNOS and COX-2 contributes to the evolution of ischemic brain injury. Both iNOS and COX-2 are expressed in the post-ischemic brain in the late stages of cerebral ischemia. Whereas delayed administration of an iNOS inhibitor attenuates focal cerebral ischemic damage and improves neurological outcome, mice lacking the iNOS gene are less susceptible to cerebral ischemic damage. Furthermore, delayed inhibition of COX-2 reduces focal cerebral ischemic damage. These observations suggest that reaction products of iNOS and COX-2 contribute to the post-ischemic evolution of brain injury. Inhibitors of iNOS and COX-2 may be useful in the treatment of cerebral ischemia because they may be effective in the late stages of ischemic injury (more than 6 h after ischemia). At this time, most treatment modalities, such as thrombolysis, glutamate receptor and calcium channel antagonists, as well as free radical scavengers, are no longer effective [20]. Therefore, treatments with iNOS or COX-2 inhibitors have the potential of filling a gap in current treatment strategies for ischemic stroke. Studies in which iNOS and COX-2 inhibitors are tested in patients with cerebral ischemia are needed to define the therapeutic value of this approach.

Acknowledgements. This study was supported by NIH grants NS31318, NS34179 and NS35806. C.I. is an Established Investigator of the American Heart Association. Dr. S. Nogawa is a Fellow of the American Heart Association (Minnesota). The editorial assistance of Ms. Karen MacEwan is gratefully acknowledged.

References

1. Baird AE, Benfield A, Schlaug G, Siewert B, Lövblad K-O, Edelman RR, Warach S (1997) Enlargement of human cerebral ischemic lesion volumes measured by diffusion-weighted magnetic resonance imaging. Ann Neurol 41: 581–589
2. Dawson V, Brahmbhatt VL, Mong JA, Dawson TM (1994) Expression of inducible nitric oxide synthase causes delayed neurotoxicity in primary mixed neuronal-glial cortical cultures. Neuropharmacology 33: 1425–1430
3. Dereski MO, Chopp M, Knight RA, Rodolosi LC, Garcia JH (1993) The heterogeneous temporal evolution of focal ischemic neuronal damage in the rat. Acta Neuropathol 85: 327–333
4. Feuerstein GZ, Wang X, Barone FC (1998) Inflammatory mediators and brain injury: the role of cytokines and chemokines in stroke and CNS diseases. In: Ginsberg MD, Bogousslavsky J (eds) Cerebrovascular diseases. Blackwell Science, Cambridge, pp 507–531
5. Furlan M, Marchal G, Viader F, Derlon J-M, Baron J-C (1996) Spontaneous neurological recovery after stroke and the fate of the ischemic penumbra. Ann Neurol 40: 216–226
6. Futaki N, Yoshikawa K, Hamasaka Y, Arai I, Higuchi S, Iizuka H, Otomo S (1993) NS-398, a novel non-steroidal anti-inflammatory drug with potent analgesic and antipyretic effects, which causes minimal stomach lesions. Gen Pharmacol 24: 105–10
7. Garcia JH, Liu KF, Yoshida Y, Lian J, Chen S, del Zoppo GJ (1994) Influx of leukocytes and platelets in an evolving brain infarct. Am J Pathol 144: 188–199
8. Garcia JH, Yoshida Y, Chen H, Li Y, Zhang ZG, Lian J, Chen S, Chopp M (1993) Progression from ischemic injury to infarct following middle cerebral artery occlusion in the rat. Am J Pathol 142: 623–635
9. Garthwaite J, Boulton CL (1995) Nitric oxide signaling in the central nervous system. Ann Rev Physiol 57: 683–706
10. Giulian D (1997) Reactive microglia and ischemic injury. In: Welsh KMA, Caplan LR, Reis DJ, Siësjo BK, Weir B (eds) Primer on cerebrovascular diseases. Academic Press, San Diego, pp 117–124

11. Griffith OW, Stuehr DJ (1995) Nitric oxide synthases: properties and catalytic mechanism. Ann Rev Physiol 57: 707–736
12. Gross SS, MS Wolin (1995) Nitric oxide: pathophysiological mechanisms. Ann Rev Physiol 57: 737–769
13. Heiss WD, Huber M, Fink GR, Herloz K, Pietrzyk U, Wagner R, Weinhard K (1992) Progressive derangement of periinfarct viable tissue in ischemic stroke. J Cereb Blood Flow Metab 12: 193–203
14. Hewett SJ, Csernansky CA, Choi DW (1994) Selective potentiation of NMDA-induced neuronal injury following induction of astrocytic iNOS. Neuron 13: 487–94
15. Hewett SJ, Muir JK, Lobner D, Symons A, Choi DW (1996) Potentiation of oxygen–glucose deprivation-induced neuronal death after induction of iNOS. Stroke 27: 1586–1591
16. Iadecola C, Zhang F, Xu X (1995) Inhibition of inducible nitric oxide synthase ameliorates cerebral ischemic damage. Am J Physiol 268: 286–292
17. Iadecola C, Zhang F, Xu X, Casey R, Ross ME (1995) Inducible nitric oxide synthase gene expression in brain following cerebral ischemia. J Cereb Blood Flow Metab 15: 378–384
18. Iadecola C, Zhang F, Casey R, Clark HB, Ross ME (1996) Inducible nitric oxide synthase gene expression in vascular cells after transient focal cerebral ischemia. Stroke 27: 1373–1380
19. Iadecola C, Zhang F, Casey R, Nagayama M, Ross ME (1997) Delayed reduction in ischemic brain injury and neurological deficits in mice lacking the inducible nitric oxide synthase gene. J Neurosci 17: 9157–9164
20. Koroshetz WJ, Moskowitz MA (1996) Emerging treatments for stroke in humans. Trends Pharmacol Sci 17: 227–233
21. MacMicking JD, Nathan C, Hom G, Chartrain N, Fletcher DS, Trumbauer M, Stevens K, Xie QW, Sokol K, Hutchinson N, Chen H, Mudgett JS (1995) Altered responses to bacterial infection and endotoxic shock in mice lacking inducible nitric oxide synthase. Cell 81: 641–650
22. MacMicking JD, Xie QW, Nathan C (1997) Nitric oxide and macrophage function. Annu Rev Immunol 15: 323–350
23. Marchal G, Beaudouin V, Rioux P, de la Sayette V, Le Doze F, Viader F, Derlon J-M, Baron JC (1996) Prolonged persistence of substantial volumes of potentially viable brain tissue after stroke. Stroke 27: 599–606
24. Nagayama M, Zhang F, Iadecola C (1998) Delayed treatment with aminoguanidine reduces focal cerebral ischemic damage and enhances neurological recovery in rats. J Cereb Blood Flow Metab (in press)
25. Nogawa S, Zhang F, Ross ME, Iadecola C (1997) Cyclo-oxygenase-2 gene expression in neurons contributes to ischemic brain damage. J Neurosci 17: 2746–2755
26. Peterson PK, Hu S, Anderson WR, Chao CC (1994) Nitric oxide production and neurotoxicity mediated by activated microglia from human versus mouse brain. J Infect Dis 170: 457–460
27. Salvemini D (1997) Regulation of cyclooxygenase enzymes by nitric oxide. Cell Mol Life Sci 53: 576–82
28. Salvemini D, Misko TP, Masferrer JL, Seibert K, Currie MG, Needleman P (1993) Nitric oxide activates cyclooxygenase enzymes. Proc Natl Acad Sci U S A 90: 7240–7244
29. Salvemini D, Seibert K, Masferrer JL, Misko TP, Currie MG, Needleman P (1994) Endogenous nitric oxide enhances prostaglandin production in a model of renal inflammation. J Clin Invest 93: 1940–1947
30. Seibert K, Masferrer J, Zhang Y, Gregory S, Olson G, Hauser S, Leahy K, Perkins W, Isakson P (1995) Mediation of inflammation by cyclooxygenase-2. Agents Actions Suppl 46: 41–50
31. Sessa W C (1994) The nitric oxide synthase family of proteins. J Vasc Res 31: 131–143
32. Smith WL, Meade EA, DeWitt DL (1994) Pharmacology of prostaglandin endoperoxide synthase isozymes-1 and -2. Ann N Y Acad Sci 714: 136–142
33. Vodovotz Y, Kwon NS, Pospischil M, Manning J, Paik J, Nathan C (1994) Inactivation of nitric oxide synthase after prolonged incubation of mouse macrophages with IFN-gamma and bacterial lipopolysaccharide. J Immunol 152: 4110–4118
34. Warach S, Gaa J, Siewert B, Wielopolski P1, Edelman RR (1995) Acute human stroke studied by whole brain echo planar diffusion-weighted magnetic resonance imaging. Ann Neurol 37: 231–241
35. Welch KMA, Windham J, Knight RA, Nagesh V, Hugg JW, Jacobs M, Peck D, Booker P, Deresky MO, Levine SR (1995) A model to predict the histopathology of human stroke using diffusion and T2-weighted magnetic resonance imaging. Stroke 26: 1983–1989
36. Yamagata K, Andreasson KI, Kaufmann WE, Barnes CA, Worley PF (1993) Expression of a mitogen-inducible cyclooxygenase in brain neurons: regulation by synaptic activity and glucocorticoids. Neuron 11: 371–386
37. Zea Longa E, Weinstein PR, Carlson S, Cummins R (1989) Reversible middle cerebral artery occlusion without craniectomy in rat. Stroke 20: 84–91

The Role of Programmed Cell Death in Cerebral Ischemia

F. Gillardon, M. Spranger, R. Hata, C. Tiesler, and K.-A. Hossmann

Summary. Following transient global cerebral ischemia, there is a progressive increase in nitric oxide (NO) synthase activity in hippocampal CA1 neurons that may be enhanced by a lack of protein inhibitor of neuronal NO synthase (*PIN*). The concomitant accumulation of NO and other reactive oxygen species causes deoxyribonucleic acid (DNA) injury, as indicated by the futile attempt to activate the DNA repair enzyme, *ref-1*, and by the expression of DNA damage-inducible, cell death-promoting *PAG608* in CA1 neurons 1 day after ischemia. Nuclear phospho-c-Jun(Ser-73) immunoreactivity becomes apparent in CA1 cells, suggesting that oxidative stress and DNA damage activate c-Jun N-terminal kinases. One day after ischemia, expression of *caspase-3* is upregulated in CA1 neurons and *caspase-3*-like proteolytic activity increases in hippocampal extracts. Intracerebroventricular infusion of the caspase inhibitor, Z-DEVD-FMK, prevents CA1 cell loss, indicating that CA1 cells die by programmed cell death. Following transient focal ischemia, *PIN* transcripts and phospho-c-Jun rapidly accumulate in neurons of the reperfused cortex. Immunoreactivity for Bcl-2-associated death protein (Bad) becomes apparent in post-ischemic cortical neurons. Furthermore, the infarct area is significantly larger in *bcl-2*-deficient mice, strongly suggesting that Bcl-2 and related proteins influence neuronal cell death after focal ischemia.

Introduction

Brief episodes of transient global cerebral ischemia lead to selective death of hippocampal CA1 pyramidal neurons 2–3 days after the initial insult. This phenomenon is referred to as selective neuronal vulnerability or delayed neuronal cell death. The underlying mechanisms of this type of ischemia-induced neurodegeneration are not yet completely understood, but preliminary evidence suggests the involvement of programmed cell death [1, 14]. In neuronal cell cultures, a temporal sequence of biochemical and genetic alterations has been described during programmed cell death [2]. Various stressful stimuli, e.g., reactive oxygen species, may activate the cell-death program. The signal is propagated by activation of c-Jun N-terminal kinases, phosphorylation of transcription factor c-Jun, and subsequent induction of gene expression [19, 20]. The death signal then reaches an apoptotic rheostat, which consists of death-inhibiting and death-promoting Bcl-2 related proteins [11]. The ratio of death antagonists to death agonists (and their phosphorylation state) seems to determine whether cellular suicide is executed. The central executioners of the cell-death program are a family of aspartate-specific cysteine proteases, termed caspases, which are

Maturation Phenomenon in Cerebral Ischemia III
U. Ito et al. (Eds.)
© Springer-Verlag Berlin Heidelberg 1999

activated by proteolytic cleavage of the inactive proenzymes [17]. Our studies were aimed at elucidating the sequence of events leading to activation of the neuronal cell-death program after cerebral ischemia and at identifying putative targets for neuro-protective intervention.

Materials and Methods

Transient global cerebral ischemia (10 min) was induced in anesthetized rats either by four-vessel occlusion with hypotension (40 mmHg) or by cardiac arrest followed by resuscitation (mechanical ventilation, external cardiac massage, i.v. epinephrine), as described in detail elsewhere [5, 6]. For induction of thromboembolic stroke, autologous blood clots were injected into the internal carotid artery [7]. After 1 h, thrombolysis was initiated by intracarotid infusion of recombinant tissue-type plas-minogen activator; control animals received saline infusion. Alternatively, transient focal cerebral ischemia was induced by intraluminal thread occlusion of the middle cerebral artery (MCA). After 1 h, the filament was withdrawn to permit reperfusion.

In situ hybridization was performed on brain cryosections, using 3' end-labeled oligonucleotide probes [7]. Mean optical density of film autoradiograms was evalu-ated by digital image analysis (NIH Image 1.60). For immunolocalization of proteins, brain sections were incubated with specific antibodies. Immunolabeling was visual-ized using the ABC-method (Vector Laboratory) [5]. For immunoblot analysis, pro-tein extracts were electrophoresed on sodium dodecyl sulfate-polyacrylamide gel electrophoresis (SDS-PAGE) gels and subsequently transferred to nitrocellulose mem-branes. Blots were incubated in primary antibody, followed by biotinylated secondary antibody and streptavidin-peroxidase. Antibody binding was visualized by enhanced chemiluminescence. Degenerating neurons were identified in brain sections by in situ end-labeling of nuclear DNA fragments (TUNEL) or by standard histological analysis using cresyl violet staining.

Results and Discussion

Mediators of Neuronal Cell Damage. The Pathophysiological Significance of Nitric Oxide Synthase in Global Cerebral Ischemia

Administration of inhibitors of neuronal nitric oxide synthase (nNOS) and deletion of the encoding gene in rodents provide evidence that nNOS activity may contribute to the neuronal cell death that occurs following global and focal cerebral ischemia [8]. Activity of nNOS is stimulated by calcium influx; this, however, does not completely explain selective neurotoxic effects on CA1 neurons following global ischemia. We investigated the expression of an endogenous inhibitor of nNOS activity, designated protein inhibitor of neuronal nitric oxide synthase (*PIN*) in the post-ischemic rat brain [10]. Following global cerebral ischemia, mRNA expression of *PIN* was rapidly induced in ischemia-resistant pyramidal neurons of the hippocampal CA3 region and in granule cells of the dentate gyrus [7]. In vulnerable CA1 pyramidal neurons, how-ever, *PIN* expression remained at baseline levels (Fig. 1). Consistently, NOS (NADPH-

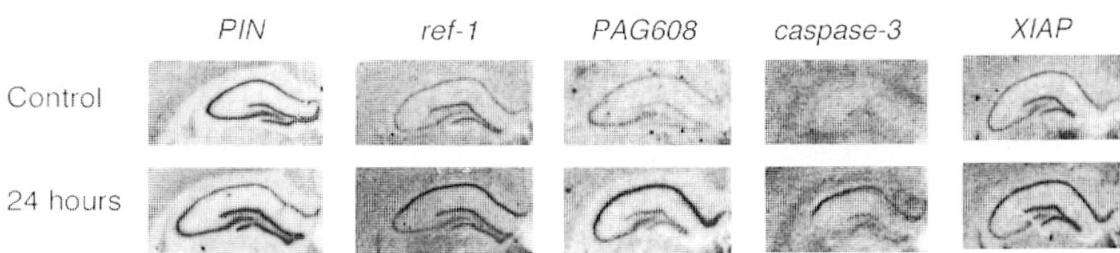

Fig. 1. Genomic response following transient global cerebral ischemia. Anesthetized rats were subjected to 10 min global cerebral ischemia. Twenty-four hours later, levels of various messenger ribonucleic acids (mRNAs) were analyzed in brain cryosections by in situ hybridization, using radioactively labeled oligonucleotide probes. Note the selective lack of induction of protein inhibitor of neuronal nitric acid synthase (nNOS) (*PIN*) in the vulnerable hippocampal CA1 cell layer. The increased mRNA expression of redox-stress sensitive deoxyribonucleic acid (DNA) repair enzyme *ref-1*, DNA damage-inducible and cell death-promoting *PAG608*, and cell death-executing *caspase-3* following ischemia points to free-radical injury in CA1 neurons leading to programmed cell death. Hippocampal expression of X-linked inhibitor of apoptosis (*XIAP*), a direct inhibitor of *caspase-3*, does not change significantly after global ischemia

diaphorase) activity was massively and selectively increased in CA1 neurons following global ischemia. Nitrotyrosine immunoreactivity became apparent in scattered CA1 neurons, indicating formation of cytotoxic peroxynitrite. Following focal cerebral ischemia induced by permanent occlusion of the middle cerebral artery (MCA), *PIN* transcripts progressively accumulated in cortical neurons bordering the infarct area [7]. After transient MCA occlusion, mRNA levels of *PIN* increased in the reperfused cortex. Our findings indicate that cerebral ischemia leads to an increase in neuronal expression of *PIN* in brain regions for which sustained or uncoupled NOS activity may be detrimental to neurons [8]. Lack of post-ischemic induction of *PIN* in CA1 pyramidal neurons may result in high levels of NO following global ischemia and may contribute to delayed neuronal cell death.

The Intracellular Signaling Cascade.
Activation of Stress-Activated Protein Kinases Following Cerebral Ischemia

Both oxidative stress (caused by NO or H_2O_2) and glutamate exposure cause phosphorylation and activation of stress-activated protein kinases/c-Jun N-terminal kinases (SAPK/JNK) in cell culture [12, 13]. JNK specifically phosphorylates transcription factor c-Jun at serines 63 and 73, leading to an increase in *trans*-activation of target genes. Transfection with dominant-negative mutants of JNK or c-Jun prevents neuronal cell death in vitro [19, 20]. Moreover, hippocampal neurons of JNK3-deficient mice are resistant to glutamate-mediated excitotoxicity, indicating that the JNK-signaling pathway may be involved in neuronal cell death [21]. The functional significance of c-Jun induction in the post-ischemic hippocampus has been debated for years, because the expression pattern does not correlate with neuronal vulnerability [14, 16]. In contrast, 1 day after global ischemia, we observed an increase in nuclear phospho-c-Jun(Ser-73) immunoreactivity that is confined to vulnerable CA1 neurons and precedes their degeneration. Six hours following permanent MCA occlusion, phospho-c-Jun immunolabeling was detectable in cortical neurons at the border of the infarcted area, whereas after transient MCA occlusion, phospho-c-Jun accumulated in neurons of the reperfused cortex. A simultaneous increase in phospho-JNK2 in cortical extracts was revealed by immunoblot analysis. Thus, the temporo-spatial distribution of phospho-c-Jun, but not of c-Jun, correlates with selective neuronal vulnerability following global cerebral ischemia and with free-radical stress following focal ischemia/reperfusion.

Gene Expression Induced by Cerebral Ischemia. Genomic Responses Indicating Neuronal DNA Damage

To identify intracellular targets for free-radical attack, we investigated the expression of the Ref-1 gene, which is inducible by oxidative stress and encodes a DNA repair enzyme [18]. Transient global cerebral ischemia activates *ref-1* mRNA expression both in the granule cells of the dentate gyrus and in CA1 pyramidal neurons of the hippocampus (Fig. 1). Confocal laser scanning microscopy revealed nuclear translocation of Ref-1 protein in granule cells of the dentate gyrus, whereas nuclear accumulation of Ref-1 was not detectable in hippocampal CA1 neurons [5]. Our data suggest that oxidative stress induced by transient global ischemia may increase neuronal Ref-1 expression. However, the prevention of *ref-1* mRNA translation and the nuclear translocation of Ref-1 protein in CA1 pyramidal neurons may inhibit repair of oxidative DNA damage, and thereby lead to delayed neuronal cell death. Lethal DNA damage in CA1 neurons is further indicated by a massive induction of *PAG608* mRNA expression 1 day after transient global ischemia (Fig. 1). *PAG608* is a p53-activated gene that is rapidly induced by DNA damage and encodes a nuclear zinc-finger protein promoting cell death [9]. Surprisingly, neither *ref-1* nor *PAG608* mRNA expression is induced following MCA occlusion. This may indicate that oxidative DNA damage is not the predominant trigger of neuronal cell death following focal cerebral ischemia or that neuronal cell death occurs too rapidly for these genes to become activated.

The Cell Death Program. I. The Pathophysiological Significance of Cell Death-preventing Bcl-2 and Related Proteins

Neuronal expression of Bcl-2 is modulated following cerebral ischemia and *bcl-2*-overexpressing mice develop smaller infarcts following permanent MCA occlusion [14, 15]. Consistently, we observed significantly larger (179±31 %) infarcts in sections from Bcl-2 gene-ablated mice compared with wild-type littermates after 1 h MCA occlusion and 24 h reperfusion, indicating that endogenous Bcl-2 protects neurons from reperfusion injury. Bcl-2-associated death protein (Bad) heterodimerizes with Bcl-2 and Bcl-X$_L$ and neutralizes their anti-apoptotic effect [4, 11]. Growth factor administration leads to phosphorylation of Bad and its dissociation from Bcl-2 and Bcl-X$_L$. By immunoblot analysis, we detected a twofold increase in death-promoting, non-phosphorylated Bad protein in the ipsilateral brain hemisphere 6 h after transient MCA occlusion. After 24 h, Bad protein migrates as a doublet, suggesting that Bad partially becomes phosphorylated by survival-promoting kinases. At the same time, cytoplasmic Bad immunoreactity becomes apparent both in neurons and in activated microglia of the infarcted cortex and putamen. Our preliminary results using phospho-specific Bad antibodies confirmed neuronal localization of phosphorylated Bad.

The Cell Death Program.
II. Ischemia-Induced Activation of Cell Death-Executing Caspases

Caspases represent the central executioners of the cell-death program and their proteolytic activation marks the beginning of programmed cell death [17]. Inhibitor studies and gene knockout point to a central role of caspase-3 in neuronal cell death. Caspase enzymatic activity is directly inhibited by members of the inhibitor of apoptosis protein (IAP) family [3]. Following transient global cerebral ischemia, levels of caspase-3 mRNA and protein immunoreactivity selectively increase in hippocampal CA1 neurons long before morphological signs of degeneration become visible (Fig. 1). Induction of *caspase-3* expression was accompanied by a nearly twofold increase in caspase-3-like proteolytic activity in post-ischemic hippocampal extracts [6]. An X-linked inhibitor of apoptosis (*XIAP*), a direct inhibitor of caspase-3 [3], was constitutively expressed in the pyramidal cell layers of the hippocampus and in the granule cell layer of the dentate gyrus. Levels of *XIAP* mRNA in hippocampal neurons did not change significantly following global ischemia (Fig. 1). Thus, an increase in the molar ratio of caspase-3 to its endogenous inhibitor, XIAP, and a concomitant increase in proteolytic activity preceded ischemia-induced CA1 cell death.

The Cell Death Program. III.
Neuroprotective Effectiveness of Synthetic Caspase Inhibitors in Cerebral Ischemia

To show a causal relationship between *caspase-3* activation and delayed CA1 cell death, the synthetic inhibitor of caspase-3-like proteases, Z-DEVD-FMK, was infused into the right lateral ventricle immediately after transient global ischemia. Continuous infusion by osmotic minipumps (50 pmol/h) significantly attenuated the increase in caspase-3-like enzymatic activity that normally follows ischemia, and prevented both DNA fragmentation and morphological signs of degeneration in ipsilateral CA1 neurons (Fig. 2). Lack of neuroprotective effectiveness on the contralateral side may be explained by slow diffusion and tissue penetration of the inhibitor following unilateral administration. Lateralized neuroprotection speaks against an effect due to systemic thermoregulatory or hemodynamic alterations. These findings indicate that caspase-3-like proteases contribute to delayed cell death of hippocampal CA1 neurons following global cerebral ischemia and that caspases may represent a target for neuroprotective therapy.

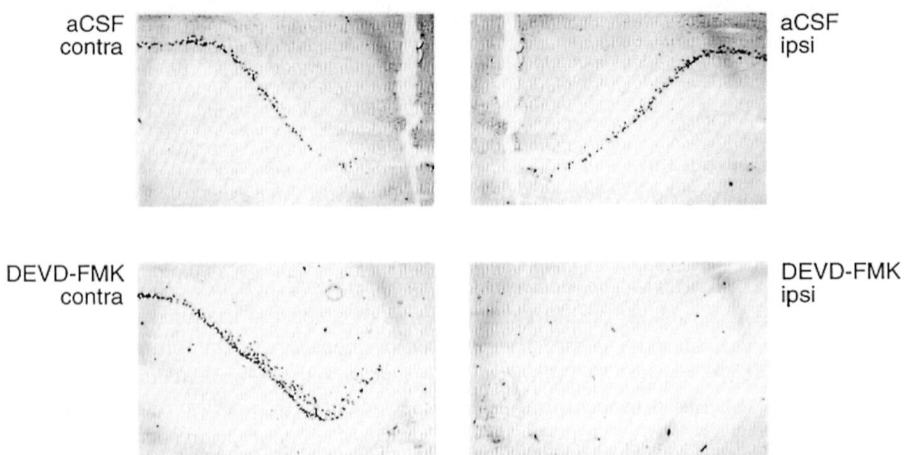

Fig. 2. Effects of caspase-3 inhibition on CA1 cell death following global cerebral ischemia. Immediately after 10 min global cerebral ischemia, the inhibitor of caspase-3-like proteases Z-DEVD-FMK was continuously infused into the right lateral ventricle using osmotic minipumps. Control animals received infusion of artificial cerebrospinal fluid (*aCSF*). Seven days after ischemia, nuclear deoxyribonucleic acid (DNA) fragmentation was analyzed in brain sections by in situ end-labeling using terminal deoxynucleotidyltransferase and biotin-dUTP. Note complete absence of nuclear DNA fragmentation in CA1 neurons of the ipsilateral hippocampus in Z-DEVD-FMK-treated animals

References

1. Abe K, Aoki M, Kawagoe J, Yoshida T, Hattori A, Kogure K, Itoyama Y (1995) Ischemic neuronal death. A mitochondrial hypothesis. Stroke 26: 1478–1489
2. Deshmukh M, Johnson EM (1997) Programmed cell death in neurons: focus on the pathway of nerve growth factor deprivation-induced death of sympathetic neurons. Mol Pharmacol 51: 897–906
3. Deveraux QL, Takahashi R, Salvesen GS, Reed JC (1997) X-linked IAP is a direct inhibitor of cell death proteases. Nature 388: 300–303
4. Gajewski TF, Thompson CB (1996) Apoptosis meets signal transduction: elimination of a bad influence. Cell 87: 589–592
5. Gillardon F, Böttiger B, Hossmann K-A (1997) Expression of nuclear redox factor *ref-1* in the rat hippocampus following global ischemia induced by cardiac arrest. Mol Brain Res 52: 194–200
6. Gillardon F, Böttiger B, Schmitz B, Zimmermann M, Hossmann K-A (1997) Activation of CPP-32 protease in hippocampal neurons following ischemia and epilepsy. Mol Brain Res 50: 16–22
7. Gillardon F, Krep H, Brinker G, Lenz C, Böttiger B, Hossmann K-A (1997) Induction of protein inhibitor of neuronal nitric oxide synthase following cerebral ischemia. Neuroscience 84: 81–88
8. Iadecola C (1997) Bright and dark sides of nitric oxide in ischemic brain injury. Trends Neurosci 20: 132–139
9. Israeli D, Tessler E, Haupt Y, Elkeles A, Wilder S, Amson R, Telerman A, Oren M (1997) A novel p53-inducible gene, *PAG608*, encodes a nuclear zinc finger protein whose overexpression promotes apoptosis. EMBO J 16: 4384–4392
10. Jaffrey SR, Snyder SH (1996) *PIN*: an associated protein inhibitor of neuronal nitric oxide synthase. Science 274: 774–777
11. Kroemer G (1997) The proto-oncogene *Bcl-2* and its role in regulating apoptosis. Nat Med 3: 614–620
12. Kyriakis JM, Avruch J (1996) Sounding the alarm: protein kinase cascades activated by stress and inflammation. J Biol Chem 271: 24313–24316
13. Lander HM, Jacovina AT, Davis RJ, Tauras JM (1996) Differential activation of mitogen-activated protein kinases by nitric oxide-related species. J Biol Chem 271: 19705–19709

14. MacManus JP, Linnik MD (1997) Gene expression induced by cerebral ischemia: an apoptotic perspective. J Cereb Blood Flow Metab 17: 815–832
15. Martinou JC, Dubois-Dauphin M, Staple JK, Rodriguez I, Frankowski H, Missotten M, Albertini P, Talabot D, Catsicas S, Pietra C, Huarte J (1994) Overexpression of *Bcl-2* in transgenic mice protects neurons from naturally occurring cell death and experimental ischemia. Neuron 13: 1017–1030
16. Neumann-Haefelin T, Wiessner C, Vogel P, Back T, Hossmann K-A (1994) Differential expression of the immediate early genes c-fos, *c-jun*, junB, and NGFI-B in the rat brain following transient forebrain ischemia. J Cereb Blood Flow Metab 14: 206–216
17. Schwartz LM, Milligan CE (1996) Cold thoughts of death: the role of ICE proteases in neuronal cell death. Trends Neurosci 19: 555–562
18. Walker LJ, Craig RB, Harris AL, Hickson ID (1994) A role for the human DNA repair enzyme HAP1 in cellular protection against DNA damaging agents and hypoxic stress. Nucleic Acids Res 22: 4884–4889
19. Watson A, Eilers A, Lallemand D, Kyriakis J, Rubin LL, Ham J (1998) Phosphorylation of *c-jun* is necessary for apoptosis induced by survival signal withdrawal in cerebellar granule neurons. J Neurosci 18: 751–762
20. Xia Z, Dickens M, Raingeaud J, Davis RJ, Greenberg ME (1995) Opposing effects of ERK and JNK-p38 MAP kinases on apoptosis. Science 270: 1326–1331
21. Yang DD, Kuan CY, Whitmarsh AJ, Rinc M, Zheng TS, Davis RJ, Rakic P, Flavell RA (1997) Absence of exitotoxicity-induced apoptosis in the hippocampus of mice lacking the Jnk3 gene. Nature 389: 865–870

The Role of Caspase-3-like Protease in the Hippocampus After Transient Global Ischemia

J. CHEN and R.P. SIMON

Summary. In the context of genetic control over cell death in brain following ischemia, we studied the functional significance of the newly described caspase-3 member of the interleukin-converting enzyme (ICE) protease family. At both message and protein levels, this gene's product was upregulated in selectively vulnerable regions following ischemia. Coincident with cell death, the precursor protein was proteolytically cleaved and the protease activity increased. In regions of neuronal death, PARP cleavage was demonstrated. Inhibition of caspase-3 protease activity decreased both neuronal death and deoxyribonucleic acid (DNA) fragmentation (TUNEL labeling) and increased survival in selectively vulnerable brain regions 1 week after ischemia. These data support the view that caspase-3 protease is an inducible modulator of cell death in ischemic brain.

Introduction

Neurons of the central nervous system that undergo delayed death following ischemia show morphologic characteristics of apoptosis. Given that a number of gene products have been shown to be involved in the regulation of apoptotic cell death, the potential modulation of this system may be relevant to future therapy for ischemic brain injury. For example, the death-inducer protein, bax, is upregulated in neurons that die following ischemia, whereas the neuroprotective gene product, bcl-2, is upregulated in cells that survive [2]. The cysteine protease genes, now referred to as caspases, constitute an important apoptosis-inducing group of gene products, of which at least 11 are now recognized [1]. These proteases are the mammalian equivalent of the *Caenorhabditis. elegans* gene, *ced-3* [11]. The caspase with the greatest degree of homology to *ced-3* is caspase-3, previously known as CPP32. Both inhibition of CPP32 and the caspase interleukin-converting enzyme (ICE) attenuate focal ischemic injury or the effects of excitotoxins in brain [7]. Thus caspase-3 and its related compounds may well be important mediators of ischemic neuronal death in brain. We, therefore, cloned and sequenced the rat *CPP32* gene from an ischemic-brain cDNA library and studied its expression at both the message and protein levels following global ischemia. We measured its protease activity and studied the effect of caspase-3 inhibition on the outcome of ischemic injury to brain.

Maturation Phenomenon in Cerebral Ischemia III
U. Ito et al. (Eds.)
© Springer-Verlag Berlin Heidelberg 1999

Methods and Results

All experiments were performed in a transient-global-ischemia model (4 VO), with monitoring of core and brain temperature, as well as electroencephalograph (EEG). The complementary deoxyribonucleic acid (cDNA) that encodes an open reading frame of 277 amino acids, was cloned from an ischemic-brain cDNA library. The sequence has 84.1 % and 92.1 % identity to the human and mouse CPP-32 sequences, respectively [5, 11]. The sequence is 99.3 % identical to the ICE-related protease reported by Ni [9] and identical to the CPP-32β cloned from rat colon cDNA [8]. We used the cloned cDNA as a template for an in vitro transcription translation assay that produced a protein of 32 kDa, which is the predicted size for caspase-3.

We studied the protein and message expression of caspase-3 in normal and ische-mic brains. Using Northern blotting, caspase-3 messenger ribonucleic acid (mRNA) is detected in normal hippocampus with a 1.8-fold increase at 8 h and a 2.3-fold increase at 24 h after 15 min global ischemia with reperfusion. Using in situ hybrid-ization, the basal expression of caspase-3 message was seen in the entire hippocam-pus. At 8 h following ischemia, the message was first increased in the dentate granule cells but had returned to baseline by 24 h. In the CA1 sector, a slight increase in mes-sage was seen at 8 h, but then a marked increase occurred at 24 h and 72 h. Using dipped-emulsion sections, the message was seen to be localized to neurons in the CA1 sector, thalamus, and dorsal lateral putamen; only rarely were labeled cells seen in cortex, however. Quantitative data are shown in Fig 1.

Caspase-3 is present in brain as an inactive precursor, which is cleaved at the C-terminus of two specific aspartate residues to form p17 and p12 subunits. We there-fore designed an antibody against the deduced C-terminal sequence of the p17 sub-unit and performed Western-blot analysis to recognize both the 32-kDa and 17-kDa proteins. The 32-kDa, but not the 17-kDa, protein was found in non-ischemic brain. Following ischemia, caspase-3 protein increased in the hippocampus and the p17 subunit markedly increased in the hippocampus and caudate putamen. No induction of caspase-3 was found in the cortex in this model. Quantitative data are shown in Fig. 2.

Immunocytochemically, basal caspase-3 was seen to be exclusively cytoplasmic in distribution. Immunoreactivity began to be detected in CA1 8 h after ischemia and was maximal at 72 h. Immunoreactivity was predominantly in the cytosol but, at 72 h, the immunoreactivity was distributed throughout the entire cell, including the nucleus. A slight increase in immunoreactivity was seen in the dentate granule cells at 8 h, but not thereafter. A marked increase in immunostaining was seen in the cau-date putamen 24–72 h after ischemia.

To assess a potential role of caspase-3 in DNA damage, double-label experiments for caspase-3 and TUNEL staining were carried out. In the CA1 sector, the majority of TUNEL-positive neurons were also shown to be immunopositive for caspase-3 at 72 h. Co-localization was also shown in the caudate putamen at 24 h and 72 h. The few scattered cortical neurons that were TUNEL-positive also co-localized caspase-3.

To study caspase-3 protease activity, cell lysates were incubated with a substrate for the protease (Ac-DEVD-pNA) and the release of *p*-nitroanilide was moni-tored. Separate experiments included addition of the caspase-3 inhibitor (DEVD-CHO). In the lysates from both the hippocampus and caudate putamen, an increase

Fig. 1. Optical density measurements from autoradiograms showing relative caspase-3 ribonucleic acid (RNA) changes in the hippocampal CA1 and CA3 sectors and in the dentate gyrus at 4, 8, 24, 72, and 96 h following ischemia ($n=3$ per group) and in sham controls. $*P<0.01; **P<0.001$ (analysis of variance and post hoc Fisher's PLSD tests)

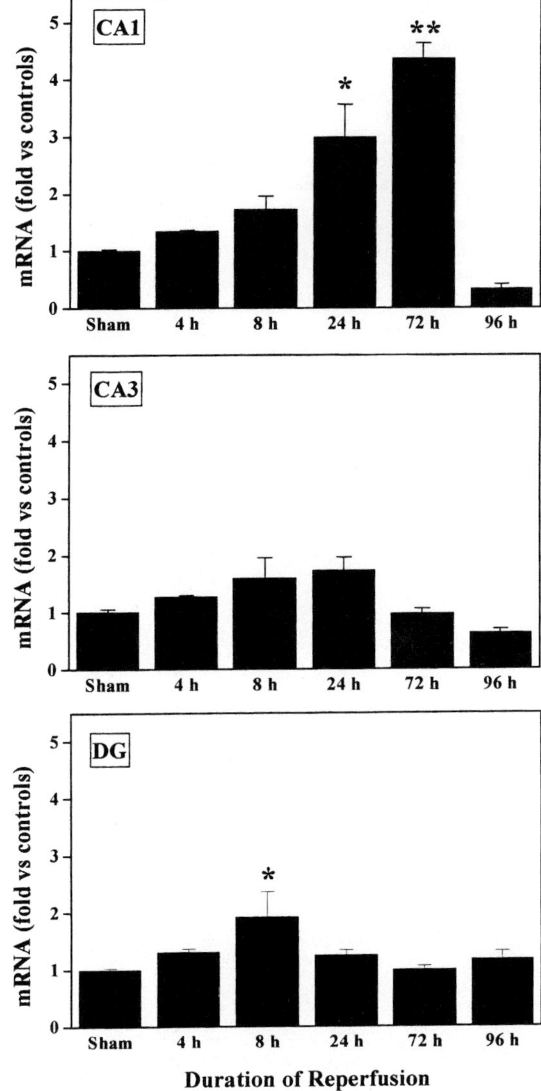

in Ac-DEVD-pNA peptide cleavage was seen at 8 h and was maximal at 24–72 h after ischemia. This increased protease activity was completely abolished by DEVD-CHO, but not by the ICE protease inhibitor, YVAD-CHO.

To study the downstream effects of caspase-3 protease activity, an analysis of poly-ADP-ribose polymerase (PARP) was investigated. With Western blotting, increased cleavage of PARP (116-kDa to an 85-kDa cleavage fragment) was seen in ischemic brain; there was a negligible amount of this fragment in non-ischemic brain. The cleaved fragment showed increased intensity on Western blotting of both the hippocampus and caudate putamen at 72 h.

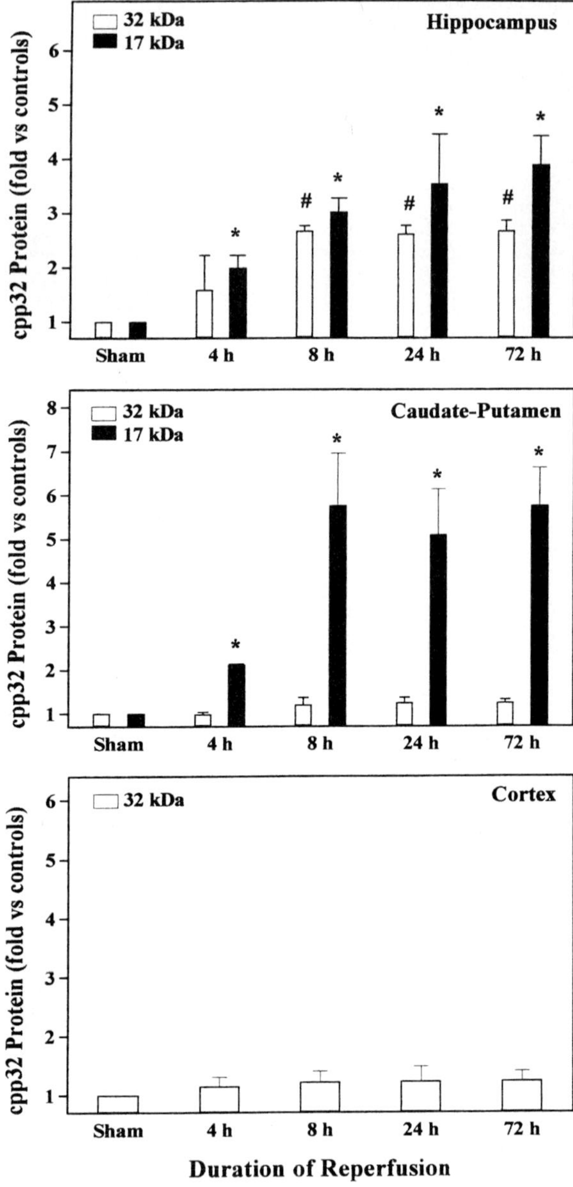

Fig. 2. Semi-quantitative changes, determined by optical density from Western blots (OD·area), of caspase-3 protein concentration (32 kDa) and the cleaved fragment (17 kDa) in hippocampus, caudate putamen and cortex from sham-operated animals and animals subjected to 4, 8, 24, and 72 h of ischemia (analysis of variance versus post hoc Fisher's PLSD tests). $n=4$ per time point. * or # $P<0.05$ versus sham controls

The caspase-3 inhibitor, Z-DVED-FMK, was studied in vivo by infusing the inhibitor into the lateral ventricles beginning 30 min before 15 min of global ischemia. At 48 h reperfusion, a dose-dependent decrease in Ac-DEVD-pNA peptide cleavage activity was seen in the hippocampus. Morphologically, there was a significant decrease in neuronal death in the CA1 sector in the inhibitor-treated animals studied at 72 h. When the inhibitor was infused 2 h after ischemia, with a second infusion

24 h later, the efficacy was similar to that of the pretreatment paradigm. TUNEL staining showed a significant decrease in labeling of CA1 neurons in the inhibitor-treated animals. The ICE inhibitor, Z-YVAD-FMK, failed to provide protection.

Discussion

Caspase-3 message and protein are found at low levels in the non-ischemic brain. Their expression is increased with ischemia. In less vulnerable regions, such as in the dentate granule cells, there is a transient increase to a low level and then resolution to normal. In selectively vulnerable regions of hippocampus and caudate putamen, there is a substantial and prolonged increase that persists for up to 72 h after ischemia. This activity appears to be localized in neurons destined to die. These data confirm and expand upon the CPP32 message expression recently reported by Gillardon [6] in a rat cardiac arrest model. The pattern of caspase-3 induction demonstrated in the current experiment is similar to that we have demonstrated previously with the pro-apoptotic gene product, bax, which is also upregulated in global ischemia [3]. Caspase-3 is upregulated in cells dying of apoptosis, as documented by the double-staining experiments showing co-localization of caspase-3 in TUNEL-positive cells.

The activation of caspase-3 and other ICE family members requires a proteolytic cleavage of a precursor protein. In the case of CPP-32, the sub-units are p17 and p12. Nearly consistent with the cleavage of caspase-3, protease activity could be measured in the same ischemic brain regions. Thus, cell death in global ischemia is associated with a post-translational activation, as well as a gene induction, of caspase-3; the proteolytic cleavage occurs slightly before gene upregulation. The mechanism of caspase-3 induction and cleavage remains unclear. The phenomenon of autoactivation is possible. In this model system ICE is probably not responsible for caspase-3 activation, given that the ICE inhibitor studies did not produce protection.

There are multiple targets for caspase-3 during apoptosis. We demonstrate here that the DNA-repair and genome-integrity-maintenance enzyme PARP is cleaved by caspase-3 into 85- and 24-kDa fragments. Other potential targets for caspase-3 include the DNA-dependent protein kinase (DNA-PK), protein kinase C and actin. Other potential mechanisms of caspase-3 cell-death induction could be activation of other caspases, such as Mch2a and Mch6 or activation of caspase-activated deoxyribonuclease (CAD) [4, 10]. Future studies will be required to identify the mechanisms of induction of this, other caspases and their specific substrates.

References

1. Bredesen DE (1995) Neural apoptosis. Ann Neurol 38: 839–851
2. Chen J, Graham SH, Nakayama M, Zhu RL, Jin K, Stetler RA, Simon RP (1997) Apoptosis repressor genes bcl-2 and bcl-x-long are expressed in the rat brain following global ischemia. J Cereb Blood Flow Metab 17: 2–10.
3. Chen J, Zhu RL, Nakayama M, Kawaguchi K, Jin K, Stetler RA, Simon RP, Graham SH (1996) Expression of the apoptosis-effector gene, Bax, is up-regulated in vulnerable hippocampal CA1 neurons following global ischemia. J Neurochem 67: 64–71
4. Enari M, Talanian RV, Wong WW, Nagata S (1996) Sequential activation of ICE-like and CPP32-like proteases during Fas-mediated apoptosis. Nature 380: 723–726

 5. Fernandes-Alnemri T, Litwack G, Alnemri ES (1994) CPP32, a novel human apoptotic protein with homology to Caenorhabditis elegans cell death protein Ced-3 and mammalian interleukin-1 beta-converting enzyme. J Biol Chem 269: 30761–30764
 6. Gillardon F, Bottiger B, Schmitz B, Zimmermann M, Hossmann KA (1997) Activation of CPP-32 protease in hippocampal neurons following ischemia and epilepsy. Brain Res Mol Brain Res 50: 16–22
 7. Hara H, Friedlander RM, Gagliardini V, Ayata C, Fink K, Huang Z, Shimizu-Sasamata M, Yuan J, Moskowitz MA (1997) Inhibition of interleukin 1beta converting enzyme family proteases reduces ischemic and excitotoxic neuronal damage. Proc Natl Acad Sci U S A 94: 2007–2012
 8. Juan TS, McNiece IK, Jenkins NA, Gilbert DJ, Copeland NG, Fletcher FA (1996) Molecular characterization of mouse and rat CPP32 beta gene encoding a cysteine protease resembling interleukin-1 beta converting enzyme and CED-3. Oncogene 13: 749–755
 9. Ni B, Wu X, Du Y, Su Y, Hamilton-Byrd E, Rockey PK, Rosteck P Jr., Poirier GG, Paul SM (1997) Cloning and expression of a rat brain interleukin-1beta-converting enzyme (ICE)-related protease (IRP) and its possible role in apoptosis of cultured cerebellar granule neurons. J Neurosci 17: 1561–1569
10. Srinivasula SM, Fernandes-Alnemri T, Zangrilli J, Robertson N, Armstrong RC, Wang L, Trapani JA, Tomaselli KJ, Litwack G, Alnemri ES (1996) The Ced-3/interleukin 1beta converting enzyme-like homolog Mch6 and the lamin-cleaving enzyme Mch2alpha are substrates for the apoptotic mediator CPP32. J Biol Chem 271: 27099–27106
11. Tewari M, Quan LT, O'Rourke K, Desnoyers S, Zeng Z, Beidler DR, Poirier GG, Salvesen GS, Dixit VM (1995) Yama/CPP32 beta, a mammalian homolog of CED-3, is a CrmA-inhibitable protease that cleaves the death substrate poly(ADP-ribose) polymerase. Cell 81: 801–809

Alterations in Translation Initiation Following Global Brain Ischemia

D. J. DeGracia, B. C. White, and G. S. Krause

Summary. Suppression of protein production has long been noted to occur in the brain following ischemia and reperfusion, and may be an important contributing factor in neuronal death [21]. It is now generally accepted that this depression of protein synthesis is due to inhibition of translation initiation. We will review data showing that phosphorylation of the eukaryotic initiation factor, eIF2, is a key event in the suppression of protein synthesis during reperfusion.

Translation Initiation

Initiation, generally believed to be the rate-limiting step in translation [6], requires the coordinated assembly of the ribosomal subunits, the messenger ribonucleic acid (mRNA) that is to be translated, and, in eukaryotic cells, the methionine-charged transfer RNA (tRNA) for the first amino acid. This process is orchestrated by a family of proteins collectively known as eukaryotic initiation factors (eIF) [23, 24]. Rates of global protein synthesis are regulated by altering the phosphorylation state of eIF2, which introduces the initiator, methionyl-tRNA, into the translation-initiation complex [30]. Phosphorylation of Ser^{51}, on the α-subunit of eIF2 [eIF2α(P)], generates a competitive inhibitor of eIF2B; this inhibitor interferes with the replenishment of guanosine triphosphate (GTP) onto eIF2, which is necessary for each round of translation initiation [32]. In several models of cellular stress, increased eIF2α(P) results in decreased protein synthesis [26].

Phosphorylation of eIF2α During Reperfusion

Hu and Wieloch [18] found that, following post-ischemic brain reperfusion, formation of the eIF2/GTP/Met-tRNA complex was diminished; they attributed this to reduced eIF2B activity. However, Burda et al. [7] presented evidence suggesting that the observed reduction in eIF2B activity could be explained by eIF2α(P). The affinity of eIF2B for eIF2α(P) is 150-fold greater than for unphosphorylated eIF2 [32], and the brain has about five times more eIF2 than eIF2B [2]. Thus, when approximately 20 % of brain eIF2α is phosphorylated, eIF2B would be effectively sequestered from participation in the GTP exchange. In agreement with this, we found 20–24 % of the eIF2α to be phosphorylated after 10 min and 90 min reperfusion; this was associated with a greater than 80 % reduction in initiation-dependent protein synthesis [10, 11].

Maturation Phenomenon in Cerebral Ischemia III
U. Ito et al. (Eds.)
© Springer-Verlag Berlin Heidelberg 1999

We utilized an antibody specific to phosphorylated eIF2α to study the regional and cellular distribution of eIF2α(P) in normal, ischemic, and reperfused rat brains [11]. Western blots of brain post-mitochondrial supernatants revealed that ~1 % of all eIF2α is phosphorylated in controls, eIF2α(P) is not reduced following up to 30 min ischemia, and eIF2α(P) is increased ~20-fold after 10 min and 90 min reperfusion. Immunostaining shows localization of eIF2α(P) to astrocytes in normal brains, a massive increase in eIF2α(P) in the cytoplasm of neurons within the first 10 min of reperfusion, accumulation of eIF2α(P) in the nuclei of selectively vulnerable neurons after 1 h reperfusion, and morphology suggesting pyknosis or apoptosis in neuronal nuclei that continue to display eIF2α(P) after 4 h reperfusion [11]. These observations, together with the fact that eIF2α(P) inhibits translation initiation, make a compelling case that eIF2α(P) is responsible for reperfusion-induced inhibition of protein synthesis in vulnerable neurons. The temporal and spatial profiles of eIF2α(P) closely follow the expected inverse relationship to post-ischemic brain protein synthesis reported by others [36]. We found gradual reduction in cytoplasmic eIF2α(P) at 60 min and 4 h reperfusion, with the dentate showing the earliest recovery; eIF2α(P) remained elevated in CA1 after 4 h reperfusion.

We were surprised to note eIF2α(P) immunostaining in nuclei of selectively vulnerable neurons after 1 h and 4 h reperfusion. Although in very early reperfusion, cytoplasmic eIF2α(P) was seen in vulnerable as well as in ischemia-resistant neurons, we never observed eIF2α(P) in the nuclei of non-vulnerable neurons. To verify that the nuclear staining was not due to a protein other than eIF2α(P), we immunoblotted unfractionated 1-h-reperfused forebrain homogenates with anti-eIF2α(P) and again observed only one band migrating at 36 kDa [11].

eIF2α Kinases

The precise identity of the enzyme that phosphorylates eIF2α following brain ischemia is unknown. There are three confirmed eIF2α kinases [8]: the double-stranded RNA-activated protein kinase (PKR); the heme-regulated inhibitor (HRI); and GCN2. GCN2 is a yeast eIF2α kinase. While a GCN2 analogue has been identified in *Drosophila* [33], a mammalian equivalent of this enzyme has not yet been reported. HRI is found predominantly in reticulocytes [26, 27]. Mellor et al. [22] cloned from a rat brain library, cDNA coding for an eIF2α kinase that had 82 % amino acid sequence homology to HRI; however, Pal et al. [27] did not find HRI in rabbit-brain sections. Because oxidized glutathione (GSSG) is known to activate HRI [9], we examined in vitro translation systems in which GSSG was added to either a rabbit reticulocyte lysate or to a normal rat-brain homogenate [10]. We obtained the expected translation inhibition in the rabbit reticulocyte system, but GSSG had no effect on translation in the rat-brain homogenate (unpublished data). This result and the studies of Pal et al. [27] argue against HRI as a major regulator of eIF2α phosphorylation in the brain.

PKR has several characteristics that led us [11] and others [3, 5] to suggest that it could be the kinase that phosphorylates eIF2α during brain reperfusion. It is widely distributed in various tissues, including the brain [16], and can be activated under conditions similar to those seen during ischemia and reperfusion. Depletion of Ca^{2+} from the endoplasmic reticulum, induced by arachidonate [14, 31] at concentrations

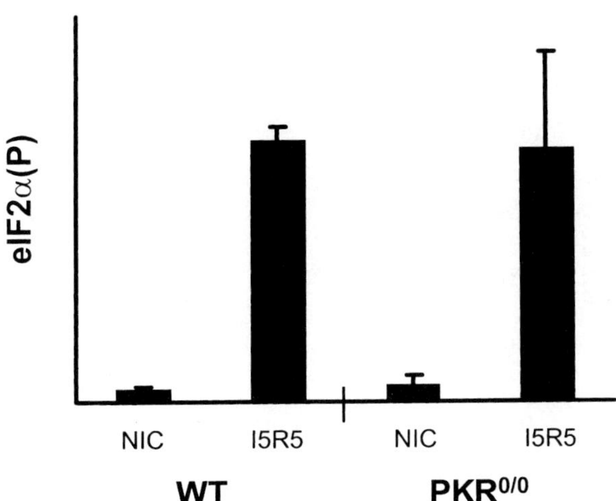

Fig. 1. An antibody specific for phosphorylated eukaryotic initiation factor (eIF)2α was utilized to examine brain homogenates (n=3 each group) obtained from wild-type (*WT*) mice or mice with a homozygous knockout of the PKR gene (*PKR$^{0/0}$*) before (*NIC*) and after a 5-min cardiac arrest that was followed by 5 min reperfusion (*I5R5*). Densitometry revealed identical 16–fold increases over control levels in brain eIF2α(P) in wild-type and PKR$^{0/0}$ mice after 5 min reperfusion

that develop during transient brain ischemia [1], can induce activation of PKR, phosphorylation of eIF2α, and inhibition of protein synthesis [4, 29, 34].

To test the possibility that PKR was the kinase responsible for the rapid phosphorylation of eIF2α during post-ischemic brain reperfusion, we utilized Western blotting to examine the effect of brain ischemia and reperfusion on eIF2α(P) in brain homogenates from wild-type and PKR-knockout C57BL6 mice (PKR$^{0/0}$ mice provided by Randal Kaufman, University of Michigan). The absence of PKR was confirmed by immunoblotting, and the abundance of eIF2α was identical in the two strains. Surprisingly, phosphorylation of eIF2α during early reperfusion was identical for the wild-type and PKR$^{0/0}$ mice (Fig. 1). Clearly, PKR is not required for phosphorylation of eIF2α during brain reperfusion and, therefore, a presently unidentified eIF2α kinase and causal pathway are involved in this process.

eIF2α(P) Phosphatases

The persistent enhancement of eIF2α phosphorylation during brain reperfusion might also reflect inappropriately low phosphatase activity against eIF2(αP). In the liver, amino acid deprivation decreases eIF2α(P) phosphatase activity, leading to increased phosphorylation of eIF2α and inhibited protein synthesis [19]. Therefore, we utilized the procedure of Kimball et al. [19] to examine the effect of brain ischemia and reperfusion on dephosphorylation of eIF2α(P). Exogenous eIF2 that contained eIF2α(^{32}P) was added to forebrain homogenates from control rats (NIC, n=3) and from rats subjected to 10 min cardiac arrest followed by 90 min reperfusion (10I/90R, n=3), and the rate of label loss was determined. Reaction aliquots were taken at 0, 10, 20 and 30 min, electrophoresed [10 % sodium dodecyl sulfate-polyacrylamide gel electrophoresis (SDS-PAGE)], and transferred to nitrocellulose. An autoradiogram of the membrane was prepared and immunoblotted for eIF2α and eIF2α(P). Ischemia and 90 min reperfusion were not associated with any loss of phosphatase activity against eIF2α(P) (Fig. 2).

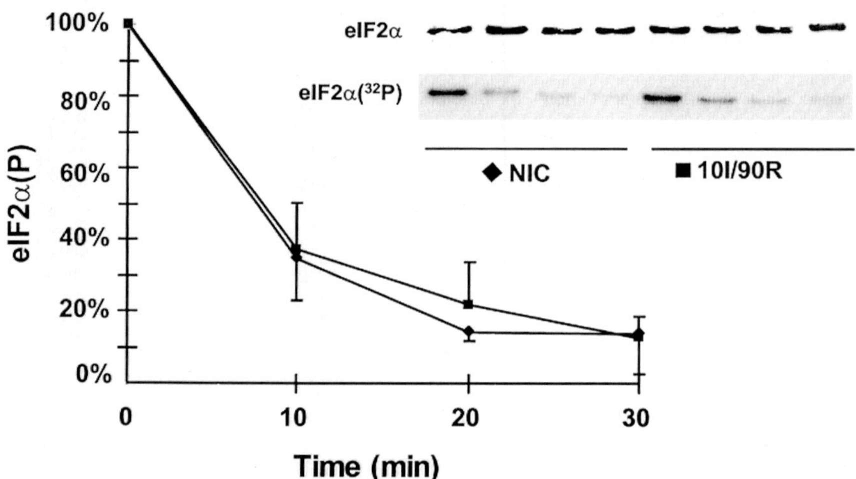

Fig. 2. Representative time courses of dephosphorylation of eukaryotic initiation factor (eIF)2α(^{32}P) in control (*NIC*) and reperfused (*10I/90R*) brain homogenates. The figure for eIF2α is an immunoblot and the figure for eIF2α(P) is an autoradiograph. The graph shows mean ±SD (*n*=3 at each point)

Nuclear eIF2α(P) and Apoptosis

The persistent presence of eIF2α(P) that we have observed in vulnerable neurons during reperfusion may be related to the induction of apoptosis [17]. Indeed, it has been hypothesized that inhibition of protein synthesis may actually trigger apoptosis [20]. Expression of the eIF2α mutant-protein Ser^{51}Ala (no phosphorylation possible) in NIH 3T3 fibroblasts blocked TNF-α-induced apoptosis, whereas conditional expression of the Ser^{51}Asp-mutant (which mimics permanent phosphorylation) induced immediate apoptosis [35]. Purified eIF2 has RNA binding properties [15]. Although DNA binding by eIF2 has yet to be demonstrated, the β-subunit of eIF2 includes a zinc finger [12] and lysine blocks [28] associated with nucleotide binding, but does not appear to be involved in binding either met-tRNA or GTP [13, 25].

The nuclear localization of eIF2α, together with the observation that apoptosis is induced by Ser^{51}Asp-mutant eIF2α makes it tempting to speculate that nuclear eIF2α(P) is involved in regulating the transcription of pro-apoptotic genes. Experimental approaches for assessing this possibility include examination of transcription of such genes as BAX and CPP32 in cells expressing the Ser^{51}Asp-mutant eIF2α.

References

1. Abe K, Yoshidomi M, Kogure K (1989) Arachidonic acid metabolism in ischemic neuronal damage. Ann NY Acad Sci 559: 259–268
2. Alcázar A, Martín ME, Soria E, Rodríguez S, Fando JL, Salinas M (1995) Purification and characterization of guanine nucleotide-exchange factor, eIF-2B, and p37 calmodulin-binding protein from calf brain. J Neurochem 65: 754–761

3. Alcázar A, de la Vega CM, Bazan E, Fando JL, Salinas M (1997) Calcium mobilization by ryanodine promotes the phosphorylation of initiation factor 2α subunit and inhibits protein synthesis in cultured neurons. J Neurochem 69: 1703–1708
4. Brostrom CO, Brostrom MA (1990) Calcium-dependent regulation of protein synthesis in intact mammalian cells. Ann Rev Physiol 52: 577–590
5. Brostrom CO, Brostrom MA (1998) Regulation of translational initiation during cellular responses to stress. Prog Nucleic Acids Res 58: 79–125
6. Brown EJ, Schreiber SL (1996) A signaling pathway to translational control. Cell 86: 517–520
7. Burda J, Martin EM, Garcia A, Alcázar A, Fando JL, Salinas M (1994) Phosphorylation of the α subunit of initiation factor 2 correlates with the inhibition of translation following transient cerebral ischaemia in the rat. Biochem J 302: 335–338
8. Clemens MJ (1996) Protein kinases that phosphorylate eIF2 and eIF2B, and their role in eukaryotic cell translational control. In: Hershey JWB, Matthews MB, Sonenberg N (eds) Translational control. Cold Spring Harbor Laboratory Press, Plainview, New York, pp 139–172
9. Clemens MJ, Safer B, Merrick WC, Anderson WF, London IM (1975) Inhibition of protein synthesis in rabbit reticulocyte lysates by double-stranded RNA and oxidized glutathione: indirect mode of action on polypeptide chain initiation. Proc Natl Acad Sci U S A 72: 1286–1290
10. DeGracia DJ, Neumar RW, White BC, Krause GS (1996) Global brain ischemia and reperfusion: modifications in eukaryotic initiation factors are associated with inhibition of translation initiation. J Neurochem 67: 2005–2012
11. DeGracia DJ, Sullivan JM, Neumar RW, Alousi SS, Hikade KR, Pittman JE, White BC, Rafols JA, Krause GS (1997) Effect of brain ischemia and reperfusion on the localization of phosphorylated eukaryotic initiation factor 2α. J Cereb Blood Flow Metab 17: 1291–1302
12. Donahue TF, Cigan AM, Pabrich EK, Valvaicius BC (1988) Mutations at a Zn(II) finger motif in the yeast eIF-2 beta gene alter ribosomal start-site selection during the scanning process. Cell 54: 621–632
13. Erickson FL, Hannig EM (1996) Ligand interactions with eukaryotic translation initiation factor 2: role of the gamma-subunit. EMBO J 15: 6311–6320
14. Fleming N, Mellow L (1995) Arachidonic acid stimulates intracellular calcium mobilization and regulates protein synthesis, ATP levels, and mucin secretion in submandibular gland cells. J Dent Res 74: 1295–1302
15. Flynn A, Shatsky IN, Proud CG, Kaminski A (1994) The RNA-binding properties of protein synthesis initation factor eIF-2. Biochim Biophys Acta 1219: 293–301
16. Haines GK, Ghadge G, Radosevich JA (1993) Expression of p68 protein kinase as recognized by the monoclonal antibody TJ4C4 during human fetal development. Tumor Biol 14: 95–104
17. Hale AJ, Smith CA, Sutherland LC, Stoneman VEA, Longthorne VL, Culhane AC, Williams GT (1996) Apoptosis: molecular regulation of death. Eur J Biochem 236: 1–26
18. Hu B, Wieloch T (1993) Stress-induced inhibition of protein synthesis initiation: modulation of initiation factor 2 and guanine nucleotide exchange factor activities following transient ischemia in the rat. J Neurosci 13: 1830–1838
19. Kimball SR, Antonetti DA, Brawley RM, Jefferson LS (1991) Mechanism of inhibition of peptide chain initiation by amino acid deprivation in perfused rat liver. J Biol Chem 266: 1969–1976
20. Koh JY, Cotman CW (1992) Programmed cell death: its possible contributions to neurotoxicity mediated by calcium channel antagonists. Brain Res 587: 233–240
21. Krause GS, Tiffany BR (1993) Suppression of protein synthesis in the reperfused brain. Stroke 24: 747–756
22. Mellor H, Flowers KM, Kimball SR, Jefferson LS (1994) Cloning and characterization of cDNA encoding rat hemin-sensitive initiation factor-2α (eIF-2α) kinase. J Biol Chem 269: 10201–10204
23. Merrick WC (1992) Mechanism and regulation of eukaryotic protein synthesis. Microbiol Rev 56: 291–315
24. Merrick WC, Hershey JWB (1996) The pathway and mechanism of eukaryotic protein synthesis. In: Hershey JWB, Matthews MB, Sonenberg N (eds) Translational control. Cold Spring Harbor Laboratory Press, New York, pp 31–69
25. Naranda T, Sirangelo I, Fabbri BJ, Hershey JW (1995) Mutations in the NKXD consensus element indicate that GTP binds to the gamma-subunit of translation initiation factor eIF2. FEBS Lett 372: 249–252
26. Pain VM (1996) Initiation of protein synthesis in eukaryotic cells. Eur J Biochem 236: 747–771
27. Pal JK, Chen JJ, London IM (1991) Tissue distribution of heme-regulated eIF-2α kinase determined by monoclonal antibodies. Biochemistry 30: 2555–2562
28. Pathak VK, Nielsen PJ, Traschel H, Hershey JWB (1988) Structure of the β subunit of translational initiation factor eIF-2. Cell 54: 633–639

29. Prostko CR, Dholakia JN, Brostrom MA, Brostrom CO (1995) Activation of the double-stranded RNA-regulated protein kinase by depletion of endoplasmic reticulum calcium stores. J Biol Chem 270: 6211–6215
30. Redpath NT, Proud CG (1994) Molecular mechanisms in the control of translation by hormones and growth factors. Biochim Biophys Acta 1220: 147–162
31. Rotman EI, Brostrom MA, Brostrom CO (1992) Inhibition of protein synthesis in intact mammalian cells by arachidonic acid. Biochem J 282: 487–494
32. Rowlands AG, Panniers R, Henshaw E (1988) The catalytic mechanism of guanine nucleotide exchange factor action and competitive inhibition by phosphorylated eukaryotic initiation factor 2. J Biol Chem 263: 5526–5533
33. Santoyo J, Alcade J, Mendez R, Pulido D, de Haro C (1997) Cloning and characterization of a cDNA encoding a protein synthesis initiation factor–2α (eIF–2α) kinase from *Drosophila melanogaster*. J Biol Chem 272: 12544–12550
34. Srivastava SP, Davies MV, Kaufman RJ (1995) Calcium deletion from the endoplasmic reticulum activates the double-stranded RNA-dependent protein kinase (PKR) to inhibit protein synthesis. J Biol Chem 28: 16619–16624
35. Srivastava SP, Kumar KU, Kaufman RJ (1998) Phosphorylation of eukaryotic translation initiation factor 2 mediates apoptosis in response to activation of the double-stranded RNA-dependent protein kinase. J Biol Chem 273: 2416–2423
36. Thilmann R, Xie Y, Kleihues P, Kiessling M (1986) Persistent inhibition of protein synthesis precedes delayed neuronal death in postischemic gerbil hippocampus. Acta Neuropathol (Berl) 71: 88–93

Studies of Neuronal Necrosis and Apoptosis after Global Cerebral Ischemia in Superoxide Dismutase Transgenic and Knockout Mutants

M. Kawase, K. Murakami, M. Fujimura, T. Kondo, Y. Morita-Fujimura, S. F. Chen, R. W. Scott, C. J. Epstein, and P. H. Chan

Summary. We have demonstrated that copper zinc-superoxide dismutase (CuZn-SOD), a cytosolic isoenzyme of SOD, has a protective role in the pathogenesis of superoxide-radical-mediated brain injury, including focal transient ischemia/reperfusion and excitotoxic neuronal injury in culture. The development of mice that overexpress and underexpress the CuZnSOD-deficient gene (*Sod1*) has provided a model for assessing the role of CuZnSOD in ischemic brain injury. Employing both *Sod1* overexpressors and knockout mutant mice, the present study is designed to clarify whether CuZnSOD plays a protective role in the pathogenesis of hippocampal injury after transient global ischemia and reperfusion. To study the role of oxidative stress on the vulnerability of hippocampal CA_1 neurons in *Sod1* transgenic (T_g) or knockout mutant mice, a reliable and reproducible model of transient global cerebral ischemia has been developed that is based on plasticity of the posterior communicating artery. Our results indicate that neuronal injury in the hippocampus was markedly reduced in *Sod1* Tg mice versus non-Tg mice 3 days after 5 min of ischemia. In contrast, significant exacerbation of neuronal injury was observed in *Sod1* (–/–) knockout mice compared with wild-type littermates. However, no difference was observed at 1 day in either *Sod1* Tg or knockout mutant mice. These data indicate that superoxide radicals play an important role in the pathogenesis of delayed neuronal death in the vulnerable hippocampus CA_1 subregion following transient global cerebral ischemia.

Introduction

Oxygen free radicals or oxidants have been proposed to be involved in the development of many neurological disorders and brain dysfunctions [15, 30]. One role of oxygen free radicals in brain injury appears to be associated with reperfusion following cerebral ischemia. Reperfusion supplies oxygen to the ischemic region of the brain; however, the oxygen could be the substrate for oxidative reactions that produce oxygen radicals. Although several antioxidant enzymes, including superoxide dismutase (SOD), glutathione peroxidase and catalase, exist, overproduction of oxygen radicals exceeds the capacity of the endogenous antioxidant enzymes and thereby causes oxidative stress or injury of brain cells in pathological conditions such as ischemia. We have demonstrated that the overexpression of copper zinc (CuZn) SOD, a cytosolic isoenzyme of SOD specific for scavenging superoxide radicals in transgenic (Tg) mice, plays a protective role in the pathogenesis of superoxide-radical-mediated brain injury, including cold-induced brain edema [4], focal transient ischemia/reperfusion [13, 34], traumatic brain injury [19], and hypoxic and excitotoxic neuronal injury in

Maturation Phenomenon in Cerebral Ischemia III
U. Ito et al. (Eds.)
© Springer-Verlag Berlin Heidelberg 1999

culture [3, 6]. In CuZnSOD Tg mice, cerebral infarction and brain edema after transient focal ischemia and reperfusion were greatly reduced. Furthermore, neurological outcome was also improved in the Tg versus non-Tg mice. However, a significant reduction of infarct size after permanent focal ischemia could not be seen in Tg mice [5]. Therefore, overexpressed CuZnSOD is mainly neuroprotective during reperfusion that follows ischemia.

The hippocampus, particularly the CA_1 subregion, is known to be one of the regions of the brain most vulnerable to transient global ischemia. Neuronal loss in the CA_1 subregion of the hippocampus has been shown to occur in a delayed fashion after transient global cerebral ischemia [14, 27], although details of the mechanism are still unclear. Recent investigations demonstrated that apoptotic neuronal death, which has different morphological and biochemical features from those of necrosis or passive cell death, contributes to neuronal injury after various brain insults, including ischemia [16, 17], trauma [29], and excitotoxicity [8, 25, 26]. Hippocampal injury after transient global ischemia also has been shown to result from apoptotic mechanisms [18, 24]. Although the mechanism of apoptosis induction is likely to be multifactorial, reactive oxygen species have been suggested as a major mediator [9, 10, 12, 33].

The present study of CuZnSOD Tg and knockout mutant mice was designed to determine whether CuZnSOD plays a protective role in the pathogenesis of hippocampal injury after transient global ischemia and, if so, which of the two pathways to neuronal cell death, apoptosis or necrosis, is ameliorated in hippocampal injury that occurs after transient global ischemia.

Materials and Methods

Global Cerebral Ischemia

We studied CuZnSOD Tg HS/SF-218/3 mice (3-month-old males, 35–45 g) that overexpress (threefold) CuZnSOD activity in brain cells [7], knockout mutant mice that are deficient in CuZnSOD activity [28], and their respective littermates or wild-type mice. Global ischemia was induced by bilateral common carotid artery (BCCA) occlusion under controlled ventilation, as detailed below.

The mice were anesthetized with chloral hydrate (350 mg/kg i.p.) and xylazine (4 mg/kg i.p.). A skin incision was made on the midline of the ventral neck, and the endotracheal intubation was performed under a surgical microscope. Respiration was controlled using an animal ventilator (rodent ventilator model 683), with inspiratory stroke volume of 0.5 ml and a respiratory rate of 120 breaths/min. Rectal temperature was maintained at 37 °C using a homeothermic blanket. BCCA bifurcations were exposed and temporary clips were applied to occlude both the external and internal carotid arteries. After 5 min or 10 min BCCA occlusion, the temporary clips were removed and the restoration of blood flow observed visually. Skin incisions were sutured, and the experimental animals were cared for in individual cages maintained at 20 °C.

Physiological Parameters

Before BCCA occlusion, the left femoral artery was cannulated to measure mean arterial blood pressure (MABP), pH, CO_2 partial pressure (PCO_2), and O_2 partial pressure (PO_2). MABP values were measured for an average of 30 s to 1 min before ischemia, during ischemia, and 1 min after blood flow restoration. Arterial blood samples for blood gas analysis were taken after post-ischemia MABP values were measured.

Plasticity of the Posterior Communicating Arteries

Given that it would influence outcome following transient global ischemia, we assessed the plasticity of the posterior communicating arteries (PcomAs) before histological evaluation of hippocampal injury. The experimental animals were anesthetized with ketamine (200 mg/kg) and xylazine (10 mg/kg) and examined for PcomA plasticity [22, 23]. The PcomA in each animal was examined independently and graded on a scale from 0–3: group 0 indicated no connection between anterior and posterior circulation; group 1, anastomosis in capillary phase; group 2, small truncal PcomA; group 3, truncal PcomA. Groups 0 and 1 were classified as having hypoplastics PcomAs and group 2 and 3 as having normal PcomAs. Groups with scores of 0 and 1 were classified as the hypoplastic PcomA group – PcomA (–) – and those with scores of 2 and 3 were classified as the normal PcomA group – PcomA (+) (Fig. 1).

Histological Analysis of Hippocampal Injury

Brain samples fixed with 3.7 % formaldehyde and evaluated for PcomA plasticity were used for evaluation of the hippocampal injury. Coronal sections 50-µm thick were taken from the brain (using a vibratome) and stained with cresyl violet. Neuronal damage in the hippocampus was qualitatively and quantitatively evaluated blindly. The qualitative evaluation was based on a scoring system of 0–4, as suggested by Møller et al. [20]. Using an image analysis system, quantitative evaluation was done by measuring the length of CA_1 neuronal loss in the brain section taken from the level of the posterior commissure. The present system was created to evaluate infarct size in focal stroke by measuring the areas of stained sections that have optical densities exceeding a threshold value [32]; it was originally applied to measure neuronal loss in CA_1 following global ischemia, without sampling error or observer bias. The ratio of CA_1 neuronal loss was calculated as (length of CA_1 neuronal loss/length of total CA_1 subregion)$\times 100$ %.

In Situ Detection and Quantification of Neurons with DNA Fragmentation in Hippocampal Injury

Deoxyribonucleic acid (DNA)-fragmented neurons were evaluated using terminal deoxynucleotidyl transferase-mediated uridine 5'-triphosphate-biotin nick end labeling (TUNEL) staining. Brain samples used for the detection of DNA fragmentation, a

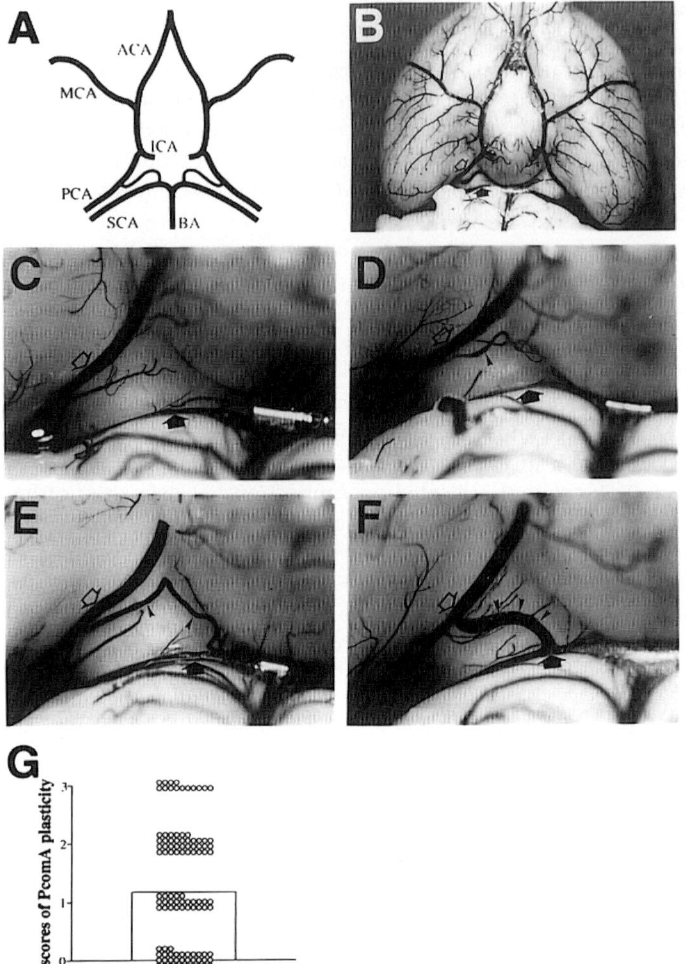

Fig. 1. A Scheme showing major blood vessels in CD1 mouse brain, including the anterior cerebral artery (*ACA*), middle cerebral artery (*MCA*), internal carotid artery (*ICA*), posterior cerebral artery (*PCA*), PcomA, superior cerebellar artery (*SCA*), and basilar artery (*BA*). Note that the PCA originates from the ICA in mice. **B** Photomicrograph showing the major blood vessels. **C–F** Photomicrographs showing the posterior communicating arteries (PcomA), graded from 0–3, respectively. **C** score 0; **D** score 1; **E** score 2; **F** score 3. *Arrowhead* PcomA; *open arrow* PCA; *arrow* SCA. **G** score of PcomA in all hemispheres used in the present study. Each *circle* and *bar* represents hemispheres graded 0–3 and the mean score of PcomAs, respectively

possible indication of apoptosis in hippocampal injury, were prepared separately. Brains were frozen in 2-methyl butane at –20 °C immediately after decapitation. Brain sections at the level of the posterior commissure were taken using a cryostat and stored at –80 °C.

Slides were fixed with 3.7 % formaldehyde in phosphate-buffered saline (PBS) for 45 min. Endogenous peroxidase was inactivated with 2 % hydrogen peroxide and

100 mM sodium azide for 30 min. After the slides were washed with PBS, they were immersed in terminal deoxynucleotidyl transferase (TdT) buffer (Gibco BRL, Gaithersburg, Md.) at room temperature for 15 min and incubated with TdT and biotin-16-uridine-5'-triphosphate (Boehringer Mannheim, Indianapolis, Ind.) at 37 °C for 60 min. The reaction was stopped by washing with 6 mM sodium citrate and 60 mM sodium chloride for 30 min; the slides were then incubated with 2 % bovine serum albumin in PBS. After washing with PBS, sections were incubated with avidin peroxidase for 30 min at room temperature, and staining was visualized with 3 mM 3, 3'-diaminobenzidine tetrahydrochloride and 18 mM hydrogen peroxide in PBS. These brain sections were also stained with methyl green.

Based on the fact that TUNEL-positive cells have extensively damaged DNA and are most likely undergoing apoptotic cell death, these cells in the CA_1 subregion were quantified blindly using a light microscope. A grid (5 mm·5 mm) was located approximately at the center of the hippocampal lesion in the CA_1 subregion. The number of TUNEL-positive neurons and total injured neurons within the grid were counted at a magnification of ×400. The ratio of the number of TUNEL-positive neurons to the total number of injured neurons was calculated and expressed as a percentage of TUNEL-positive cells in each group.

Results

PcomA Plasticity in CD1 Mice

Given that the CD1 mouse strain has been used for making *SOD1* Tg mice and for cross-breeding of *SOD1* knockout mutants (CD1/129), we first examined the PcomA plasticity in wild-type CD1 mice. The PcomAs were evaluated in each hemisphere and graded on a scale from 0–3 (Fig. 1C–F). The mean score of the PcomAs was 1.18 (Fig. 1G). In the present study, PcomAs with scores of 0 and 1 were classified into the PcomA(–) group, and those with scores of 2 and 3 were classified into the PcomA(+) group. In this latter classification, the PcomAs were patent on both sides in 25.4 % (15/59) of mice and on either side in 33.9 % (20/59) of mice. Thus, 40.7 % (24/59) of mice lacked the patent PcomA on both sides. There was no significance in PcomA plasticity between the wild-types, *SOD1* overexpressors and knockout mutants. In our subsequent ischemia studies, only animals with PcomA patency grades of 0–1 were employed.

Hippocampal Injury after Global Ischemia

Injured neurons in the hippocampus showed various levels of severity following global ischemia. The hemisphere with the hypoplastic PcomA was therefore employed to normalize the anatomic background (which could affect the ischemic condition induced by BCCA occlusion). Several types of damaged neurons were observed in hippocampal injury. Some of these neurons had a slightly condensed nucleus. The most frequently observed neurons in the injured hippocampus had an oval or triangular nucleus. The neurons with an oval nucleus, in particular, occasion-

Fig. 2. A Qualitative analysis of neuronal damage of the hippocampal injury in non-transgenic (Tg) and Tg mice at 1 day and 3 days after global ischemia. White and black *dots* show the score of the injury in the hemisphere used in non-Tg and Tg mice, respectively, and each *column* shows mean score of the hippocampal injury of each group. *$P<0.05$, Mann-Whitney U test. Hippocampal injury was ameliorated in Tg mice, in the 5- and 10-min ischemia groups, and at both 1 day and 3 days. The tendency for delayed development of the hippocampal injury was demonstrated in the 5-min group, and the injury was significantly milder in Tg than non-Tg mice at 3 days. However, this injury was near the peak at 1 day after 10 min of ischemia in non-Tg mice, although it progressed at 3 days in Tg mice. In the 10-min group, a significant difference was obtained at 1 day rather than at 3 days. **B** Qualitative analysis of neuronal damage of the hippocampus in *Sod1 (–/–)* mutant and wild-type mice at 1 day and 3 days after global ischemia. Open and closed *circles* show the scores for the injury in the hemisphere used in the wild-type and *Sod1 (–/–)* mice, and each *column* shows the mean scores of the hippocampal injury in each group. *$P<0.05$, Mann-Whitney U test. The hippocampal injury was exacerbated in the *Sod1 (–/–)* mice at 3 days after 5 min of ischemia compared with the wild-type mice. No significant difference in hippocampal injury was observed between *Sod1 (–/–)* mutant mice and wild-type mice at 1 day after 5 min of ischemia

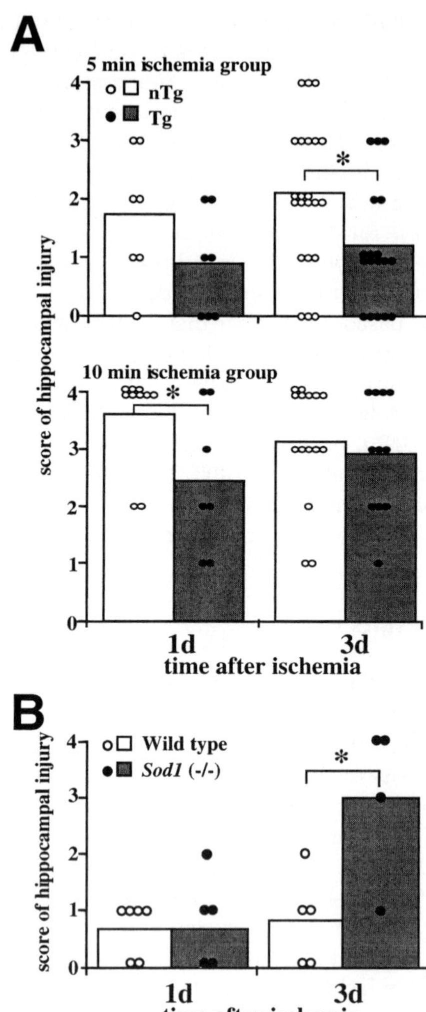

ally displayed small particles that appeared to be apoptotic bodies in the cytosol. These compact neurons were observed to coexist in the same hippocampal lesion. However, hippocampal neurons with different morphology displayed a swollen cell body or cell lysis.

Injury in the hippocampus ipsilateral to the hypoplastic PcomA was evaluated. These data demonstrate that hippocampal injury was reduced in Tg mice, compared with non-Tg mice (Fig. 2A). In addition to the reduction of injury in Tg mice, hippocampal injury progressed from 1–3 days after ischemia in the 5-min ischemia group, although a statistical difference was not seen between 1 day and 3 days. The mean score was 1.71 in non-Tg ($n=7$) mice and 0.86 in Tg ($n=7$) mice at 1 day and no significant difference was seen between non-Tg and Tg mice. At 3 days, however, the hippocampal injury score of Tg mice was significantly lower than that of non-Tg mice ($P<0.05$, Mann-Whitney U test). The mean score was 2.09 in non-Tg ($n=22$) mice and 1.17 in Tg ($n=18$) mice at 3 days (Fig. 2A).

In the 10-min ischemia group, hippocampal injury was also reduced in Tg mice. The hippocampal injury at 1 day was also significantly more severe in non-Tg than in Tg mice. Mean scores were 3.60 in non-Tg ($n=8$) mice and 2.43 in Tg ($n=9$) mice at 1 day, and hippocampal injury was significantly reduced in Tg mice compared with non-Tg mice ($P<0.05$, Mann-Whitney U test). Hippocampal injury was likely to progress only in Tg mice and was maximal at 1 day in non-Tg mice, although a statistical significance was not obtained. Scores were 3.13 in non-Tg ($n=15$) animals and 2.91 in Tg ($n=11$) mice at 3 days after ischemia (Fig. 2A).

DNA Fragmentation in Hippocampal Neurons after Global Ischemia

On the basis of these biochemical and morphological features of ischemic neurons in the hippocampal CA_1 subregion, the ratio of TUNEL-positive neurons to total ischemic neurons was investigated at 1 day or 3 days after global ischemia. In the 5-min ischemia group, the ratio was significantly lower in the non-Tg than the Tg mice at 1 day ($P<0.05$, analysis of variance). These TUNEL-positive neurons represented $21.9\pm11.4\%$ ($n=4$) and $44.2\pm20.0\%$ ($n=5$) of total injured neurons in non-Tg and Tg mice, respectively. At 3 days after 5 min of ischemia, this ratio was $34.1\pm9.2\%$ in non-Tg mice and $42.5\pm2.1\%$ in Tg mice. In the 10-min group, this ratio was $38.6\pm20.5\%$ in non-Tg ($n=7$) and $35.0\pm24.2\%$ in Tg ($n=4$) mice at 1 day, and $38.2\pm20.9\%$ in non-Tg ($n=5$) and $31.1\pm20.4\%$ in Tg ($n=2$) mice, respectively.

Hippocampal Injury after Global Ischemia in *Sod1 (–/–)* Mutant Mice

Injury in the hippocampus ipsilateral to the hypoplastic PcomA was evaluated in *Sod1* (–/–) mutant mice. Unlike in Tg mice, the hippocampal injury was exacerbated in the *Sod1* (–/–) mice, with a score of 3 ($n=4$) at 3 days after 5 min of ischemia, compared with the wild-type mice ($n=5$). No significant difference in hippocampal injury was observed between the *Sod1* (–/–) mutant and wild-type mice at 1 day following 5 min of ischemia (Fig. 2B). The study of global ischemia in *Sod1* (–/–) mice is still in progress. Therefore, the DNA fragmentation in *Sod1* (–/–) mutant mice has not yet been evaluated. The mitochondrial viability assay using rhodamine 123 (Rh123) revealed that the fluorescent signals of Rh123 were reduced in the hippocampal CA_1 subregion in *Sod1*-deficient mutant mice compared with wild-types 1 day after 5 min of ischemia.

Discussion

The present study demonstrated that endogenously overexpressed CuZnSOD plays a protective role in the development of hippocampal injury following transient global ischemia. This protective role was observed both in acute injury induced by relatively intense ischemia and in delayed-progress injury induced by relatively mild ischemia. In situ detection of DNA fragmentation by TUNEL staining demonstrated that apoptotic neuronal death partly contributes to hippocampal injury following transient global ischemia in mice. Furthermore, neuroprotective action by overexpressed CuZnSOD is also involved in the apoptotic process that follows global ischemia.

In the study of global and focal ischemia, both physiological and anatomical backgrounds affected the outcome of neuronal injury, especially when genetically different animals were used. In this study, physiological conditions, including MABP and arterial blood gas, were not significantly different for non-Tg mice, Tg mice and the knockout mutants. Other factors, including plasticity of the PcomA, are probably the most important components of the anatomic background affecting the outcome in global ischemia [1]. Because of the lack of a PcomA connection between anterior and posterior circulation, gerbils have been widely used for global ischemia studies, on the basis that BCCA occlusion can induce almost complete forebrain ischemia without a reduction in collateral blood flow from posterior circulation, including hemorrhagic hypotension [31], bilateral vertebral artery occlusion [27], and basilar artery occlusion, as seen in rats [11]. We have previously reported that the residual regional cortical blood flow is correlated with plasticity of the PcomA in BCCA occlusion [21]. Furthermore, hippocampal injury was occasionally observed following brief ischemia, usually in either hemisphere. Therefore, we evaluated plasticity of the PcomA and selected the hippocampus ipsilateral to the hypoplastic PcomA (on the basis that complete ischemia was induced). This method might be useful for the investigation of global ischemia in mice.

Hippocampal injury was determined both qualitatively and quantitatively after relatively mild and intense global ischemia produced by 5 min and 10 min periods of BCCA occlusion, respectively. In the quantitative evaluation, an image analysis system was used to detect neuronal loss in the CA_1 subregion. Qualitative evaluation clearly demonstrated the protective role of CuZnSOD in global ischemia. The development and occurrence of hippocampal injury appeared to depend on the duration of ischemia, which is strongly correlated with the intensity of the ischemic insult. Hippocampal injury after 5 min of ischemia tended to progress in a delayed fashion, although statistical significance was not achieved. The injury was reduced in Tg mice and exacerbated in knockout mutants at both 1 day and 3 days after global ischemia, and was significant at 3 days. In contrast, for the 10-min ischemia group, hippocampal injury was maximized as early as 1 day after ischemia in non-Tg mice; the mean score was higher at 1 day than 3 days. This discrepancy may be due to the fact that the severely injured mice died 1–3 days after ischemia, and thus were excluded from the evaluation.

Recent studies have demonstrated that apoptosis, in addition to necrosis, is involved in hippocampal injury after global ischemia [18, 24]. Therefore, we used TUNEL staining to determine the role of overexpressed CuZnSOD in DNA fragmentation – a process that might precede apoptosis. The present study demonstrated that DNA fragmentation also contributes to hippocampal injury following global ischemia in mice. Hippocampal injury was revealed by several types of morphological feature in ischemic neurons. These neurons were observed in both ischemia groups and in both groups of mice. Not all of the neurons displaying the morphological features of apoptosis were labeled by TUNEL staining. Therefore, in the present study, the contribution of DNA-fragmented neurons was evaluated as the ratio of TUNEL-positive neurons in the hippocampal injury. In the 5-min ischemia group, the percentage of TUNEL-positive neurons was increased at 1 day in Tg mice relative to non-Tg mice, although the total injury to the hippocampus was reduced in Tg mice. However, in the 10-min ischemia group, this ratio was almost the same for non-Tg and Tg mice. This discrepancy in the ratio of TUNEL-positive neurons between the 5-min and 10-min ischemia groups might result from a difference in the intensity of the ischemic insult. A decrease of TUNEL-positive neurons means that TUNEL-negative cells, which might also include necrotic cells, were increased in non-Tg mice after 5 min of ischemia. Thus, the increased TUNEL-positive neurons in Tg mice following 5 min of ischemia may reflect TUNEL-positive neurons that were unmasked by necrotic neurons. It has been demonstrated that excitotoxicity mediated by the N-methyl-D-aspartate receptor induces calcium overload and generates superoxide anions, thereby causing neuronal injury. Two distinct pathways to neuronal death, apoptosis and necrosis, have been demonstrated, depending on the intensity of the insult [2]. We have demonstrated that oxygen deprivation, but not in combination with substrate, induces DNA degradation in cortical neurons [6]. Considering these findings together with the present results, overexpressed CuZnSOD effectively detoxifies abnormally overproduced superoxide anions and reduces oxidative stress to neurons; this might also alter apoptosis and necrosis in Tg mice. Following intense ischemia by 10 min of BCCA occlusion, the ratio was not altered by overexpressed CuZnSOD in Tg mice. Oxidative stress might be partly detoxified by overexpressed CuZnSOD and the hippocampal injury thereby reduced in Tg mice (as shown in histological analysis).

We conclude that overexpressed CuZnSOD plays a protective role in the pathogenesis of hippocampal injury, either in an acute or delayed fashion. Furthermore, we postulate that the alternation of the pathway to neuronal death might depend on the intensity of oxidative stress and that CuZnSOD possibly ameliorates both types of neuronal death in hippocampal injury that follows transient global ischemia.

Acknowledgements. This study was supported by National Institutes of Health grants P 50 NS 14543, NS 25372, P 01 AG 08938, N O1 NS 52334, NS 36147 and NO1-NS 8–2386. The authors thank Liza Reola and Bernard Calagui for their technical assistance and Cheryl Christensen for her editorial assistance.

References

1. Barone FC, Knudsen DJ, Nelson AH, Feuerstein GZ, Willette RN (1993) Mouse strain differences in susceptibility to cerebral ischemia are related to cerebral vascular anatomy. J Cereb Blood Flow Metab 13: 683–692
2. Bonfoco E, Krainc D, Ankarcrona M, Nicotera P, Lipton SA (1995) Apoptosis and necrosis: two distinct events induced, respectively, by mild and intense insults with N-methyl-d-aspartate or nitric oxide/superoxide in cortical cell cultures. Proc Natl Acad Sci U S A 92: 7162–7166
3. Chan PH, Chu L, Chen SF, Carlson EJ, Epstein CJ (1990) Reduced neurotoxicity in transgenic mice overexpressing human copper-zinc-superoxide dismutase. Stroke 21[Suppl III]:80-82
4. Chan PH, Yang GY, Chen SF, Carlson E, Epstein CJ (1991) Cold-induced brain edema and infarction are reduced in transgenic mice overexpressing CuZn-superoxide dismutase. Ann Neurol 29: 482–486
5. Chan PH, Kamii H, Yang G, Gafni J, Epstein CJ, Carlson E, Reola L (1993) Brain infarction is not reduced in SOD-1 transgenic mice after a permanent focal cerebral ischemia. Neuroreport 5: 293–296

6. Copin J-C, Reola LF, Chan TYY, Li Y, Epstein CJ, Chan PH (1996) Oxygen deprivation but not a combination of oxygen, glucose, and serum deprivation induces DNA degradation in mouse cortical neurons in vitro: attenuation by transgenic overexpressing of CuZn-superoxide dismutase. J Neurotrauma 13: 233–244

7. Epstein CJ, Avraham KB, Lovett M, Smith S, Elroy-Stein O, Rotman G, Bry C, Groner Y (1987) Transgenic mice with increased Cu/Zn-superoxide dismutase activity: animal model of dosage effects in Down syndrome. Proc Natl Acad Sci U S A 84: 8044–8048

8. Ferrer I, Martin F, Serrano T, Reiriz J, Perez-Navarro E, Alberch J, Macaya A, Planas AM (1995) Both apoptosis and necrosis occur following intrastriatal administration of excitotoxins. Acta Neuropathol (Berl) 90: 504–510

9. Greenlund LJ, Deckwerth TL, Johnson EM Jr (1995) Superoxide dismutase delays neuronal apoptosis: a role for reactive oxygen species in programmed neuronal death. Neuron 14: 303–315

10. Hockenbery DM, Oltvai ZN, Yin XM, Milliman CL, Korsmeyer SJ (1993) Bcl-2 functions in an antioxidant pathway to prevent apoptosis. Cell 75: 241–251

11. Kameyama M, Suzuki J, Shirane R, Ogawa A (1985) A new model of bilateral hemispheric ischemia in the rat – three vessel occlusion model. Stroke 16: 489–493

12. Kane DJ, Sarafian TA, Anton R, Hahn H, Gralla EB, Valentine JS, Ord T, Bredesen DE (1993) Bcl-2 inhibition of neural death: decreased generation of reactive oxygen species. Science 262: 1274–1277

13. Kinouchi H, Epstein CJ, Mizui T, Carlson E, Chen SF, Chan PH (1991) Attenuation of focal cerebral ischemic injury in transgenic mice overexpressing CuZn superoxide dismutase. Proc Natl Acad Sci U S A 88: 11158–11162

14. Kirino T (1982) Delayed neuronal death in the gerbil hippocampus following ischemia. Brain Res 239: 57–69

15. Kontos HA (1985) George E. Brown memorial lecture. Oxygen radicals in cerebral vascular injury. Circ Res 57: 508–516

16. Li Y, Chopp M, Jiang N, Yao F, Zaloga C (1995) Temporal profile of in situ DNA fragmentation after transient middle cerebral artery occlusion in the rat. J Cereb Blood Flow Metab 15: 389–397

17. Linnik MD, Miller JA, Sprinkle-Cavallo J, Mason PJ, Thompson FY, Montgomery LR, Schroeder KK (1995) Apoptotic DNA fragmentation in the rat cerebral cortex induced by permanent middle cerebral artery occlusion. Brain Res Mol Brain Res 32: 116–124

18. MacManus JP, Buchan AM, Hill IE, Rasquinha I, Preston E (1993) Global ischemia can cause DNA fragmentation indicative of apoptosis in rat brain. Neurosci Lett 164: 89–92

19. Mikawa S, Kinouchi H, Kamii H, Gobbel GT, Chen CF, Carlson E, Epstein CJ, Chan PH (1996) Attenuation of acute and chronic damage following traumatic brain injury in copper, zinc-superoxide dismutase transgenic mice. J Neurosurg 85: 885–891

20. Møller A, Axelsson O, Christoffersen P, Drejer J, Jensen LH, Nielsen EO (1994) Results with calcium antagonists. In: Kuhl P (ed) New strategies to prevent neuronal damage from ischemic stroke. CHI Press, Cambridge, pp 125–133

21. Murakami K, Kondo T, Honkaniemi J, Mikawa S, Chan T, Chen S, Sharp FR, Epstein CJ, Chan PH (1995) Expression of hsp70 mRNA following transient bilateral common carotid artery occlusion in transgenic mice overexpressing CuZn-superoxide dismutase. Soc Neurosci Abstr 3: 1730

22. Murakami K, Kondo T, Epstein CJ, Chan PH (1997) Overexpression of CuZn-superoxide dismutase reduces hippocampal injury after global ischemia in transgenic mice. Stroke 28: 1797–1804

23. Murakami K, Kondo T, Kawase M, Chan PH (1998) The development of a new mouse model of global ischemia: focus on the relationships between ischemia duration, anesthesia, cerebral vasculature, and neuronal injury following global ischemia in mice. Brain Res 780: 304–310

24. Nitatori T, Sato N, Waguri S, Karasawa Y, Araki H, Shibanai K, Kominami E, Uchiyama Y (1995) Delayed neuronal death in the CA1 pyramidal cell layer of the gerbil hippocampus following transient ischemia is apoptosis. J Neurosci 15: 1001–1011

25. Pollard H, Charriaut-Marlangue C, Cantagrel S, Represa A, Robain O, Moreau J, Ben-Ari Y (1994) Kainate-induced apoptotic cell death in hippocampal neurons. Neuroscience 63: 7

26. Portera-Cailliau C, Hedreen JC, Price DL, Koliatsos VE (1995) Evidence for apoptotic cell death in Huntington disease and excitotoxic animal models. J Neurosci 15: 3775–3787

27. Pulsinelli WA, Brierley JB, Plum F (1982) Temporal profile of neuronal damage in a model of transient forebrain ischemia. Ann Neurol 11: 491–498

28. Reaume AG, Elliott JL, Hoffman EK, Kowall NW, Ferrante RJ, Siwek DF, Wilcox HM, Flood DG, Beal MF, Brown RH Jr (1996) Motor neurons in Cu/Zn superoxide dismutase-deficient mice develop normally but exhibit enhanced cell death after axonal injury. Nat Genet 13: 43–47

29. Rink A, Fung KM, Trojanowski JQ, Lee VM, Neugebauer E, McIntosh TK (1995) Evidence of apoptotic cell death after experimental traumatic brain injury in the rat. Am J Pathol 147: 1575–1583

30. Siesjö BK, Agardh CD, Bengtsson F (1989) Free radicals and brain damage. Cerebrovasc Brain Metab Rev 1: 165–211
31. Smith ML, Bendek G, Dahlgren N, Rosen I, Wieloch T, Siesjö BK (1984) Models for studying long-term recovery following forebrain ischemia in the rat. 2. A 2-vessel occlusion model. Acta Neurol Scand 69: 385–401
32. Swanson RA, Morton MT, Wu GT, Savalos R, Davidson C, Sharp FR (1990) A semi-automated method for measuring brain infarct volume. J Cereb Blood Flow Metab 10: 290–293
33. Troy CM, Shelanski ML (1994) Down-regulation of copper/zinc superoxide dismutase causes apoptotic death in PC12 neuronal cells. Proc Natl Acad Sci U S A 91: 6384–6387
34. Yang G, Chan PH, Chen J, Carlson E, Chen SF, Weinstein P, Epstein CJ, Kamii H (1994) Human copper-zinc superoxide dismutase transgenic mice are highly resistant to reperfusion injury after focal cerebral ischemia. Stroke 25: 165–170

Apoptosis-Related Genes Are Expressed in the Rat Model of Subarachnoid Hemorrhage

K. Yamada, M. Nakatsuka, A. Masago, and H. Taki

Summary. Apoptosis in neurons can be induced by mild cerebral ischemia. We developed a rat model of subarachnoid hemorrhage that caused mild ischemic stress to the brain and detected expression of apoptosis-related genes in the hippocampus. Intracranial carotid bifurcation of the rat was perforated by a 3–0 nylon and subarachnoid hemorrhage induced. The intracranial pressure rose immediately to a level similar to systemic arterial pressure for 30 s to 1 min and returned to baseline by 20 min. We detected mRNA expression of *bax*, *bcl-2*, *bcl-x*, *ice*, *p53* and *p21*(Waf1) using an in situ hybridization technique. With this model, about one-third of the CA1 neurons were TUNEL-positive at 48 h after perforation, and histological findings were compatible with apoptotic cell changes. The *bax*, *bcl-2*, and *bcl-x* mRNA were expressed transiently at CA1 pyramidal neurons, with a peak at 12 h. The *bax* tended to be expressed for a longer period than *bcl-2*. The CA3 pyramidal neurons showed *bax*, *bcl-2*, and *bcl-x* mRNA expression as well, but transiently and with an intensity that was about half that at CA1. The *ice* mRNA, the key enzyme for protease cascade, was upregulated at CA1 neurons with a peak at 12–18 h. The *p53* mRNA expression was transient with maximum levels at 12 h, indicating that *p53* is located upstream of *bax* expression. The *p21*(Waf1) expression, however, reached maximum levels at 48 h and lasted until 120 h, suggesting no relation to *bax* or *bcl-2* expression. The results may relate to delayed ischemic neurological deficit, which is often observed as a result of subarachnoid hemorrhage and vasospasm.

Introduction

Mild cerebral ischemia may induce apoptotic changes in neurons. We developed a rat model of subarachnoid hemorrhage that caused mild ischemic stress to the hippocampal and cortical neurons [2]. With this model, we detected expression of apoptosis-related genes in the hippocampus. The results are related to a delayed ischemic neurological deficit, which is often observed as a result of subarachnoid hemorrhage and vasospasm.

Materials and Methods

Wistar rats weighing 280–400 g were subjected to the model of subarachnoid hemorrhage. A 3–0 nylon thread was inserted into the right internal carotid artery through the external carotid artery. The intracranial carotid bifurcation was perforated by the

Maturation Phenomenon in Cerebral Ischemia III
U. Ito et al. (Eds.)
© Springer-Verlag Berlin Heidelberg 1999

thread, and subarachnoid hemorrhage was produced. The intracranial pressure rose transiently to the level close to systemic arterial pressure for 30 s to 1 min after perforation, and returned to baseline by 20 min [2]. Although we did not measure blood flow, a previous study reported that blood flow was reduced to below 30 ml/100 g/min for 2 h [7]. We detected mRNA expression of *bax, bcl-2, bcl-x, ice, p53* and *p21*(Waf1) using an in situ hybridization technique [2–5]. The oligonucleotide probes complementary to these mRNAs were synthesized and used for this study. TUNEL staining was done at selected times after subarachnoid hemorrhage.

Results and Discussion

The animals became inactive and showed signs of meningismus: hunching their backs and ruffling their hair. This appearance was similar to the meningismus in animals with meningeal carcinomatosis [6]. The rat showed massive subarachnoid hem-

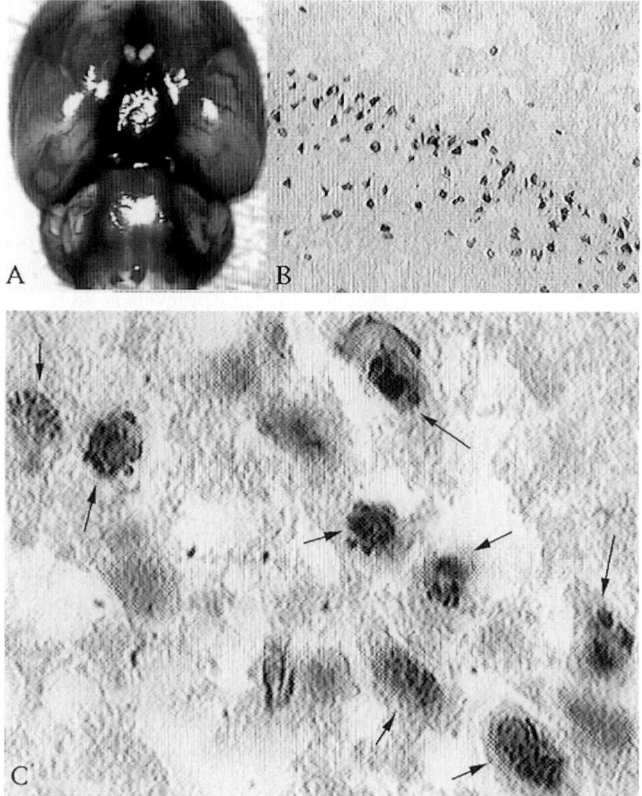

Fig. 1A–C. TUNEL-proven apoptosis in the rat model of subarachnoid hemorrhage. Subarachnoid hemorrhage was induced by endovascular perforation and diffuse hemorrhage was noted (A). The CA1 pyramidal neurons showed TUNEL-positive 48 h after subarachnoid hemorrhage (B), and higher magnification revealed nuclear fragmentation in the TUNEL-positive neurons (C; *arrows*)

orrhage in the basal and prepontine cistern (Fig. 1A). There was no apparent laterality in the distribution of subarachnoid hemorrhage. The *hsp70* mRNA was, however, expressed mainly on the side of the arterial puncture, suggesting the importance of arterial tear and subsequent local thrombosis [2]. The *hsp70* mRNA was expressed in the puncture-side hippocampus from 1–24 h after arterial penetration [2], suggesting mild ischemic stress to the hippocampus.

The TUNEL staining revealed that about one-third of CA1 neurons were TUNEL-positive at 48 h after perforation (Fig. 1B). Some of the nuclei showed fragmented and condensed chromatin, which is compatible with apoptotic cell changes (Fig. 1C). The result suggests that mild ischemia to the hippocampus by subarachnoid hemorrhage was enough to induce apoptotic changes to the CA1 pyramidal neurons of the hippocampus. Therefore, this model is suitable for studying apoptosis induced by mild ischemia.

The mRNA expression of *bax*, *bcl-2*, and *bcl-x* increased transiently at CA1 pyramidal neurons with a peak at 12 h after perforation (Fig. 2). The *bax* tended to express for a longer period than *bcl-2*. The CA3 pyramidal neurons also showed expression of *bax*, *bcl-2*, and *bcl-x* mRNA, but it was transient and the intensity was about half of the intensity at CA1(Fig. 2). When *bax* and *bcl-2* mRNA expression were compared, *bax* expression started at 6 h whereas *bcl-2* expression was delayed until 12 h. The *bcl-2* expression was weaker than *bax* and faded out at 48 h. These data indicate that the ratio of *bax/bcl-2* is higher at 6–48 h, and this might be a key factor in indicating that CA1 pyramidal neurons became apoptotic (as seen using TUNEL staining). Apoptosis, indeed, occurred in the hippocampus after subarachnoid hemorrhage.

We then studied caspase activity by detecting expression of interleukin-1 converting enzyme (ice), which is one of the key enzymes for protease cascade of apoptosis.

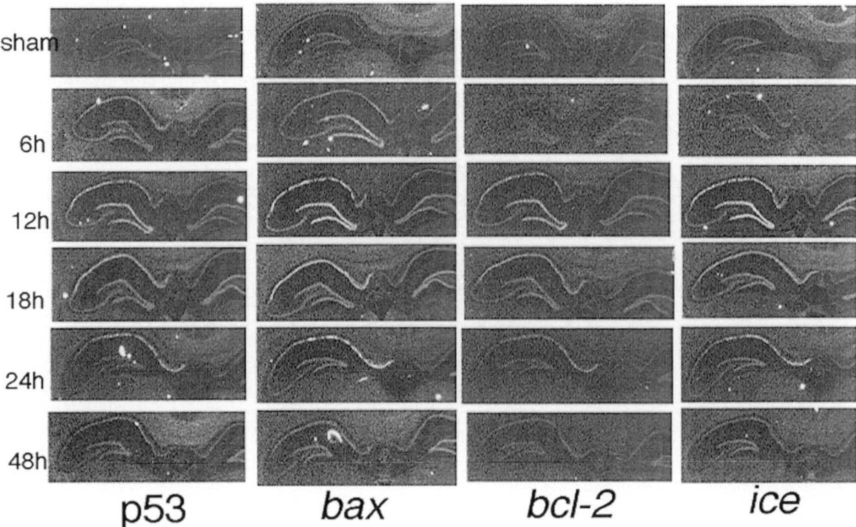

Fig. 2. Expression of apoptosis-related genes in the rat model of subarachnoid hemorrhage. The *left* side is the side of arterial puncture

The *ice* mRNA was upregulated at CA1 pyramidal neurons and dentate gyrus with a peak at 12–18 h after perforation. The data indicated that caspase cascade was also involved in this apoptosis.

Many cascades induce *bax* and *bcl-2* expression. Among those, we detected expression of *p53* and *p21*(Waf1) mRNAs. The *p53* is related to apoptosis induced by radiation, chemotherapy drugs, growth factor depletion, etc. In this model, *p53* was expressed transiently, starting at 6 h and reaching maximum levels at 12 h (Fig. 2). It is, therefore, reasonable to conclude that *p53* expression induced *bax* expression. The *p21*(Waf1) expression, however, was different from *p53* expression. The *p21*(Waf1) expression reached a maximum level at 48 h after perforation and lasted until 120 h (data not shown). Therefore, *p21* expression may not be related to *bax* or *bcl-2* expression, but may relate to regenerative processes by arresting cell cycles [1].

The present data indicate that apoptosis plays an important role in the neuronal dysfunction and neuronal death that follows subarachnoid hemorrhage and which is commonly thought to be related solely to vascular factors (vasospasm).

Acknowledgement. This study is supported in part by Grant-in-Aid from Ministry of Education and Welfare.

References

1. Fuse T, Yamada K, Asai K, Kato T, Nakanishi M (1996) Heat shock-mediated cell cycle arrest is accompanied by induction of p21 CKI. Biochem Biophys Res Commun 225: 759–763
2. Harada S, Kamiya K, Masago A, Iwata A, Yamada K (1997) Subarachnoid hemorrhage induces c-fos, c-jun and hsp70 mRNA expression in rat brain. Neuroreport 8: 3399–3404
3. Iwata A, Masago A, Yamada K (1997) Expression of basic fibroblast growth factor mRNA after transient focal ischemia: comparison with expression of c-fos, c-jun and hsp70 mRNA. J Neurotrauma 14: 201–210
4. Katano H, Masago A, Yamada K (1997) Marked alteration of c-fos and c-jun but not hsp70 messenger RNA expression in rat brain after cold-induced trauma: an in situ hybridization study. Res Neurol Neurosci 11: 153–160
5. Masago A, Shimada S, Minami Y, Inoue K, Morimura H, Otori Y, Miyai A, Tohyama M, Yamada K (1996) GLAST mRNA expression in the periventricular area of experimental hydrocephalus. Neuroreport 7: 2565–2570
6. Ushio Y, Chernik NL, Posner JB, Shapiro WR (1977) Meningeal carcinomatosis: development of an experimental model. J Neuropathol Exp Neurol 36: 228–244
7. Veelken JA, Laing RJ, Jakubowski J (1995) The Sheffield model of subarachnoid hemorrhage in rats. Stroke 26: 1279–1284

No Morphological Evidence of Apoptosis Following Mild to Severe Episodes of Four-Vessel-Occlusion Ischemia in Rats

F. Colbourne, H. Li, and A. Buchan

Summary. Severe, but brief forebrain ischemia in rat leads to a loss of hippocampal CA1 neurons 24–72 h post-ischemia. Whereas the ultrastructural features of this cell loss have been repeatedly described as necrotic, recent biochemical studies implicate apoptosis. In this study, we examined the consequences of 5-min and 15-min periods of four-vessel-occlusion (4-VO) ischemia using light and electron microscopy. Because slower maturation follows the 5-min insult, it is possible that such injury might have morphological features of apoptosis. We also examined whether caspase inhibition by z-VAD and z-DEVD would reduce injury following 10 min of ischemia. In the first experiment, CA1 cells were examined under light and electron microscopy following 5 (14-day survival) or 15 min (7-day survival) of 4-VO ischemia in rats. In the second experiment, CA1 injury (7-day survival) was quantified in rats occluded for 10 min and given an immediate 320 ng i.c.v. injection of z-VAD, z-DEVD or 3 % dimethylsulfoxide (DMSO) as a control. Five minutes and 15 min of ischemia resulted in 78 % and 81 % CA1 damage at 14 days and 7 days, respectively. Ultrastructural examination revealed extensive necrosis, with pre-lethal signs of injury in many of the surviving neurons, including dilated organelles, e.g., mitochondria, rough endoplasmic reticulum, and numerous vacuoles in the cytoplasm and nucleus. Extensive gliosis was also noted. No qualitative differences were noted between the groups and no evidence of apoptosis was observed. In the second experiment, z-VAD (76±14 % dead) and z-DEVD (72±17 % dead) failed to reduce injury compared with control (84 %±11 % SD). Thus, no morphological or pharmacological evidence of apoptosis was evident following transient forebrain ischemia that produced either typical or more delayed CA1 injury.

Introduction

A striking, but selective loss of hippocampal CA1 neurons follows brief forebrain ischemia. Because CA1 cell death matures over 24–72 h post-ischemia [22, 32, 35], this effect has been named delayed neuronal death (DND) [22]. Electron microscopic studies have revealed several early ultrastructural changes in CA1 cells destined to die, e.g., disaggregation of polyribosomes, dilated organelles [8, 22–23]. However, while pre-lethal and lethal morphological findings, e.g., mitochondrial flocculent densities, clumped tigroid chromatin, indicate a necrotic mode of cell death [3, 8, 23, 39, 42], the finding of oligonucleosomal deoxyribonucleic acid (DNA) fragmentation following global ischemia suggests a role for apoptosis [11, 18, 21, 26–28, 37]. In addition, CA1 neuroprotection that occurs through the use of protein synthesis inhibitors,

Maturation Phenomenon in Cerebral Ischemia III
U. Ito et al. (Eds.)
© Springer-Verlag Berlin Heidelberg 1999

such as cycloheximide or anisomycin [14, 30, 38, 40], also suggests apoptosis given that it often depends on new protein synthesis [19]. However, results with cycloheximide have been inconsistent [8, 30] and there is a possibility that side effects have contributed to the observed protection.

It must be noted that the findings of oligonucleosomal DNA fragmentation following global ischemia is not definitive proof of an apoptotic mode of cell death, because such DNA fragmentation can occur in necrotic cells [6]. Indeed, Petito et al. [33] recently observed that DNA fragmentation (TUNEL staining) occurred at the time of, or after, CA1 cellular disintegration. Finally, because procedures such as TUNEL labeling also tag necrotic neurons [7, 13, 15], they cannot be used solely to indicate apoptosis.

It has been suggested that apoptosis is more prevalent after mild ischemia [2, 4, 9, 10], as is the case following hyperthermia-induced injury [17] and ultraviolet irradiation [12]. While the ultrastructural morphology of typical DND in CA1 is clearly necrotic, the possibility exists that a milder insult would produce apoptosis. A brief period of four-vessel-occlusion (4-VO) ischemia in rats will result in a slower maturation of CA1 cell death [24]. Thus, we compared the light and ultrastructural morphology of CA1 DND following brief and extended episodes of 4-VO ischemia, looking specifically for signs of apoptosis. Because a prolonged expression of the caspase-3 messenger ribonucleic acid (mRNA) has been found following severe 4-VO ischemia [29], we tested whether inhibition of apoptosis-promoting caspases [26] by z-VAD and z-DEVD would reduce injury when given following global ischemia, as they have following focal ischemia [10, 16, 25].

Materials and Methods

4-VO Preparative Surgery

Adult male Wistar rats were obtained from Charles River (Montreal, Quebec, Canada) and used when they reached a weight of 175–255 g. Forebrain ischemia was induced by using a modification [36] of the 4-VO model described by Pulsinelli and Brierley [34]. Rats were anesthetized with 3 % halothane and subsequently maintained with 1–2 % halothane in a 28 % O_2, 70 % N_2 mixture. The vertebral arteries were electrocauterized and then both common carotid arteries were isolated using a loop of 2–0 silk. An 18-gauge needle was used to guide a 1–0 silk thread through the neck at a location posterior to the trachea, esophagus, external jugular veins, carotid arteries, and vagal nerves. The silk was anterior to the cervical and paravertebral musculature.

Ischemia

The following day, under direct vision, aneurysm clips were used to occlude both carotid arteries for various durations, during which core temperature was regulated at 37.5±0.5 °C by a feedback-controlled infrared lamp. Rats (no anesthesia) that became unresponsive, had initial running behavior, lost righting reflexes and showed pupil dilation were included in the study. Rats that ceased to remain in coma or that developed righting reflexes or seizure activity either during or after ischemia were excluded from the study.

Experimental Paradigms

In the ultrastructure study, rats were subjected to 5 min ($n=5$) or 15 min ($n=5$, with one death) of ischemia and allowed to survive for 14 days or 7 days, respectively. Sections of the anterior dorsal hippocampus at ≈-3.8 mm to bregma [31] were used for transmission electron microscopy. In the neuroprotection study, rats were subjected to 10 min of ischemia and subsequently given i.c.v. z-VAD (320 ng; $n=11$), z-DEVD (320 ng; $n=10$ with one post-ischemic death), or 3 % dimethylsulfoxide (DMSO) as a control ($n=9$). These animals survived for 7 days.

Assessment of Hippocampal Injury

Rats in the electron microscopy study were perfused with Karnovsky's fixative (3 % glutaraldehyde, 4 % formaldehyde) and their brains were left in situ overnight prior to removal. Thin sections of the hippocampal CA1 region were taken at ≈-3.8 mm and processed for electron microscopy. Ultra-thin sections of CA1, stained with uranyl acetate and lead citrate, were taken based on toluidine blue stained semi-thin (1-µm) sections. Many thousands of neurons per group were examined with a Hitachi M600 electron microscope. The remaining anterior tissue block from the TEM study was immersed in 10 % formalin for several days before paraffin embedding. In the second study, rats were perfusion fixed with 10 % formalin prior to paraffin embedding. Coronal sections (6-µm) were cut at 3.3 mm posterior to bregma [31] and stained with hematoxylin and eosin. Normal cells (normal appearance, not eosinophilic) were counted in the entire hippocampal CA1 band and expressed as percentage dead based on previous counts of normal tissue. Data presented as mean ± SD were compared by means of independent t-tests, using either the pooled or separate test depending on heterogeneity of variance.

Results

The same amount of CA1 injury was observed in rats subjected to 5 min (14-day survival; 77.6±17.7 % damage) and 15 min of ischemia (7-day survival; 80.6±14.7 % damage). Light and ultrastructural features of ischemic injury in both the 5-min and 15-min occlusion groups were qualitatively similar. Pre-lethal signs of injury were common in surviving neurons. These included: dispersal of Golgi apparatus, rough endoplasmic reticulum and mitochondria dilations, as well as cytoplasmic and intranuclear vacuoles. Typical signs of lethal injury included mitochondrial flocculent densities, nuclear and plasma membrane breaks, and clumped tigroid chromatin. Notably, cytoplasmic changes (organelle dilations) preceded nuclear changes (clumped chromatin). Aggregates of necrotic chromatin were of various sizes and had a punctate appearance under light microscopy (LM). Signs of apoptosis (apoptotic bodies) were never observed under transmission electron microscopy (TEM). Notably, large chromatin clumps that could be confused with apoptotic bodies were seen under LM, but were clearly from necrotic neurons when observed under TEM.

In the second experiment, both z-VAD (76±14 % damage) and z-DEVD (72±17 % damage) given as a 320-ng i.c.v. dose failed to significantly reduce injury compared with DMSO controls (84±11 %); differences between groups were not statistically significant [$F(2,26)=1.86$, $P=0.1755$].

Discussion

Both 5-min and 15-min periods of 4-VO ischemia produced severe CA1 injury, which we have shown previously to mature at different rates [24]. While injury progresses more slowly following the 5-min insult, our light and ultrastructural findings were similar in the 5-min and 15-min groups. That is, there was clear evidence of necrosis and no unequivocal evidence of apoptosis, e.g., apoptotic bodies containing chromatin. Ultrastructural features of CA1 necrosis were quite consistent with those reported by others for CA1 neurons that died over a 72-h period [3, 8, 23, 39, 42]. The observation that a 5-min period of 4-VO ischemia, which produces a slower progression, i.e., 1 week versus 3 days, of CA1 injury than a 15-min insult, results in morphologically similar CA1 death is in contrast to the findings in liver. In liver, mild ischemia results in marked atrophy due to extensive apoptosis (originally called shrinkage necrosis), while severe ischemia results in coagulation necrosis [20, 41]. However, the present results of global cerebral ischemia in rat are supported by recent findings in gerbil which showed that treatment with delayed post-ischemic hypothermia produced a very slow (months) DND in some CA1 cells and resulted in necrosis, not apoptosis [5]. Thus, while milder insults favor an apoptotic mode of cell death in liver, this is apparently not the case for CA1 neurons following global ischemia.

Supporting the lack of morphological evidence for apoptosis in CA1 was the failure of z-VAD and z-DEVD to reduce ischemic injury. However, it remains possible that other dosing regimens, such as continuous infusion, would be more efficacious. Both z-VAD and z-DEVD have been shown to reduce focal ischemic injury [10, 16, 25]. Indeed, recent experiments in our lab have confirmed a protective effect with administration of z-VAD and z-DEVD prior to transient middle cerebral artery occlusion. Given that caspase-I [interleukin converting enzyme (ICE)] inhibition would reduce inflammation and perhaps fever, the mechanism of action is not necessarily related to apoptosis.

In summary, our morphological findings indicate a necrotic mode of cell death in CA1 following either mild or severe 4-VO ischemia. Inhibition of caspase 1 and caspase 3 did not significantly attenuate CA1 injury. Thus, the elevation of caspase-1 mRNA [1] and caspase-3 mRNA [29] in CA1 following global ischemia, which should be attenuated by z-VAD and z-DEVD [16, 26], appears not to be essential for CA1 death. Our results do not support a role for programmed cell death in the CA1 zone following global ischemia.

References

1. Bhat RV, DiRocco R, Marcy VR, Flood DG, Zhu Y, Dobrzanski P, Siman R, Scott R, Contreras PC, Miller M (1996) Increased expression of IL-β converting enzyme in hippocampus after ischemia: selective localization in microglia. J Neurosci 16: 4146
2. Bonfoco E, Krainc D, Ankarcrona M, Nicotera P, Lipton SA (1995) Apoptosis and necrosis: two distinct events induced, respectively, by mild and intense insults after N-methyl-D-aspartate or nitric oxide/superoxide in cortical cell cultures. Proc Natl Acad Sci U S A 92: 7162
3. Bonnekoh P, Barbier A, Oschlies U, Hossmann K-A (1990) Selective vulnerability in the gerbil hippocampus: morphological changes after 5 min ischemia and long survival times. Acta Neuropathol (Berl) 80: 18
4. Choi DW (1996) Ischemia-induced neuronal apoptosis. Curr Opin Neurobiol 6: 667
5. Colbourne F, Sutherland GR, Auer RN (1997) New features of delayed neuronal death in gerbils treated with prolonged postischemic hypothermia. Soc Neurosci Abstr 23: 1917
6. Collins RJ, Harmon BV, Gobé GC, Kerr JFR (1992) Internucleosomal DNA cleavage should not be the sole criterion for identifying apoptosis. Int J Radiat Biol 61: 451
7. de Torres C, Munell F, Ferrer I, Reventós J, Macaya A (1997) Identification of necrotic cell death by the TUNEL assay in the hypoxic–ischemic neonatal rat brain. Neurosci Lett 230: 1
8. Deshpande J, Bergstedt K, Lindén T, Kalimo H, Wieloch T (1992) Ultrastructural changes in the hippocampal CA1 region following transient cerebral ischemia: evidence against programmed cell death. Exp Brain Res 88: 91
9. Du C, Hu R, Csernansky CA, Hsu CY, Choi DW (1996) Very delayed infarction after mild focal cerebral ischemia: a role for apoptosis? J Cereb Blood Flow Metab 16: 195
10. Endres M, Namura S, Shimizu-Sasamata M, Waeber C, Zhang L, Gómez-Isla T, Hyman BT, Moskowitz MA (1998) Attenuation of delayed neuronal death after mild focal ischemia in mice by inhibition of the caspase family. J Cereb Blood Flow Metab 18: 238
11. Ferrer I, Tortoise A, Macaya A, Sierra A, Moreno D, Munell F, Blanco R, Squier W (1994) Evidence of nuclear DNA fragmentation following hypoxia–ischemia in the infant rat brain, and transient forebrain ischemia in the adult gerbil. Brain Pathol 4: 115
12. Fukuda K, Kojiro M, Chiu J-F (1993) Demonstration of extensive chromatin cleavage in transplanted morris hepatoma 7777 tissue: apoptosis or necrosis? Am J Pathol 142: 935
13. Gold R, Schmied M, Giegerich G, Breitschopf H, Hartung HP, Toyka KV, Lassmann H (1994) Differentiation between cellular apoptosis and necrosis by the combined use of in situ tailing and nick translation techniques. Lab Invest 71: 219
14. Goto K, Ishige A, Sekiguchi K, Iizuka S, Sugimoto A, Yuzurihara M, Aburada M, Hosoya E, Kogure K (1990) Effects of cycloheximide on delayed neuronal death in rat hippocampus. Brain Res 534: 299
15. Grasl-Kraupp B, Ruttkay-Nedecky B, Koudelka H, Bukowska K, Bursch W, Schulte-Hermann R (1995) In situ detection of fragmented DNA (TUNEL assay) fails to discriminate among apoptosis, necrosis, and autolytic cell death: a cautionary note. Hepatology 21: 1465
16. Hara H, Friedlander RM, Gagliardini V, Ayata C, Fink K, Huang Z, Shimizu–Sasamata M, Yuan J, Moskowitz MA (1997) Inhibition of interleukin 1β converting enzyme family proteases reduces ischemic and excitotoxic neuronal damage. Proc Natl Acad Sci U S A 94: 2007
17. Harmon BV, Corder AM, Collins RJ, Gobe GC, Allen J, Allan DJ, Keff JF (1990) Cell death induced in a murine mastocytoma by 42 °C heating in vitro: evidence that the form of death changes from apoptosis to necrosis above a critical heat load. Int J Radiat Biol 53: 845–858
18. Heron A, Pollard H, Dessi F, Moreau J, Lasbennes F, Ben-Ari Y, Charriaut-Marlangue C (1993) Regional variability in DNA fragmentation after global ischemia evidenced by combined histological and gel electrophoresis observations in the rat brain. J Neurochem 61: 1973
19. Johnson EM Jr., Deckwerth TL (1993) Molecular mechanisms of developmental neuronal death. Ann Rev Neurosci 16: 31
20. Kerr JFR (1971) Shrinkage necrosis: a distinct mode of cellular death. J Pathol 105: 13
21. Kihara S, Shiraishi T, Nakagawa S, Toda K, Tabuchi K (1994) Visualization of DNA double strand breaks in the gerbil hippocampal CA1 following transient ischemia. Neurosci Lett 175: 133
22. Kirino T (1982) Delayed neuronal death in the gerbil hippocampus following ischemia. Brain Res 239: 57
23. Kirino T, Sano K (1984) Fine structural nature of delayed neuronal death following ischemia in the gerbil hippocampus. Acta Neuropathol (Berl) 62: 209
24. Li H, Buchan AM (1995) Progressive loss of hippocampal CA1 neurons following transient forebrain ischemia. J Cereb Blood Flow Metab 15[Suppl 1]: S246
25. Loddick SA, MacKenzie A, Rothwell NJ (1996) An ICE inhibitor, z-VAD-DCB attenuates ischaemic brain damage in the rat. Neuroreport 7: 1465

26. MacManus JP, Linnik MD (1997) Gene expression induced by cerebral ischemia: an apoptotic perspective. J Cereb Blood Flow Metab 17: 815
27. MacManus JP, Buchan AM, Hill IE, Rasquinha I, Preston E (1993) Global ischemia can cause DNA fragmentation indicative of apoptosis in rat brain. Neurosci Lett 164: 89
28. MacManus JP, Hill IE, Preston E, Rasquinha I, Walker T, Buchan AM (1995) Differences in DNA fragmentation following transient cerebral or decapitation ischemia in rats. J Cereb Blood Flow Metab 15: 728
29. Ni B, Wu X, Su Y, Stephenson D, Smalstig EB, Clemens J, Paul SM (1998) Transient global forebrain ischemia induces a prolonged expression of the caspase-3 mRNA in rat hippocampal CA1 pyramidal neurons. J Cereb Blood Flow Metab 18: 248
30. Papas S, Crépel V, Hasboun D, Jorquera I, Chinestra P, Ben-Ari Y (1992) Cyclohemimide reduces the effects of anoxic insult in vivo and in vitro. Eur J Neuro 4: 758
31. Paxinos G, and Watson C (1982) The rat brain in stereotaxic coordinates. Academic Press, New York
32. Petito CK, Feldmann E, Pulsinelli WA, Plum F (1987) Delayed hippocampal damage in humans following cardiorespiratory arrest. Neurology 37: 1281
33. Petito CK, Torres–Munoz J, Roberts B, Olarte J–P, Nowak TS, Pulsinelli WA (1997) DNA fragmentation follows delayed neuronal death in CA1 neurons exposed to transient global ischemia in the rat. J Cereb Blood Flow Metab 17: 967
34. Pulsinelli WA, Brierley JB (1979) A new model of bilateral hemispheric ischemia in the unanesthetized rat. Stroke 10: 267
35. Pulsinelli WA, Brierley JB, Plum F (1982) Temporal profile of neuronal damage in a model of transient forebrain ischemia. Ann Neurol 11: 491–
36. Pulsinelli WA, Buchan AM (1988) The four–vessel occlusion rat model:method for complete occlusion of vertebral arteries and control of collateral circulation. Stroke 19: 913
37. Sei Y, Von Lubitz KJ, Basile AS, Borner MM, Lin RC, Skolnick P, Fossom LH (1994) Internucleosomal DNA fragmentation in gerbil hippocampus following forebrain ischemia. Neurosci Lett 171: 179
38. Shigeno T, Yamasaki Y, Kato G, Kusaka K, Mima T, Takakura K, Graham DI, Furukawa S (1990) Reduction of delayed neuronal death by inhibition of protein synthesis. Neurosci Lett 120: 117
39. Tomimoto H, Yamamoto K, Homburger HA, Yanagihara T (1993) Immunoelectron microscopic investigation of creatine kinase BB-isoenzyme after cerebral ischemia. Acta Neuropathol 86: 447
40. Tortosa A, Rivera R, Ferrer I (1994) Dose-related effects of cycloheximide on delayed neuronal death in the gerbil hippocampus after bilateral transitory forebrain ischemia. J Neurol Sci 121: 10
41. Wyllie AH, Kerr JFR, Currie AR (1980) Cell death: the significance of apoptosis. Int Rev Cytol 68: 251
42. Yamamoto K, Hayakawa T, Mogami H, Akai F, Yanagihara T (1990) Ultrastructural investigation of the CA1 region of the hippocampus after transient cerebral ischemia in gerbils. Acta Neuropathol (Berl) 80: 487

II Factors and Mechanisms Enhancing Susceptibility or Tolerance (Growth Factors)

Stimulation of β_2-Adrenoceptors Induces Nerve Growth Factor and Inhibits Apoptosis in Rat Brain After Ischemia

J. Krieglstein, C. Culmsee, Y. Zhu, and I. Semkova

Summary. Stimulation of β_2-adrenoceptors in primary mixed cultures of rat hippocampal cells clearly protects neurons against glutamate-induced damage by an increased expression of nerve growth factor (NGF), since the neuroprotective effect of clenbuterol, a β_2-adrenergic drug, was abolished, or at least reduced, by a β-blocker, NGF antibodies, p75 antibodies and NGF antisense oligodeoxynucleotide (ODN). Clenbuterol also reduced the infarct volume after occlusion of the middle cerebral artery in the rat and it decreased the number of damaged neurons after 10 min forebrain ischemia in the CA1 subfield of the rat. Simultaneously, the synthesis of NGF, as well as the synthesis of basic fibroblast growth factor (bFGF) and transforming growth factor-beta 1 (TGF-β1), was upregulated in various regions of the brain. In the rat model of global forebrain ischemia, DNA fragmentation and terminal deoxynucleotidyl transferase-mediated dUTP nick-end labeling(TUNEL)-positive cells were diminished by clenbuterol, suggesting an anti-apoptotic potency of this drug. In addition, we could demonstrate an upregulation of the anti-apoptotic oncogenes Bcl-2 and Bcl-xl caused by clenbuterol, an effect, which could also contribute to the neuroprotection caused by stimulation of β_2-adrenoceptors.

Introduction

Evidence has been provided that neurotrophic factors can protect neurons from acute injury due to brain ischemia or trauma [16]. Particularly, the nerve growth factor (NGF) has been shown to exert neuroprotective properties in the hippocampus and cortex [3, 26, 35], regions which are highly vulnerable to cerebral ischemia. Therefore, administering neurotrophic factors could represent a promising strategy for the treatment of both acute and chronic brain disorders. However, the therapeutic application of these compounds seems to be complicated because of their chemical properties. Neurotrophic factors are large protein molecules that cannot easily pass the blood–brain barrier and do not distribute properly after systemic administration. One approach to enhance the amounts of neurotrophic factors available to neurons is to stimulate their endogenous synthesis in affected brain regions by lipophilic drugs.

Stimulation of β-Adrenoceptors Causes NGF Synthesis and Neuroprotection

β-Adrenoceptor activation has been shown to stimulate endogenous NGF synthesis in cultured glial cells as well as in brain tissue in vivo [6, 9, 10]. The stimulation of these receptors has been shown to modulate a wide range of astrocyte functions, including

Maturation Phenomenon in Cerebral Ischemia III
U. Ito et al. (Eds.)
© Springer-Verlag Berlin Heidelberg 1999

expression of early-response genes [1], alteration in glial-cell morphology [13], and the synthesis and release of cytokines [20] and neurotrophic substances such as NGF [31]. We have found that the stimulation of β-adrenoceptors with clenbuterol, a lipophilic β$_2$-adrenoceptor agonist, increased NGF gene expression in primary cultures of rat cortical astrocytes [32]. The effect seemed to be mediated via activation of β-adrenergic receptors on astrocytes and subsequent elevation of the intracellular cyclic adenosine monophosphate (cAMP) level, since it was completely blocked by propranolol. Furthermore, isoproterenol, forskolin, and lipophilic cAMP derivatives were also able to induce NGF synthesis under our experimental conditions.

Therefore, we tried to find out whether clenbuterol could protect cultured hippocampal neurons from excitotoxic damage by stimulation of NGF synthesis. First, however, we wanted to see whether NGF itself could protect hippocampal neurons against damage and we found neuroprotection caused by NGF at concentrations ranging between 0.15 ng/ml and 10 ng/ml added to the culture medium 4 h before and left in contact with the cells up to 18 h after the induction of damage [33, 34]. Our results are in agreement with the previously reported neuroprotective activity of NGF in cultured hippocampal neurons against damage caused by hypoglycemia, excitotoxicity and iron [5, 22, 45]. In vivo, NGF has also been shown to rescue hippocampal neurons from ischemic insult [3, 26, 35, 43]. However, the exact mechanism by which NGF protected hippocampal neurons against excitotoxic injury is not clear, since these neurons do not express TrkA, the high-affinity receptor for NGF [14]. However, the expression of p75, the low-affinity NGF receptor, has been demonstrated in the hippocampal formation after transient ischemia [17] or environmental damage [44]. Increasing data indicate that p75 is linked to the ceramide signal-transducing pathway, resulting in activation of the transcriptional factor nuclear factor kappa B (NFϰB), and increased the activity of antioxidant enzymes, such as manganese superoxide dismutase [4, 41]. Therefore, the activation of this signal-transduction pathway may trigger neuroprotective stimuli.

In line with this hypothesis, we found that monoclonal antibody directed against p75 (10 ng/ml) completely abolished the neuroprotective activity of NGF (1 ng/ml). Moreover, the inhibition of NFϰB with pyrrolidinedithiocarbamate (PDTC), known as an inhibitor of NFϰB, blocked the protective effect of NGF under our experimental conditions. Therefore, we suggest that activation of NFϰB through the p75-receptor pathway mediates the neuroprotective activity of NGF. In addition, agents capable of activating NFϰB, such as C2-ceramide, mimicked the rescuing effect of NGF in hippocampal cultures. Our results are in agreement with previously reported excitoprotective and antioxidant actions of NGF and tumor necrosis factor (TNF), mediated via activation of p75 and NFϰB [4, 23, 38].

The next step was to investigate the potency of clenbuterol to induce NGF synthesis in hippocampal cultures. We found that clenbuterol significantly enhanced the content of NGF protein secreted into the culture medium (33.3±3.4 pg/ml in the control cultures vs 147±20.6 pg/ml in clenbuterol-treated cultures) [33, 34]. Furthermore, we attempted to determine whether clenbuterol could protect hippocampal neurons against glutamate-induced damage by increasing NGF synthesis. We were able to demonstrate that this drug (1–100 μM) significantly reduced the number of damaged neurons and preserved cell morphology, similar to NGF. The neuroprotective activity of clenbuterol was shown at the same concentration range that increased the NGF content in the culture medium, suggesting a relationship between NGF induction and neuroprotection. In addition, the neuroprotective activity of clenbuterol was completely blocked by co-administration of monoclonal anti-NGF antibody, demonstrating that the neuroprotective effect was mediated by NGF.

NGF Antisense Oligonucleotide

We attempted to find out whether the neuroprotective effect of clenbuterol against glutamate-induced excitotoxicity could be blocked by antisense-mediated NGF knock down. To this end, we used a NGF antisense oligodeoxynucleotide (ODN) complementary to the binding site between the intron and exon 3 of the NGF pre-messenger ribonucleic acid (mRNA) versus a random control ODN, which had no complementarity with the NGF mRNA, but the same base composition as the antisense ODN. The ODNs were diluted in culture medium to final concentrations of 0.3–1 µM in primary astrocyte cultures and 1 µM in mixed hippocampal cultures. The ODNs were repeatedly added with the medium exchange every 24 h for 3 days in astrocytes and 30 h before NGF-protein measurement in hippocampal cells, respectively. The NGF-protein content of the medium was determined by means of enzyme-linked immunosorbent assay (ELISA).

Preincubation of primary cortical astrocytes with phosphothioated NGF antisense ODN (0.3–1 µM) for 3 days reduced the concentration of NGF in the culture medium concentration dependently. The most pronounced effect was observed at a concentration of 1 µM antisense, which reduced the NGF concentration to 20 % of control levels. The viability of astrocytes was not affected by exposure to the different concentration of NGF antisense ODN. NGF antisense ODN (1 µM, 30 h) also reduced the NGF content in the medium of hippocampal cultures to 55 % ($P<0.05$) of control sister cultures treated with vehicle or random ODN. The random ODN did not influence the concentration of NGF in the culture medium compared with controls. Neither the antisense nor the random ODN affected the neuronal viability in mixed hippocampal cells.

Primary mixed hippocampal cultures were preincubated with 1 µM NGF antisense ODN 30 h before exposure to glutamate (0.5 mM, 1 h) to investigate the effect of the suppression of NGF-protein synthesis on the neuroprotective effect of clenbuterol (10 µM) in vitro. Excitotoxic injury was induced in rat hippocampal neurons after 14 days in vitro. The cultures were exposed to serum-free medium containing 0.5 mM L-glutamate for 1 h. The glutamate-containing medium was replaced with serum-free medium for 18 h. Control sister cultures not exposed to L-glutamate were also cultured with serum-free medium. The percentage of damaged neurons was determined 18 h later by trypan-blue exclusion.

Approximately 40 % of neurons lost their membrane integrity and became stained with trypan blue. The neuronal damage observed 18 h after glutamate exposure was not affected by incubation with NGF antisense ODN or random ODN (1 µM, 30 h each). In contrast, the neuroprotective effect of clenbuterol pretreatment (10 µM, 6 h) was only found to be affected by the NGF antisense ODN. Clenbuterol significantly reduced the percentage of damaged neurons to 17 % (p < 0.01) evaluated 18 h after exposure to glutamate in the cultures preincubated with random ODN. This neuro-

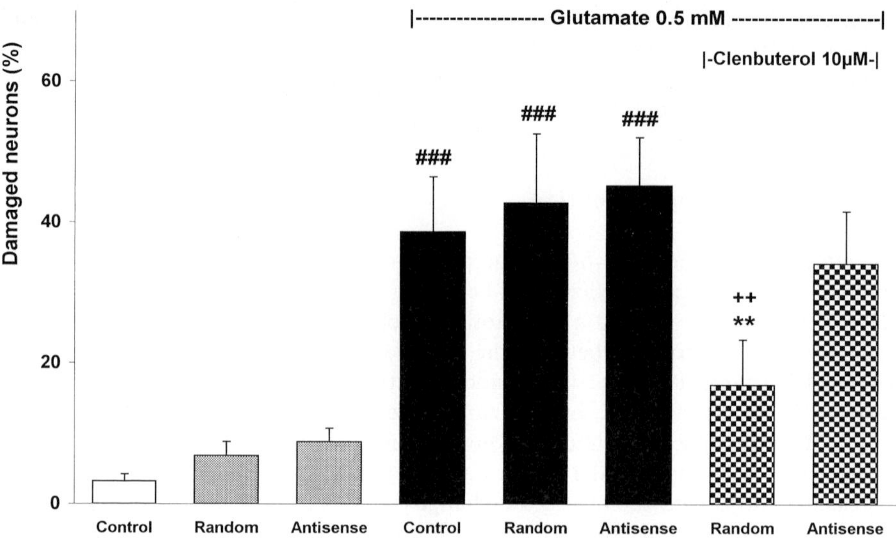

Fig. 1. Nerve growth factor (NGF)-antisense oligonucleotide (ODN) suppresses neuroprotective effect of clenbuterol in mixed hippocampal cultures. Mixed hippocampal cultures from neonatal rats (*P1*) were treated with 1 µM NGF-antisense ODN for 30 h before and for up to 18 h after 1 h of 0.5 mM L-glutamate exposure. Clenbuterol (10 µM) was added to the cultures 6 h before glutamate exposure. Control cultures received vehicle (control), antisense and random ODN respectively. Different from vehicle control ### $P<0.001$; different from glutamate-exposed controls **$P<0.01$; different from clenbuterol- and glutamate-treated antisense group ++$P<0.01$ by Scheffé's test

protective effect was blocked by NGF antisense ODN (Fig. 1; percentage of damaged neurons: 35 %, p < 0.01).

As reported previously, the β_2-adrenergic drug clenbuterol has been shown to increase NGF synthesis in mixed hippocampal cultures [33, 34]. Investigating the effect of NGF antisense ODN in the present study, we could confirm the neuroprotective effect of clenbuterol against glutamate-induced damage of cultured hippocampal neurons. The suppression of NGF synthesis by pretreatment with a newly designed NGF antisense ODN abolished the protective activity of clenbuterol, suggesting that NGF mediates the neuroprotective effect.

The stimulation of β_2-adrenergic receptors in vivo leads to an induction of growth factor synthesis in the brain tissue, similar to that discussed for the in vitro experiments [9, 10, 33, 34]. There is evidence from our work that drugs that increase the content of NGF in the CNS sufficiently, also reduce the damage of brain tissue after cerebral ischemia [33, 34]. However, it remains to be clarified whether NGF is the only, or at least the main, mediator of the neuroprotective activity of clenbuterol in vivo. To further investigate this issue, the specific inhibition of either NGF expression or NGF activity in the central nervous system (CNS) regions of interest would be necessary.

Rat Model of Focal Cerebral Ischemia: Induction of Growth Factors and Neuroprotection

Based on our in vitro studies, we attempted to find out whether the induction of NGF or other growth factors were involved in the protective effects of clenbuterol against ischemic brain damage in vivo. Furthermore, we examined the effect of clenbuterol on the activation of astrocytes after the ischemic brain lesion. Clenbuterol (0.001–0.1 mg/kg) was administered intraperitoneally 3 h before permanent MCA occlusion in male Long-Evans rats. The brains were removed for histological evaluation of the infarct volume 7 days after ischemia. The changes in the mRNA levels of NGF, basic fibroblast growth factor (bFGF) and transforming growth factor beta 1 (TGF-β_1) induced by clenbuterol (0.1 mg/kg) in cortical and hippocampal tissue were determined by reverse-transcription polymerase chain reaction (RT-PCR) up to 9 h after the induction of permanent focal cerebral ischemia. At 6 h after ischemia, in situ hybridization was performed to analyze the effects of clenbuterol (0.1 mg/kg) on NGF and glial fibrillary acidic protein (GFAP) expression.

Clenbuterol (0.01 mg/kg and 0.1 mg/kg) reduced the cortical infarct volume in a dose-dependent manner to 82 % ($P<0.01$) and 59 % ($P<0.001$) of control values [33, 34]. At 9 h after ischemia, an increase in NGF mRNA in cortex and hippocampus was measured by means of RT-PCR. However, this increase in NGF mRNA occurred earlier, i.e., at 3–6 h after ischemia, and was more pronounced in animals treated with clenbuterol. After 6 h of ischemia, in situ hybridization revealed an increase in NGF mRNA by clenbuterol to 180 % ($P<0.05$) in the cortical penumbra, to 170 % ($P<0.05$) in the contralateral cortex, and to 300 % ($P<0.001$) in the CA1 region of the hippocampus. A similar time course of upregulation of bFGF mRNA after ischemia was observed in the cortex and hippocampus. Again, clenbuterol-treated animals showed an enhanced expression of bFGF mRNA compared with controls as early as 3–6 h after ischemia. These results are in line with previous observations showing an upregulation of NGF and bFGF mRNA by 10 mg/kg clenbuterol under physiological conditions [9, 10, 33, 34].

In contrast to the cerebroprotective doses (0.01–0.1 mg/kg) used in the present study, 10 mg/kg clenbuterol did not reduce the infarct volume after focal cerebral ischemia due to side effects, such as an increase in blood glucose and a decrease of mean arterial blood pressure [33, 34].

Furthermore, TGF-β_1 mRNA was found to be enhanced in hippocampal tissue 3 h after clenbuterol treatment. This early mRNA induction, in particular, suggests that TGF-β_1 could also contribute to the protective effect of clenbuterol against brain damage [33, 34, 46]. Although the role of endogenous TGF-β_1 expression after ischemic lesions of brain tissue is still unclear, there is growing evidence for neuroprotective activities of this cytokine [15]. It has been shown previously that TGF-β_1 protects cultured neurons against excitotoxic damage induced by glutamate agonists and also against staurosporine-induced apoptosis [11, 27, 28]. Interestingly, TGF-β_1 significantly reduced the amount of neuronal damage in the CA1 subfield of the hippocampus after 10 min of global cerebral ischemia at relatively low concentrations, compared with neuroprotective doses of other growth factors investigated in similar models. NGF, for example, ameliorated neuronal degeneration after transient global cerebral ischemia in gerbils at a dose of 150 µg/kg [35], while TGF-β_1 was effective at doses 10,000 times less, i.e., at 15 ng/kg after transient global ischemia in the rat [11].

It has been suggested that neurons are the source of enhanced NGF synthesis after stimulation of β-adrenoceptors by clenbuterol [9]. This might be true under physiological conditions. However, the situation is totally different in lesioned brain tissue as, for example, after ischemia when astrocytes and microglial cells are activated and their pattern of cytokine expression has changed. Astrocytes have been widely discussed as a possible source of neuroprotective factors that support neuronal survival under lesioning conditions [18, 21, 25, 29]. It has been suggested that specific manipulation of cytokine expression in glial cells by so-called astrocyte-kinetic drugs could become a new therapeutic strategy for neurodegenerative diseases [2, 13, 18]. Astrocytes in culture, as well as in various regions of the mammalian CNS, have been shown to express β_2-adrenergic receptors [21, 30, 37]. Furthermore, there is evidence that expression of β-receptors increased in astrocytes in response to CNS injury or disease [13]. In line with these findings, in situ hybridization revealed an enhanced expression of GFAP mRNA in clenbuterol-treated animals compared with controls at 6 h after focal cerebral ischemia, indicating an activation of astrocytes by the β-mimetic drug.

Rat Model of Global Cerebral Ischemia: Anti-Apoptotic Effect of Clenbuterol

We further investigated whether clenbuterol was able to prevent neuronal apoptosis induced in a rat model of global ischemia. Global ischemia was induced in male Wistar rats for 10 min by clamping both common carotid arteries and reducing the mean arterial blood pressure to 40 mmHg. Clenbuterol was administered 3 h before ischemia (0.1 mg/kg, 0.5 mg/kg and 1.0 mg/kg, i.p.) or immediately after ischemia (0.5 mg/kg, i.p.). The brains were removed 7 days after ischemia for histological evaluation. The neuronal damage in CA1 subfield was unaffected by 0.1 mg/kg clenbuterol. Both 0.5 mg/kg and 1.0 mg/kg clenbuterol pretreatment resulted in a reduced neuronal loss. The immediate injection of 0.5 mg/kg clenbuterol after ischemia (posttreatment) showed a similar neuroprotective effect ($P<0.05$).

Apoptosis is described by the morphological changes of dying cells, including cell shrinkage, nuclear and plasma membrane blebbing, chromatin condensation and the formation of apoptotic bodies. The accumulation of intracellular free calcium after global ischemia [7, 8] has been suggested to activate the Ca^{2+}/Mg^{2+}-dependent endonucleases, resulting first in the fragmentation of the DNA into 180–300 Kbp and, subsequently, into oligonucleosomal cleavage products, which appear as a DNA ladder in electrophoresis [36, 39]. Therefore, DNA laddering is considered as a biochemical hallmark of apoptosis [12, 19]. To evaluate the anti-apoptotic effect of clenbuterol, gel electrophoresis and terminal deoxynucleotidyl transferase (TdT)-mediated dUTP nick- end labeling (TUNEL) staining were used to measure DNA laddering and to detect DNA fragmentation in situ, respectively, 3 days after global ischemia.

The DNA in the hippocampus, striatum and occipital cortex was individually extracted from ischemic, untreated animals and ischemic, clenbuterol-treated animals (0.5 mg/kg, i.p., 3 h before ischemia). The extracted total DNA underwent electrophoresis in a 2 % agarose gel, containing ethidium bromide, for 3 h. The effect of

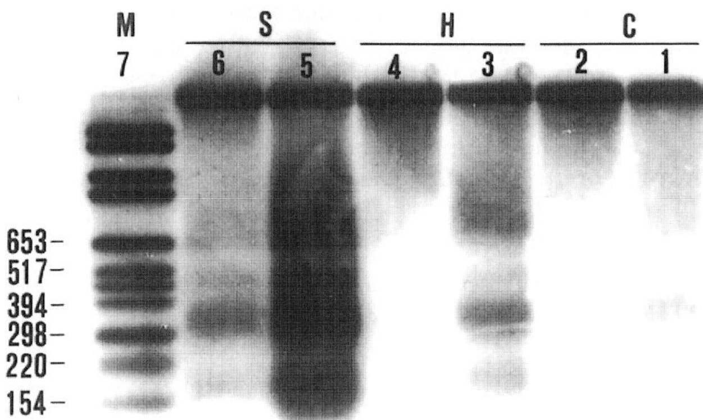

Fig. 2. Clenbuterol prevents deoxyribonucleic acid (DNA) fragmentation in hippocampus (*H*), striatum (*S*) and cortex (*C*) after 10 min transient forebrain ischemia in the rat. Clenbuterol (0.5 mg/kg) was intraperitoneally administered 3 h before ischemia. Brains were removed 3 days after ischemia and DNA was extracted from hippocampus, striatum and cortex, respectively. Control group received saline only. *Lane 7* digoxigenin-labeled marker; *lanes 2, 4 and 6* clenbuterol-treated ischemic animals; *lanes 1, 3 and 5* untreated, ischemic animals

clenbuterol against DNA degradation is shown in Fig. 2. The typical DNA ladders of approximately 180 bp and its multiples were observed in the control group, as shown in Fig. 2, lanes 1, 3, and 5. In the hippocampus, the DNA fragmentation was nearly abolished after the treatment with clenbuterol (Fig. 2, lane 4). Clenbuterol partially blocked the DNA fragmentation in the occipital cortex and striatum (Fig. 2, lane 2 and lane 6).

To confirm the results obtained from gel electrophoresis, the rats were treated in another series of experiments with either saline or clenbuterol (0.5 mg/kg, i.p.) 3 h prior to ischemia, and the brains were removed 3 days after ischemia. Coronal paraffin sections (0.5 mm) were cut from the hippocampus, striatum and occipital cortex (–3.6 mm, –1.00 mm and –6.30 mm to bregma, respectively) for the evaluation of cellular DNA fragmentation in situ. TUNEL was performed using the ApopTag Kit. In the control group, which was subjected to 10 min global ischemia followed by 3 days of recovery, there were extensive positively stained neurons localized in the CA1 subfield of the hippocampus and in the striatum. In comparison, the number of positively stained neurons in the clenbuterol-treated group was smaller than in the corresponding region of the controls and the intensity of staining was much weaker than in the control group.

These results indicate that clenbuterol can efficiently antagonize apoptosis in all three brain regions after global ischemia. We further attempted to find out whether clenbuterol could elevate the NGF-protein content in the brain subjected to transient forebrain ischemia and whether induction of NGF synthesis by clenbuterol is associated with its anti-apoptotic effect in a rat model of global ischemia.

The two-site NGF ELISA was used for measuring NGF protein in the hippocampus, cortex and striatum 3 days after the onset of global ischemia. One series of rats was treated with clenbuterol (0.5 mg/kg, i.p.) 3 h prior to ischemia and the brains were removed 6 h or 3 days after ischemia. A second series of rats received clenbuterol (0.5 mg/kg, i.p.) 3 h before ischemia and a daily injection for 3 days after ischemia. Clenbuterol (0.5 mg/kg) injected 3 h before global ischemia elevated the NGF protein by 33.1 % ($P<0.05$) in the hippocampus and 44.4 % ($P<0.05$) in the cortex, compared with the control group when measured 6 h after ischemia. However, no significant increase in the NGF level was found in the striatum. The NGF levels in both clenbuterol-treated groups (0.5 mg/kg and 0.5 mg/kg·4) were not different from controls 3 days after ischemia. These results indicate that the NGF synthesis increased by clenbuterol during the first hours after ischemia might be important for the prevention of DNA degradation and neuronal survival. NGF induction may be involved in the anti-apoptotic effect of clenbuterol, at least in the hippocampus and cortex. However, an increase in NGF expression induced by clenbuterol was not seen in the striatum. We argued, therefore, that other mechanisms might be involved in the anti-apoptotic effect of clenbuterol.

Apoptosis is an active suicide process of the cell, requiring the activation of the genetic programs. Recently, several families of molecules that regulate apoptosis have been identified [40, 42]. The Bcl-2 family of genes is one of the best characterized [24]. Some family members, including Bcl-2 and Bcl-xl, inhibit apoptosis, whereas other members, such as Bax, Bcl-xs and Bak, promote apoptosis. Cell death or survival can be regulated by the balance between the levels of pro- and anti-apoptotic members of the Bcl-2 family. We tried to demonstrate that the apoptosis-associated genes, including Bcl-2, Bcl-xl and Bax, could be induced after global ischemia and, furthermore, whether expression of these genes could be influenced by clenbuterol. To address this issue, Western blotting was performed to measure these proteins in ischemic, untreated animals and ischemic, clenbuterol-treated-animals (0.5 mg/kg, i.p., 3 h before ischemia).

The expression of these oncogenes was upregulated in the hippocampus and striatum after 10 min of global ischemia. In the hippocampus, the upregulation of Bcl-2 was found at 24 h, while the increase in Bax and Bcl-xl expression appeared as early as 6 h and 24 h after the onset of ischemia. In the striatum, only a slight increase in Bcl-2 and Bcl-xl expression was found at 6 h and 24 h after ischemia, whereas Bax signals were markedly enhanced. Clenbuterol further increased the expression of Bcl-2 in the hippocampus and the striatum at 6 h and 24 h after ischemia. In contrast, Bax-protein levels were downregulated by clenbuterol at 6 h and 24 h after ischemia. Clenbuterol also upregulated the expression of Bcl-xl in the striatum at 6 h and 24 h, but the effect of clenbuterol on the Bcl-xl in the ischemic hippocampus varied among the different tested animals. These results suggest that transient global ischemia induces oncogenes and, therefore, we assume that genetic programs, which mediate apoptotic cell death, are activated after ischemia. Clenbuterol did not only increase Bcl-2 expression, but also downregulated Bax expression in the ischemic hippocampus and the striatum; this may contribute to its anti-apoptotic effect. The mechanism of action of clenbuterol regulating oncogene-protein expression is still unknown.

References

1. Arenander AT, De Vellis J, Herschman HR (1989) Induction of c-fos and TIS genes in cultured astrocytes by neurotransmitters. J Neurosci Res 24: 107–114
2. Biagini G, Frasoldati A, Fuxe K, Agnati LF (1994) The concept of astrocyte-kinetic drugs in the treatment of neurodegenerative diseases: evidence for 1-deprenyl-induced activation of reactive astrocytes. Neurochem Int 25: 17–22
3. Buchan AM, Williams L, Bruederlin B (1990) Nerve growth factor: pretreatment ameliorates ischemic hippocampal neuronal injury. Stroke 21: 177
4. Carter BD, Kaltschmidt C, Kaltschmidt B, Offenhäuser N, Böhm-Matthaei R, Baeuerle PA, Barde Y-A (1996) Selective activation of NFϰB by nerve growth factor through the neurotrophin receptor p75. Science 272: 542–545
5. Cheng B, Mattson MP (1991) NGF and bFGF protect rat hippocampal and human cortical neurons against hypoglycemic damage by stabilizing calcium homeostasis. Neuron 7: 1031–1041
6. Dal Toso R, De Bernardi MA, Brooker G, Costa E, Mocchetti I (1988) Beta-adrenergic and prostaglandine receptor activation increases nerve growth factor mRNA content in C6-2B rat astrocytoma cells. J Pharmacol Exp Ther 246: 1190–1193
7. Deshpande JK, Siesjö BK, Wieloch T (1987) Calcium accumulation and neuronal damage in the rat hippocampus following cerebral ischemia. J Cereb Blood Flow Metab 7: 89–95
8. Dux E, Mies G, Hossmann K-A, Siklos L (1987) Calcium in the mitochondria following brief ischemia of gerbil brain. Neurosci Lett 78: 295–300
9. Follesa P, Mocchetti I (1993) Regulation of basic fibroblast growth factor and nerve growth factor mRNA by β-adrenergic receptor activation and adrenal steroids in rat central nervous system. Mol Pharmacol 43: 132–138
10. Hayes VY, Isackson PJ, Fabrazzo M, Follesa P, Mocchetti I (1995) Induction of nerve growth factor and basic fibroblast growth factor mRNA following clenbuterol: contrasting anatomical and cellular localization. Exp Neurol 132: 33–41
11. Henrich-Noack P, Prehn JHM, Krieglstein J (1996) TGF-β₁ protects hippocampal neurons against degeneration caused by transient global ischemia: dose-response relationship and potential neuroprotective mechanism. Stroke 27: 1609–1615
12. Heron A, Pollard H, Dessi F, Moreau J, Labennes F, Ben-Ari Y, Charriaut-Marlangue C (1993) Regional variability in DNA fragmentation after global ischemia evidenced by combined histological and gel electrophoresis observations in the rat brain. J Neurochem 61: 1973–1976
13. Hodges-Savola C, Rogers SD, Ghilardi JR, Timm DR, Mantyh P (1996) β-adrenergic receptors regulate astrogliosis and cell proliferation in the central nervous system in vivo. Glia 17: 52–62
14. Ip NY, Li Y, Yancopoulos GD, Lindsay RM (1993) Cultured hippocampal neurons show responses to BDNF, NT-3, and NT-4, but not NGF. J Neurosci 13: 3394–3405
15. Krieglstein K, Krieglstein J (1998) TGF-β signaling and neuroprotection: relevance to ischemic brain injury, Alzheimer's and Parkinson's disease. In: Mattson MP (ed) Neuroprotective signal transduction. Humana Press, Totowa, pp 119–144
16. Krieglstein J, Oberpichler-Schwenk H, Prehn JHM (1998) Alternative approaches to the pharmacotherapy of ischemia. In: Ginsberg M, Bogousslavsky J (eds) Cerebrovascular disease: pathophysiology, diagnosis and management. Blackwell Science, Cambridge MA, pp 733–757
17. Lee T-H, Abe K, Kogure K, Itoyama Y (1995) Expressions of nerve growth factor and p75 low affinity receptor after transient forebrain ischemia in gerbil hippocampal CA1 neurons. J Neurosci Res 41: 684–695
18. Lu B, Yokoyama M, Dreyfus CF, Black IB (1991) NGF-gene expression in actively growing brain glia. J Neurosci 11: 318–326
19. MacManus JP, Hill IE, Preston E, Rasquinha I, Walker T, Buchan AM (1995) Differences in DNA fragmentation following transient cerebral or decapitation ischemia in rats. J Cereb Blood Flow Metab 15: 728–737
20. Maimone D, Cioni C, Rosa S, Macchia G, Aloisi F, Annunziata P (1993) Norepinephrine and vasoactive intestinal peptide induce IL-6 secretion by astrocytes: synergism with IL-1β and TNF. J Neuroimmunol 47: 73–82
21. Mantyh PW, Rogers SD, Allen CJ, Catton MD, Ghilard JR, Levin LA, Maggio JE, Vigna SR (1995) β₂-Adrenergic receptors are expressed by glia in vivo in the normal and injured central nervous system in the rat, rabbit, and human. J Neurosci 15: 152–164
22. Mattson MP, Lovell MA, Furukawa K, Markesbery WR (1995) Neurotrophic factors attenuate glutamate-induced accumulation of peroxides, elevation of intracellular Ca^{2+} concentration, and neurotoxicity and increase antioxidant enzyme activities in hippocampal neurons. J Neurochem 65: 1740–1751

23. Mattson MP, Goodman Y, Luo H, Fu W, Furukawa K (1997) Activation of NFϰB protects hippocampal neurons against oxidative stress-induced apoptosis: evidence for induction of manganese superoxide dismutase and suppression of peroxynitrate production and protein tyrosine nitration. J Neurosci Res 49: 681–697

24. Merry DE, Korsmeyer SJ (1997) Bcl-2 gene family in the nervous system. Ann Rev Neurosci 20: 245–267

25. Nieto-Sampedro M, Lewis ER, Cotman CW, Manthorpe M, Skaper SD, Barbin G, Longo FM, Varon S (1982) Brain injury causes a time-dependent increase in neuronotrophic activity at the lesion site. Science 217: 860–861

26. Pechan TA, Yoshida T, Panahian N, Moskowitz MA, Breakefield XO (1995) Genetically modified fibroblasts producing NGF protect hippocampal neurons after ischemia in the rat. Neuroreport 6: 669–672

27. Prehn JHM, Peruche B, Unsicker K, Krieglstein J (1993) Isoform-specific effects of transforming growth factors-β on degeneration of primary neuronal cultures induced by cytotoxic hypoxia or glutamate. J Neurochem 60: 1665–1672

28. Prehn JHM, Bindokas VP, Marcuccilli CJ, Krajewski S, Reed JC, Miller RJ (1995) Regulation of neuronal bcl-2 protein expression and calcium homeostasis by transforming growth factor β_1 confers wide ranging protection on rat hippocampal neurons. Proc Natl Acad Sci U S A 91: 12599–12603

29. Rudge RS (1993) Astrocyte-derived neurotrophic factors. In: Murphy S (ed), Astrocytes: pharmacology and function. Academic Press, New York, pp 267–305

30. Salm AK, McCarthy LD (1989) Expression of β-adrenergic receptors by astrocytes isolated from adult rat cortex. Glia 2: 346–352

31. Schwartz JP, Mishler K (1990) Beta-adrenergic receptor regulation, through cyclic AMP, of nerve growth factor expression in rat cortical and cerebellar astrocytes. Cell Mol Neurobiol 10: 447–457

32. Semkova I, Krieglstein J (1995) Induction of NGF in rat cortical astrocytes by isoproterenol, clenbuterol and selegiline (abstract). J Cereb Blood Flow Metab 15[Suppl 1]:573

33. Semkova I, Culmsee C, Krieglstein J (1996a) Neuroprotection caused by NGF and NGF-inducing drugs. In: Krieglstein J (ed) Pharmacology of Cerebral Ischemia 1996. Medpharm Scientific Publishers, Stuttgart, pp 477–493

34. Semkova I, Schilling M, Henrich-Noack P, Rami A, Krieglstein J (1996b) Clenbuterol protects mouse cerebral cortex and rat hippocampus from ischemic damage and attenuates glutamate neurotoxicity in cultured hippocampal neurons by induction of NGF. Brain Res 717: 44–54

35. Shigeno T, Mima T, Takaura K, Graham DI, Kato G, Hashimoto Y, Furukawa S (1991) Amelioration of delayed neuronal death in the hippocampus by nerve growth factor. J Neurosci 11: 2914–2919

36. Siesjö BK, Katsura K-I, Zhao Q, Folbergrová J, Pahlmark E, Siesjö P, Smith M-L (1995) Mechanisms of secondary brain damage in global and focal ischemia: a speculative synthesis. J Neurotrauma 12: 943–955

37. Sutin J, Shao Y (1992) Resting and reactive astrocytes express adrenergic receptors in the adult rat brain. Brain Res Bull 29: 277–284

38. Taglialatela G, Robinson R, Perez-Polo R (1997) Inhibition of nuclear factor kappa B (NFϰB), activity induces nerve growth factor-resistant apoptosis in PC12 cells. J Neurosci Res 47: 155–162

39. Tominaga T, Kure S, Narisawa K, Yoshimito T (1993) Endonuclease activities following focal ischemic injury in the rat brain. Brain Res 608: 21–26

40. White E (1996) Life, death, and the pursuit of apoptosis. Genes Dev 10: 1–15

41. Wiegmann K, Schutze S, Machleidt T, Witte D, Kronke M (1994) Functional dichotomy of neutral and acidic sphingomyelinases in tumor necrosis factor signaling. Cell 78: 1005–1015

42. Yakovlev AG, Faden AI (1995) Molecular strategies in CNS injury. J Neurotrauma 12: 767–777

43. Yamamoto S, Yoshimine T, Fujita T, Kuroda R, Irie T, Fujioka K, Hayakawa T (1992) Protective effect of NGF atelocollagen mini-pellet on the hippocampal delayed neuronal death in gerbils. Neurosci Lett 141: 161–162

44. Yankner BA, Caceres A, Duffy LK (1990) Nerve growth factor potentiates the neurotoxicity of beta amyloid. Proc Natl Acad Sci U S A 87: 9020–9023

45. Zhang Y, Tatsuno T, Carney JM, Mattson MP (1993) Basic FGF, NGF, and IGFs protect hippocampal and cortical neurons against iron-induced degeneration. J Cereb Blood Flow Metab 13: 378–388

46. Zhu Y, Culmsee C, Semkova I, Krieglstein J (1998) Stimulation of β_2-adrenoceptors inhibits apoptosis in rat brain after transient forebrain ischemia. J Cereb Blood Flow Metab 18: 1032–1039

Ischemia-Induced Dynamic Cellular Response in the Brain

M. Matsumoto, K. Kitagawa, M. Hori, and T. Yanagihara

Summary. To clarify the molecular mechanisms underlying the complex and dynamic cellular responses in the ischemic brain, it seems quite important to establish reproducible brain ischemia models in mice, which are often bred as transgenic or knock-out animals to identify the physiological or pathophysiological roles of specific candidate genes. In the present study, first, we developed a prediction method for selecting mice that lack functional anastomosis between the carotid and vertebrobasilar circulations. This method involves observing the relationship between the patency of the posterior communicating artery and the decrease of cortical microperfusion, as measured by means of laser Doppler flowmetry during a 1-min occlusion of both common carotid arteries. Using this prediction method, we could establish reproducible brain ischemia models in mice, whether produced by bilateral carotid occlusion or by intraluminal suture occlusion. Second, we investigated the role of Bcl-2 family proteins, which have multiple functions, including maintenance of mitochondrial homeostasis. Using both focal and global ischemia models in mice, our results suggest important roles of Bcl-2 family proteins in apoptosis-like neuronal cell death induced by transient ischemia. Third, using intercellular adhesion molecule-1 (ICAM-1) knock-out mice with prediction as a model for permanent or transient focal ischemia, we have documented a pivotal role of inflammatory responses, including expression of adhesion molecules such as ICAM-1 in the microcirculatory disturbances that follow brain ischemia. Through the establishment and adequate application of reproducible brain ischemia models in mice, the present investigation strongly suggested crucial roles of ischemia-induced dynamic cellular responses, including alteration of Bcl-2 family proteins in neuronal cells and ICAM-1 expression in the microcirculatory system, in the pathophysiology of ischemic stroke.

Introduction

Since the first documentation of heat-shock-protein (HSP) induction following transient cerebral ischemia [21], much experimental evidence has suggested that all of the cellular elements in the central nervous system show dynamic stress responses, depending on the degree of environmental change induced by ischemia and reperfusion. Using rodent models of transient brain ischemia and in vitro culture models of ischemia and reperfusion, we have demonstrated several intriguing phenomena, such as ischemic tolerance [9], delayed opening of the blood–brain barrier [10], apoptosis-like cell death [20, 22] and induction of stress proteins and cytokines by ischemia and reperfusion [5, 6, 14, 17]. To elucidate the molecular mechanism underlying these

Maturation Phenomenon in Cerebral Ischemia III
U. Ito et al. (Eds.)
© Springer-Verlag Berlin Heidelberg 1999

complex phenomena, several newly developed strategies, including the use of transgenic or knock-out mouse as models for brain ischemia, have been enthusiastically employed with great success.

In the present report, our research is focused initially on the importance of establishing reproducible models for brain ischemia in mice. We examined species differences in the susceptibility of cerebral ischemia induced by bilateral common carotid and intraluminal suture occlusion, and developed a prediction method for reducing variability of the ischemic lesions in both global and focal ischemia models. Then, using these reproducible brain ischemia models in mice, we investigated the pathophysiological roles of Bcl-2 family proteins and inflammatory responses in ischemia-induced apoptosis-like neuronal cell death and in microcirculatory disturbances, respectively.

Establishment of Reproducible Brain-Ischemia Models in Mice

To investigate the complex and dynamic cellular responses, cerebral ischemia models using mice have drawn increasing attention, particularly because of the availability of transgenic animals. However, the variability of intracranial vasculature at the circle of Willis in mice can influence the degree of ischemia in both the global and focal brain ischemia models, as documented in the gerbil model of experimental brain ischemia [3, 8, 19]. As for the global forebrain ischemia model in mice, clear strain differences have been observed [2, 26]; of seven commonly used mouse strains, including C57BL/6, ICR, BALB/c, C3H, CBA, ddY and DBA/2, the C57BL/6 strain was most susceptible to cerebral ischemia [26].

Previously [26], we identified strain differences in the patency of the posterior communicating artery (Pcom) at the circle of Willis as a major cause of differences in the susceptibility. This variability in the degree of anastomosis can also cause the variability in the degree and extent of the focal brain ischemia produced in the intraluminal suture occlusion model [13]. We have therefore developed a method to predict the extent of this anastomosis that measures cortical microperfusion with laser Doppler flowmetry during a 1-min occlusion of both common carotid arteries. When animals showed residual cortical perfusion of less than 12 % of the baseline value during bilateral carotid occlusion, the mice developed subsequent adenosine triphosphate (ATP) depletion in the frontal cortex and – as revealed in a separate experiment using India-ink perfusion – an absence of functional Pcom.

In the absence of collateral circulation through a functional Pcom, the territory supplied by the posterior cerebral artery (PCA), including the hippocampus and the thalamus, was expected to experience ischemia during the intraluminal suture occlusion. Autoradiography with C-14 iodoantipyrine of mice with and without functional Pcom showed clear differences in the ischemic territory during the intraluminal suture occlusion. The effect of this variation of the anastomosis was also confirmed histologically and immunohistochemically. Two days after intraluminal suture occlusion for 30 min, clear ischemic lesions, with loss of immunostaining for microtubule-associated protein 2 (MAP-2), were observed in the ipsilateral hippocampus of mice that showed less than 12 % of baseline cortical microperfusion during 1-min bilateral common carotid occlusion; other mice with functional anastomosis showed the

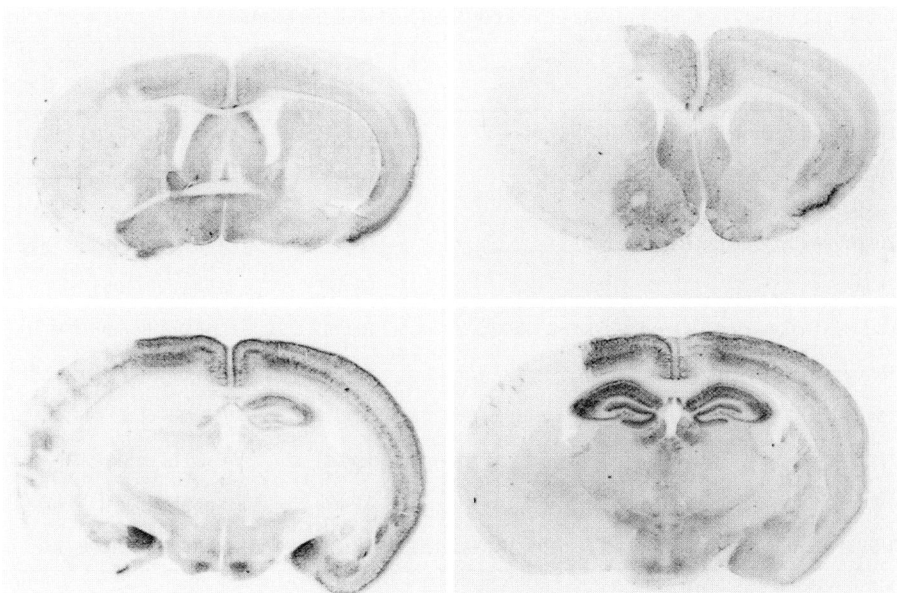

Fig. 1. Representative immunohistochemical findings following intraluminal suture occlusion in mice with or without functional Pcom. The *upper* and *lower* panels show immunoreactivity to microtubule-associated protein 2 (MAP2) in coronal sections taken from the level of the caudoputamen and hippocampus, respectively. In the C57BL/6 mouse brain without functional posterior communicating artery (Pcom; *left panel*), ischemic lesions with loss of MAP2 immunoreactivity are seen not only in the caudoputamen and cerebral cortex, but also in the hippocampus, whereas in the DBA/2 mouse with functional Pcom (*right panel*), ischemic lesions are confined to the caudoputamen and cerebral cortex

ischemic lesions only in the cerebral cortex and the caudoputamen (Fig. 1). These results strongly suggest the importance of assessing patency of Pcom in each animal, whether cerebral ischemia is produced by bilateral carotid occlusion or by intraluminal suture occlusion; our prediction method would be useful for the reproducible induction of cerebral ischemia in transgenic mice.

Ischemia-Induced Stress Responses in the Brain

Through several lines of experimental studies on cellular responses to brain ischemia, the existence of positive and negative responses of neuronal cells to ischemic stress (induction of stress proteins, or ischemic-tolerance phenomenon, and apoptosis-like selective neuronal cell death, respectively) have been well documented. A variety of stress proteins are so far known to be induced in ischemic brain (Table 1), although the specific roles of these stress proteins need to be clarified. In a previous study [11], using a reproducible unilateral ischemia model and prediction in gerbils, we could clearly show that ischemic tolerance was induced by ischemic stress, not by systemic changes caused by preconditioning ischemia, and was augmented by repetition, with-

Table 1. A variety of stress proteins induced by brain ischemia/reperfusion

Classification of stress proteins	Experimental animal	Reference
Hsp70 family proteins (Hsc70,GRP78, etc.)	Gerbil	Nowak 1985 [21]
Ubiquitin	Gerbil	Magnusson and Wieloch 1989 [18]
Hsp90 family proteins (GRP94, etc.)	Gerbil	Kawagoe et al. 1993 [7]
Hsp60	Gerbil	Abe et al., 1993 [1]
Glucose transporters (a kind of GRPs*, GLUT)	Rat	Lee and Bondy 1993 [15]
Heme oxygenase (HO-1; Hsp32, ORP33)	Rat	Takeda et al. 1994 [24]
Hsp20 family proteins (Hsp27, a-crystallin, etc.)	Rat	Higashi et al. 1994 [4]
Hsp47	Rat	Higashi et al. 1994 [4]
ORP150	Mouse	Kuwabara et al. 1996 [14]
HSP110 family proteins (Hsp110, Hsp105, IRP94, etc.)	Rat	Yagita et al. 1998 [25]

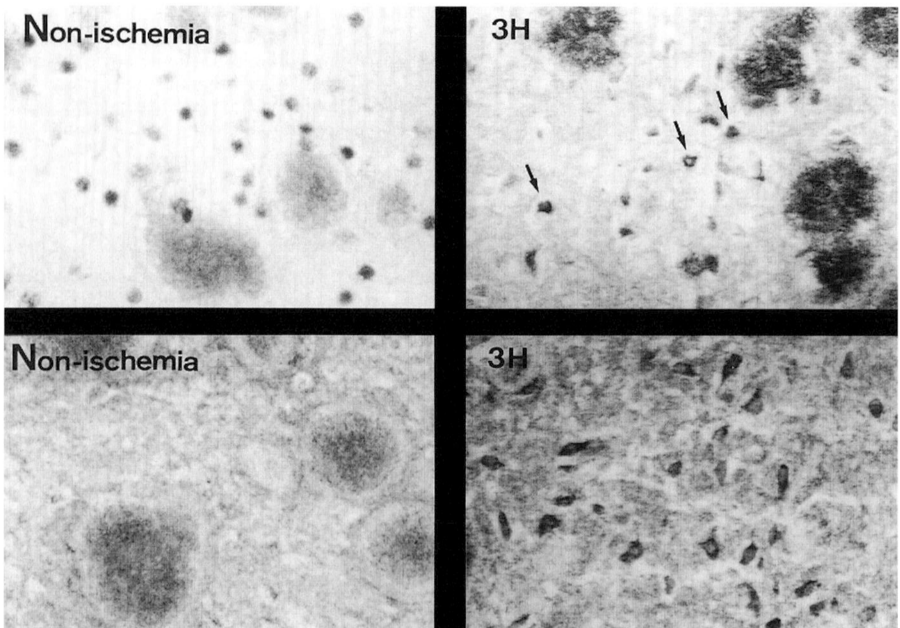

Fig. 2. Bcl-2 (*upper panel*) and Bax (*lower panel*) immunoreactivity in the non-ischemic control cau-doputamen (*left panel*) and in the ischemic caudoputamen (*right panel*), with 30 min intraluminal suture occlusion and 3-h reperfusion. Compared with the non-ischemic side, in the ischemic side, a reduction of Bcl-2 immunoreactivity and an increase of Bax immunoreactivity are clearly observed. *Arrows* indicate the location of Bcl-2 protein in dying neurons

out further increases of HSP70. We also demonstrated the beneficial role of improved mitochondrial oxygen metabolism during transient forebrain ischemia, by measuring intracerebral oxygenation state with near-infrared spectroscopy in gerbils with preconditioning ischemia [16].

In the apoptotic process, the key role of mitochondrial dysfunction has also been suggested in conjunction with the protective role of ced-9 homologous gene, Bcl-2 with multiple functions [23]. In a recent study [20], we examined sequential changes of Bcl-2 family proteins, using the intraluminal-suture occlusion model in mice. In the striatum, following 30 min occlusion and 3 h reperfusion (Fig. 2), Bcl-2 and Bcl-X proteins were reduced concomitantly with the reduction of MAP-2 antigenicity, and increased Bax protein levels were clearly observed in the cytosol of the dying neurons. This contrasted with the non-ischemic caudoputamen, for which Bcl-2 and Bcl-X proteins were strongly positive and Bax protein was only mildly positive in the cytosol of neurons. These changes preceded the appearance of terminal deoxynucleotidyltransferase (TdT)-mediated dUTP-biotin nick-end labeling (TUNEL)-positive cells in the same lesion at 6–12 h recirculation, suggesting crucial roles for these Bcl-2 family proteins in apoptosis-like cell death induced by transient focal ischemia.

We have also investigated the role of Bcl-2 in selective neuronal death induced by transient forebrain ischemia in Bcl-2 transgenic animals. Compared with littermate wild mice with the same ischemic stress, both the frequency of ischemic lesions and the severity of neuronal damage in the hippocampus were reduced significantly but mildly in Bcl-2 transgenic mice exposed to 7-day recirculation following 12 min forebrain ischemia. These results suggested that beneficial effects of increased Bcl-2 protein might be weak and limited in apoptosis-like neuronal cell death induced by transient global ischemia.

Pathophysiological Roles of Cellular Cross-Talk in Brain Ischemia

In parallel with the ischemia-induced apoptosis-like cell death, brain ischemia is known to trigger microcirculatory disturbances through the inflammatory response that is thought to be initiated by expression of adhesion molecules, such as P-selectin and intracellular adhesion molecule-1 (ICAM-1), and cytokines such as tumor necrosis factor (TNF) and interleukins 1 and 6 (IL-1 and IL-6). In our recent studies, we have examined the effect of ICAM-1 elimination on the lesion size induced by permanent or transient focal ischemia in the ICAM-1 knock-out mice [13].

In selecting experimental animals, we have applied the prediction method to eliminate variations of lesion size caused by variability of anastomosis. This enabled us to detect a significant decrease of ischemic lesions in the ICAM-1 knock-out mouse, especially in the transient focal ischemia model that employed 30 min ischemia and 48 h recirculation. The differences in lesion size between ICAM-1 knock-out and wild mice decreased when the duration of transient ischemia was increased from 30 min to 45 min. The depletion of neutrophils by intraperitoneal injections of RB6-8c5, a monoclonal antibody against granulocytes, 24 h before induction of ischemia showed a clear protective effect even in the 45-min transient focal ischemia model that used ICAM-1 knock-out mice. These results clearly suggested an important role of ICAM-1 expression in microcirculatory failure and subsequent development and expansion of infarction after transient focal ischemia. As for the accumulation of granulocytes and their detrimental effects, factors other than ICAM-1 should be further investigated.

References

1. Abe K, Kawagoe J, Aoki M, Kogure K (1993) Changes of mitochondrial DNA and heat shock protein gene expression in gerbil hippocampus after transient forebrain ischemia. J Cereb Blood Flow Metab 13: 773–780
2. Barone FC, Knudsen DJ, Nelson AH, Feuerstein GZ, Willette RN (1993) Mouse strain differences in susceptibility to cerebral ischemia are related to cerebral vascular anatomy. J Cereb Blood Flow Metab 13: 683–692
3. Berry K, Wisniewski HM, Svarzbein L, Baez S (1975) On the relationship of brain vasculature to production of neurological deficit and morphological changes following acute unilateral common carotid artery ligation in gerbils. J Neurol Sci 25: 75–92
4. Higashi T, Takechi H, Uemura Y, Kikuchi H, Nagata K (1994) Differential induction of mRNA species encoding several classes of stress proteins following focal cerebral ischemia in rats. Brain Res 650: 239–248
5. Hori 0, Matsumoto M, Maeda Y, Ueda H, Ohtsuki T, Stern DM, Kinoshita T, Ogawa S, Kamada T (1994) Metabolic and biosynthetic alterations in cultured astrocytes exposed to hypoxia/reoxygenation. J Neurochem 62: 1489–1495
6. Hori 0, Matsumoto M, Kuwabara K, Maeda Y, Ueda H, Ohtsuki T, Kinoshita T, Ogawa S, Stern DM, Kamada T (1996) Exposure of astrocytes to hypoxia/reoxygenation enhances expression of glucose-regulated protein 78 facilitating astrocyte release of the neuroprotective cytokine interleukin 6. J Neurochem 66: 973–979
7. Kawagoe J, Abe K, Aoki M, Kogure K (1993) Induction of HSP90 alpha heat shock mRNA after transient global ischemia in gerbil hippocampus. Brain Res 621: 121–125
8. Kitagawa K, Matsumoto M, Handa N, Fukunaga R, Ueda H, Isaka Y, Kimura K, Kamada T (1989) Prediction of stroke-prone gerbils and their cerebral circulation. Brain Res 479: 263–269
9. Kitagawa K, Matsumoto M, Tagaya M, Hata R, Ueda H, Niinobe M, Handa N, Fukunaga R, Mikoshiba Y, Kamada T (1990) Ischemic tolerance phenomenon found in the brain. Brain Res 528: 21–24
10. Kitagawa K, Matsumoto M, Ohtsuki T, Tagaya M, Okabe T, Hata R, Ueda H, Handa N, Sobue K, Kamada T (1992) The characteristics of blood–brain barrier in three different conditions – infarction, selective neuronal death and selective loss of presynaptic terminals –following cerebral ischemia. Acta Neuropathol 84: 378–386
11. Kitagawa K, Matsumoto M, Mabuchi T, Yagita Y, Mandai K, Matsushita K, Hori M, Yanagihara T (1997) Ischemic tolerance in hippocampal CA1 neurons studied using contralateral controls. Neuroscience 81: 989–998
12. Kitagawa K, Matsumoto M, Mabuchi T, Yagita Y, Ohtsuki T, Hori M, Yanagihara T (1998) Deficiency of intercellular adhesion molecule 1 attenuates microcirculatory disturbance and infarction size in focal cerebral ischemia. J Cereb Blood Flow Metab 18: 1336–1345
13. Kiatagawa Y, Matsumoto M, Yang G, Mabuchi T, Yagita Y, Hori M, Yanagihara T (1998) Cerebral ischemia after bilateral carotid artery occlusion and intraluminal suture occlusion in mice: evaluation of the patency of the posterior communicating artery. J Cereb Blood Flow Metab 18: 570–579
14. Kuwabara K, Matsumoto M, lkeda J, Hori 0, Ogawa S, Maeda Y, Kitagawa K, Imuta N, Kinoshita T, Stern DM, Yanagi H, Kamada T (1996) Purification and characterization of a novel stress protein, the 150 kDa oxygen-regulated protein (ORP150), from cultured rat astrocytes and its expression in ischemic mouse brain. J Biol Chem 271: 5025–5032
15. Lee WH, Bondy CA (1993) Ischemic injury induces brain glucose transporter gene expression. Endocrinology 133: 2540–2544
16. Li J-Y, Ueda H, Seiyama A, Nakano M, Matsumoto M, Yanagihara T (1997) A near-infrared spectroscopic study of cerebral ischemia and ischemic tolerance in gerbils. Stroke 28: 1451–1457
17. Maeda Y, Matsumoto M, Hori O, Kuwabara K, Ogawa S, Yan SD, Ohtsuki T, Kinoshita T, Kamada T, Stern D (1994) Hypoxia-reoxygenation mediated induction of interleukin-6 in cultured rat astrocytes and expression in ischemic gerbil brain: a paracrine mechanism enhancing neuron survival. J Exp Med 180: 2297–2308
18. Magnusson K, Wieloch T (1989) Impairment of protein ubiquitination may cause delayed neuronal death. Neurosci Lett 96: 264–270

19. Matsumoto M, Hatakeyama T, Yamamoto K, Yanagihara T (1988) Prediction of stroke before and after unilateral occlusion of the common carotid artery in gerbils. Stroke 19: 490–497
20. Matsushita K, Matsuyama T, Kitagawa K, Matsumoto M, Yanagihara T, Sugita M (1998) Alterations of BCL-2 family proteins precede cytoskeltal proteolysis in the penumbra, but not in infarct centers following focal cerebral ischemia in mice. Neuroscience 83: 439–448
21. Nowak TSJR (1985) Synthesis of a stress protein following transient ischemia in the gerbil. J Neurochem 45: 1635–1641
22. Okamoto M, Matsumoto M, Ohtsuki T, Taguchi A, Mikoshiba K, Yanagihara T, Kamada T (1993) Internucleosomal DNA cleavage involved in ischemia-induced neuronal death. Biochem Biophys Res Commun 196: 1356–1362
23. Reed JC (1997) Double identity for proteins of the Bcl-2 family. Nature 387: 773–776
24. Takeda A, Onodera H, Sugimoto A, Itoyama Y, Kogure K, Shibahara S (1994) Increased expression of heme oxygenase mRNA in rat brain following transient forebrain ischemia. Brain Res 666: 120–124
25. Yagita Y, Kitagawa K, Taguchi A, Ohtsuki T, Kuwabara K, Mabuchi T, Matsumoto M, Yanagihara T, Hori M (1998) Molecular cloning of a novel member of HSP110 family gene, ischemia responsive protein 94 kDa (irp94), expressed in rat brain after transient forebrain ischemia. J Neurochem (in press)
26. Yang G, Kitagawa K Matsushita K, Mabuchi T, Yagita Y, Yanagihara T, Matsumoto M (1997) C57BL/6 strain is most susceptible to cerebral ischemia following bilateral common carotid occlusion among seven mouse strains: selective neuronal death in the murine forebrain ischemia. Brain Res 752: 209–218

Oxygen Free Radicals and Ischaemic Preconditioning in the Brain: Preliminary Data and a Hypothesis

P. Schumann, K. Prass, F. Wiegand, M. Ahrens, D. Megow, and U. Dirnagl

Summary. The mechanisms by which a sublethal preconditioning stress increases the resistance of the brain to a subsequent ischaemic event are not fully elucidated. This phenomenon seems to involve the neo-synthesis of proteins, but little is known about the signalling cascade and the nature of the protective proteins that are involved. Two experimental paradigms were used to induce tolerance to focal cerebral ischaemia achieved by middle cerebral-artery occlusion in the rat: first, metabolic inhibition by a single dose of 3-nitropropionic acid (NPA), an inhibitor of the succinate dehydrogenase, was induced 3 days before transient focal cerebral ischaemia (90 min); second, hyperbaric oxygenation (1 h, 100 % oxygen at 2 atm) was performed daily for the 5 days preceding permanent focal cerebral ischaemia. Neither stimuli caused any detectable brain damage. The 3-NPA pretreatment, and 2 atm hyperbaric oxygen (HBO) pre-exposition led to infarct volumes, which were smaller than in control animals by approximately 30 %. Both preconditioning stimuli induced the generation of oxygen free radicals (OFR) as measured by chemiluminescence in the 3-NPA group, and malondialdehyde (MDA) production in the HBO group. Furthermore, tolerance induction was abolished in both groups when animals were pretreated with the free-radical scavenger, dimethyl-thiourea (DMTU). These data argue for a critical role of OFRs in tolerance induction by metabolic inhibition or HBO. Since most of the known preconditioning stimuli lead to OFRs, we forward the hypothesis that OFRs may constitute a common signal, triggering the induction of tolerance to ischaemia. This hypothesis is further supported by the effects of free radicals on transcription factors, such as nuclear factor (NF)-$\varkappa$B. Their possible interaction in tolerance, as well as the nature of the putative neuroprotective proteins, will be discussed. Hyperbaric oxygenation seems to be a useful and safe way to induce tolerance to focal cerebral ischaemia, which may lead to clinical applications.

Introduction

Ischaemic tolerance, a phenomenon whereby a sublethal preconditioning stress may increase the resistance of the brain to a subsequent ischaemic event, may be induced by various stimuli, including short periods of ischaemia itself [5], metabolic inhibition [29], cortical spreading depression [21] or cytokines [26]. There is a growing body of evidence suggesting that tolerance induction may involve the neo-synthesis of endogenous neuroprotective proteins; among others, upregulation of heat-shock proteins [18], antiapoptotic protein [40] and antioxidant enzymes [17, 36] have been described. However, the exact role of these proteins and, more generally, the cascade of cellular events leading to tolerance, are not fully elucidated.

Maturation Phenomenon in Cerebral Ischemia III
U. Ito et al. (Eds.)
© Springer-Verlag Berlin Heidelberg 1999

It is noteworthy that most of the above-mentioned preconditioning stimuli can induce the formation of oxygen-free radicals (OFRs). Indeed, OFRs are produced during ischaemia/reperfusion [28], hypoxia/reoxygenation [29], exposition to cytokines [14] and, potentially, by cortical spreading depression [20]. It may, thus, be speculated that formation of OFRs is a critical step in tolerance induction. Furthermore, OFRs are known to activate transcription factors [32] (for review [33]), which may ultimately lead to the expression of neuroprotective proteins. In particular, several arguments speak for the involvement of an antioxidant enzyme, the superoxide dismutase (SOD), in tolerance induction. An increase in SOD activity has been reported after ischaemic preconditioning in the rat [36], and the loss of SOD after a lethal global-ischaemic challenge is attenuated by ischaemic preconditioning [17].

Regarding the existing literature, two major issues need to be addressed: first, it is necessary to further analyse the sequence of events at the molecular level leading to ischaemic tolerance in order to better understand the endogenous ability of brain neuroprotection; this may, second, help to develop clinically relevant protocols of ischaemic tolerance. Here, we present some recent experimental data arguing for the involvement of OFRs in the induction of tolerance against focal cerebral ischaemia, induced by metabolic inhibition or hyperbaric oxygen (HBO) in the rat. In addition, these results point to the usefulness of HBO as a new stimulus for ischaemic tolerance induction, which may lead to clinical applications.

Materials and Methods

Focal Cerebral Ischaemia

In male Wistar rats, the right ipsilateral common carotid artery and the middle cerebral artery were transiently [90 min, 3-nitropropionic acid (NPA) group] or permanently (HBO group) occluded under halothane anaesthesia [4]. In addition to the right common carotid artery, the left one was temporarily occluded for 1 h. All relevant physiological and biochemical parameters (blood pressure, temperature, blood gases, etc.) were monitored throughout surgery. Animals were sacrificed 4 days after ischaemia, and brain infarct volume was assessed by quantitative histology using vanadium acidic fuchsin for staining.

Ischaemic Tolerance

Tolerance was induced by two different means in two distinct groups of rats. In the 3-NPA group, ischaemic tolerance was induced by 3-NPA, an irreversible inhibitor of succinate dehydrogenase [13], administered once as a single dose (20 mg/kg, i.p.) at different time points (7, 5, 3 and 2 days and 24 h, 12 h and 15 min, $n>10$ in each group) before ischaemia.

In a second group, the HBO group, rats were repeatedly exposed to a HBO environment (pure oxygen at 2 atm, 1 h/day) during a 5-day pretreatment period. Cerebral ischaemia was then induced on the following (sixth) day.

Free-Radical Measurements

To evaluate whether 3-NPA induces the generation of free radicals, a lucigenin-enhanced chemiluminescence technique [10] was used to record the OFR production of acute brain slices superfused with 3-NPA in a dose equivalent to the in vivo experiments (300 µM), over a 5-h period.

In the HBO group, OFR production was assessed by the MDA production using the thiobarbituric-acid technique [38] on the first and fifth day of preconditioning.

Pharmacological Manipulation of the Free-Radical Production

In order to evaluate the involvement of free radicals in 3-NPA-tolerance induction, DMTU (750 mg/kg, i.p.) was given shortly prior to each 3-NPA stimulus, and the effect of this OFR scavenging on tolerance induction was examined.

Likewise, in the HBO group, OFRs were exogenously scavenged during the HBO treatment by pretreating animals with the OFR-scavenger DMTU (750 mg/kg, i.p.) prior to each HBO preconditioning.

Evaluation of the Protein-Synthesis Involvement in Tolerance Induction

The implication of protein synthesis in the establishment of tolerance induced by 3-NPA was assessed by the administration of an inhibitor of protein synthesis, cycloheximide (1 mg/kg, i.p.) 15 min prior to 3-NPA treatment.

Results

Both Metabolic Inhibition and HBO Lead to Ischaemic Tolerance

As illustrated in Fig. 1, preconditioning with 3-NPA decreases the infarct volume by 36 %, when compared with the control group subjected to focal ischaemia alone. Furthermore, this neuroprotective effect was maximal when ischaemia was achieved on the third day of preconditioning (other time points not shown). Likewise, the 2 atm-HBO pretreatment reduced infarct volume by 29 % (Fig. 2).

Free Radicals are Generated During 3-NPA- and HBO-Induced Tolerance

The 3-NPA induced a burst of free radicals, detected with lucigenin-enhanced chemiluminescence, commencing 1 h after the application of the drug and reaching a maximum 2 h later (data not shown). MDA measurements performed 1 day and 5 days after HBO treatment indicated a significant production of OFRs at both time points of preconditioning (data not shown). Moreover, this phenomenon seemed to be attenuated on the fifth day, when compared with the first day of HBO. In both cases, administration of DMTU prevented OFR production.

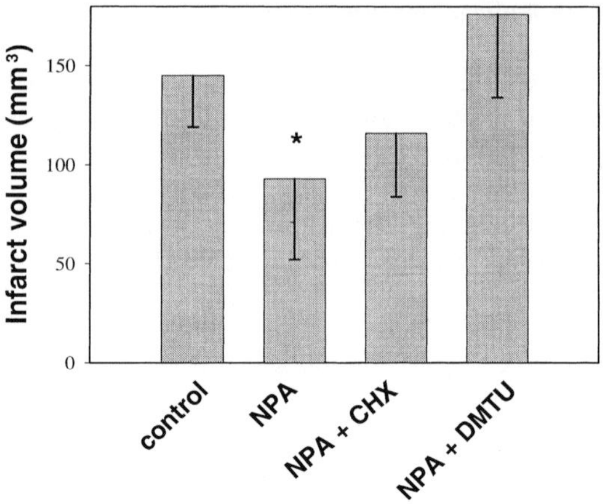

Fig. 1. A single dose of 3-nitropropionic acid (NPA), (20 mg/kg, i.p., 3 days prior to induction of focal cerebral ischaemia) induces tolerance to 90 min of ipsilateral common carotid and middle cerebral-artery occlusion, followed by reperfusion. Quantitative infarct volume determination by histology 4 days after induction of ischaemia. Cycloheximide or dimethylthiourea (CHX, 1 mg/kg i.p.; dimethylthiourea (DMTU), 750 mg/kg, 15 min prior to 3-NPA) blocked tolerance induction. Data [mean (SD)] are analysed by an one-way ANOVA followed by Student-Newman-Keuls post-hoc test (* $P<0.01$)

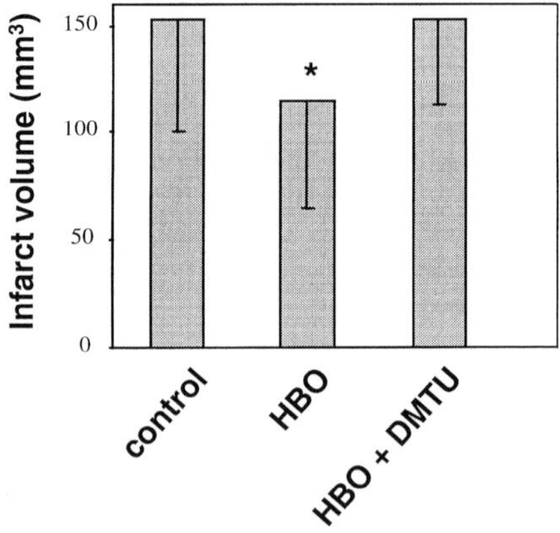

Fig. 2. Effect of pre-exposure to hyperbaric oxygen (HBO) (1 h/day, 5 days, 2 atm) on brain damage following permanent focal cerebral ischaemia achieved by middle cerebral-artery occlusion on day 6 in the rat. Infarct volume, determined 4 days after ischaemia, is significantly reduced in the hyperbaric group (*HBO*) when compared with the control group (one-way ANOVA followed by Student-Newman-Keuls post-hoc test, * $P<0.05$). Administration of the free-radical scavenger dimethylthiourea (DMTU, 750 mg/kg, intraperitoneally) abolishes the preconditioning effect of HBO

Free-Radical Scavenging Blocks Tolerance Induction

Pretreatment with DMTU completely blocked preconditioning by either 3-NPA (Fig. 1) or HBO (Fig. 2), whereas DMTU alone did not modify the extent of cerebral infarction (not shown).

Protein-Synthesis Inhibition Prevents 3-NPA-Tolerance Induction

Inhibition of protein synthesis by cycloheximide given at the time of 3-NPA administration completely inhibited preconditioning (Fig. 1).

Discussion

In this study, we have presented two new paradigms to induce tolerance to focal cerebral ischaemia in the rat: metabolic inhibition and HBO. The efficiency of HBO as a preconditioning stimulus has already been reported against global ischaemia in the gerbil [37], whereas 3-NPA was shown to be effective in inducing tolerance in an in vitro brain-slice hypoxia paradigm [29]. By chemiluminescence or MDA production, we demonstrated that both stimuli lead to the generation of OFRs. The question arises whether OFR production in these models is only an epiphenomenon in the induction of tolerance, or whether it is a common trigger for tolerance induction. The abolition of tolerance by the free-radical scavenger, DMTU, strongly suggests that OFR generation is a necessary step in the establishment of ischaemic tolerance in both models.

The concept of a beneficial role of OFR, by stimulating endogenous neuroprotective mechanisms, is somewhat conflicting with the well-known deleterious role of these molecules in the development of brain injury (for review, see Siesjö et al. [34]). Indeed, OFRs are involved in the pathophysiology of numerous brain insults, including global [7] or focal [19, 28] cerebral ischaemia and several neurodegenerative processes [3, 12]. It is thought that OFRs contribute to ischaemic neuronal death during the reoxygenation period following reperfusion [7, 28, 41], when the antioxidant defence mechanisms are overloaded. This so-called oxidative stress is the consequence of the overproduction of OFRs and the consumption of antioxidants, which are not replenished in ischaemic tissue. These unscavenged OFRs can then react with a number of target molecules, including proteins, lipids and DNA, thereby initiating lipid peroxidation, protein oxidation or glycation, DNA damage and, ultimately, disruption of cellular functions and integrity.

The occurrence of oxidative stress depends on both the amount of OFR produced and the antioxidant capacity of the tissue. It may, thus, be speculated that the preconditioning stimuli used in this study do not critically perturb the balance between each parameter and, therefore, remain safe for the brain. This duality of OFRs in inducing either toxicity or protection according to the antioxidant state of the brain is further illustrated by comparing the studies of Mizui and colleagues [22], and Ohtsuki and co-workers [25]. Indeed, both authors reduced the levels of endogenous antioxidant agents (reduced glutathione and SOD, respectively [22, 25]) and, thereafter, induced cerebral ischaemia. Depletion of reduced glutathione shortly before ischaemia exacerbated the severity of the insult [22], while inhibition of SOD 4 days before ischaemia elicited neuroprotection [25]. Therefore, deliberately increasing the level of OFRs induced two different responses of the brain. In one case [22], antioxidant capacity of the brain was exhausted by ischaemia itself and OFRs displayed their deleterious effects, while in the other case [25], the antioxidant state of the brain was unaltered and OFR only exhibited their beneficial role, i.e. delayed neuroprotection, i.e. ischaemic tolerance. Likewise, no brain damage or systemic injury has been observed after administration of 3-NPA or HBO preconditioning. In contrast, as suggested by the effectiveness of DMTU in preventing tolerance, OFR production may be beneficial for the brain by protecting it against a following ischaemic insult.

The mechanisms of 3-NPA-tolerance induction seem to involve the synthesis of new proteins, since this phenomenon is maximal on the third day (time course not shown) and is abolished by cycloheximide. We believe that such an adaptive response also takes place in the HBO group between the first and fifth day of preconditioning. Indeed, the amount of OFR detected on the last, i.e. fifth, day of HBO, is lower than the amount measured on the first day (data not shown). This finding could be explained by a synthesis of antioxidant proteins, induced at the beginning of the HBO treatment and, thereafter, scavenging or eliminating part of the OFRs generated on the last, fifth, HBO session. However, this hypothesis needs to be further explored. These findings are in line with the reported delay required for tolerance induction by other stimuli [6, 21].

Therefore, both OFR production and, at least in the 3-NPA group, protein synthesis seem to be a necessary step for tolerance induction. Considering the cascade of events leading to tolerance, two hypotheses may be advanced: either OFR generation precedes and induces protein neo-synthesis or OFR production and protein synthesis are unrelated events, both of which lead to tolerance by distinct pathways. However, the latter proposal is unlikely, since blocking the synthesis of OFR by DMTU, or proteins by cycloheximide, may partially or completely prevent tolerance, suggesting that they share at least one common pathway in tolerance induction. In addition, it is known that OFRs modulate gene expression through activation of transcription factors, such as nuclear factor (NF)-$\varkappa$B or activator protein (AP)-1 (for review, see [27]). The constitutive form of NF-$\varkappa$B is restricted to a few cell types, including mature B cells, certain T cells, monocytes and neurons [16]. Target genes activated by NF-$\varkappa$B include those involved in viral activation, adhesion and inflammatory responses (cytokines, nitric-oxide synthase) and other genes containing a $\varkappa$B regulatory element, such as SOD [8] (for review, see [2]). It has been reported that the addition of H_2O_2 directly into the culture medium activated NF-$\varkappa$B in several cell lines [32]. Further support for the role of OFRs as NF-$\varkappa$B activators comes from experiments showing that antioxidant compounds prevent NF-$\varkappa$B activation [30, 31]. The exact mechanisms by which OFRs may activate NF-$\varkappa$B are not fully elucidated, but several transduction pathways may be involved [33]. NF-$\varkappa$B consists of a heterodimer of two proteins and is found in the cytoplasm of unstimulated cells in an inactive form, i.e. bound to an inhibitory subunit I$\varkappa$B. Activation of NF-$\varkappa$B implicates the phosphorylation of I$\varkappa$B, leading to the dissociation of NF-$\varkappa$B from I$\varkappa$B. NF-$\varkappa$B then translocates into the nucleus while I$\varkappa$B is rapidly degraded. Therefore, all the activators of NF-$\varkappa$B ultimately lead to a phosphorylation of I$\varkappa$B. Several candidate kinases (mostly serine but also tyrosine) may mediate phosphorylation of I$\varkappa$B (39).

Interestingly, it has been reported that tyrosine-kinase inhibitors impaired the ultraviolet (UV) response, which may involve OFR formation, mediated by NF-$\varkappa$B [9] or the OFR-mediated NF-$\varkappa$B activation [1]. There is increasing evidence that free radicals, mostly H_2O_2, may control, directly or indirectly, kinases and phosphatases involved in phosphorylation of I$\varkappa$B [33]. It is also possible that an oxidative modification of either NF-$\varkappa$B or I$\varkappa$B may cause the dissociation of the NF-$\varkappa$B/I$\varkappa$B complex. Regulation of gene expression by OFR could also take place downstream of NF-$\varkappa$B activation, i.e. on the DNA NF-$\varkappa$B binding site, which is redox sensitive [35]. All these data support the possibility of an OFR-mediated activation of NF-$\varkappa$B mediating the induction of ischaemic tolerance. However, this hypothesis should be further tested by several experiments, including assaying the activation of NF-$\varkappa$B after 3-NPA- or HBO preconditioning.

32. Schreck R, Rieber P, Baeuerle PA (1991) Reactive oxygen intermediates as apparently widely used messengers in the activation of the NF-kappa B transcription factor and HIV-1. EMBO J 10: 2247–2258
33. Sen CK, Packer L (1996) Antioxidant and redox regulation of gene transcription. FASEB J 10: 709–720
34. Siesjö BK, Agardh CD, Bengtsson F (1989) Free radicals and brain damage. Cerebrovasc Brain Metab Rev 1: 165–211
35. Suzuki YJ, Mizuno M, Tritschler HJ, Packer L (1995) Redox regulation of NF-kappa B DNA binding activity by dihydrolipoate. Biochem Mol Biol Int 36: 241–246
36. Toyoda T, Kassell NF, Lee KS (1997) Induction of ischemic tolerance and antioxidant activity by brief focal ischemia. Neuroreport 8: 847–851
37. Wada K, Ito M, Miyazawa T, Katoh H, Nawashiro H, Shima K, Chigasaki H (1996) Repeated hyperbaric oxygen induces ischemic tolerance in gerbil hippocampus. Brain Res 740: 15–20
38. Wong SH, Knight JA, Hopfer SM, Zaharia O, Leach CN, Sunderman FW (1987) Lipoperoxides in plasma as measured by liquid-chromatographic separation of malondialdehyde-thiobarbituric acid adduct. Clin Chem 33: 214–220
39. Woronicz JD, Gao X, CaoZ, Rothe M, Goeddel DV (1997) IϰB kinase-β: NF-ϰB activation and complex formation with IϰB kinase-α and NIK. Science 278: 866–869
40. Xu DG, Crocker SJ, Doucet JP, St-Jean M, Tamai K, Hakim AM, Ikeda JE, Liston P, Thompson CS, Korneluk RG, MacKenzie A, Robertson GS (1997) Elevation of neuronal expression of NAIP reduces ischemic damage in the rat hippocampus. Nat Med 3: 997–1004
41. Yang GY, Betz AL (1994) Reperfusion-induced injury to the blood–brain barrier after middle cerebral artery occlusion in rats. Stroke 25: 1658–1664
42. Zhou X, Zhai X, Ashraf M (1996) Direct evidence that initial oxidative stress triggered by preconditioning contributes to second window of protection by endogenous antioxidant enzyme in myocytes. Circulation 93: 1177–1184

Ischemic Tolerance in the Maturation of Disseminated Selective Neuronal Necrosis and Cerebral Infarction After Repetitive Ischemia

S. Hanyu, U. Ito, T. Kuroiwa, Y. Hakamata, and I. Nakano

Summary. We examined whether a brief non-lethal ischemia could induce ischemic tolerance to subsequent ischemia as well as reduce infarct size in gerbils subjected to repeated transient cerebral ischemia. Gerbils subjected to a repeated occlusion of the left common carotid artery (two occlusions separated by a 5-h interval) developed infarction (infarct size 2.28±0.75 % of the hemisphere, mean ± SEM) in the frontal cortex. A total of 8 min of unilateral carotid-artery occlusion, experienced 48–72 h prior to the repeated ischemia, reduced the infarct size (0.11±0.04 % in the 60-h group, $P<0.05$). Reduction of succinic dehydrogenase activity examined 48 h after the repeated ischemic insults was significantly milder in the preconditioned animal. Thus, preconditioning by a brief non-lethal ischemia experienced 48 h or more, prior to repeated ischemia, induced tolerance and significantly reduced infarct size. Impairment of mitochondrial function in a non-neuronal cell is probably important in the observed ischemic tolerance.

Introduction

It has been shown that neural tissue subjected to a brief non-lethal ischemia acquires tolerance to subsequent ischemia. An understanding of the involved mechanism would be clinically important, as it may define new therapeutic strategies for the treatment of cerebral ischemia. However, experimental data have also shown exaggeration, rather than amelioration, of postischemic injury by the repetition of ischemia.

We were interested in the different outcomes following similar repeated episodes of ischemia. Gerbils subjected to repeated ischemia, separated by 3-h to 48-h intervals, slowly developed disseminated selective neuronal necrosis (DSNN) and infarction in the postischemic cortex [4–6]. Ischemic injury varied in intensity, depending on the interval between the ischemia as well as the duration of ischemia. Using this model, we examined: (1) the change of infarction size by ischemic preconditioning given at different time intervals, and (2) changes in levels of succinic dehydrogenase (SDH), a mitochondrial respiratory enzyme, following ischemic preconditioning.

Materials and Methods

Adult Mongolian gerbils ($n=28$) weighing 60–80 g were used in the following experiment. In the ischemic preconditioning group, the animals were anesthetized with halothane, the left common carotid artery occluded and the animal allowed to recover

Maturation Phenomenon in Cerebral Ischemia III
U. Ito et al. (Eds.)
© Springer-Verlag Berlin Heidelberg 1999

from anesthesia. Stroke symptom-positive animals [10] were selected and the blood flow was restored after 8 min of ischemia. After 48, 60 or 72 h of recirculation, the animals were subjected to two episodes of 10-min ischemia by occlusion of the left common carotid artery, separated by 5-h intervals. At 7 days after the repeated ischemia, the animal was transcardially perfused. Brain sections at the stereotactic level of the chiasma were prepared for light-microscopic examination. The size of infarction was measured as the percentage of the area of the ipsilateral hemisphere and was expressed as the mean ± SEM.

Regional SDH activity was measured for the evaluation of mitochondrial respiration. The animals were sacrificed at 48 h after repeated ischemia, and the brains immediately removed and sectioned coronally at the chiasma level. Sections were submerged for 3 min in 1 % triphenyl tetrazolium solution kept at 35 °C. The speed of formazan accumulation on the coronal surface was quantified with the use of an image-analyzing system, and a map of SDH activity was generated (NIH Image 1.57) [9]. In the no-preconditioning group, the animals were subjected only to repeated ischemia (two 10-min periods of ischemia separated by a 5-h interval).

Results

Histological examination revealed cortical infarction in the no-preconditioning group. The infarction was located in the left dorsolateral part of the cortex, and the size was 2.28±0.75 % of the ipsilateral hemisphere. In the adjacent cortex, many neurons showing cytoplasmic eosinophilia (ischemic change) were scattered among neurons with a normal appearance. The ischemic neurons were distributed throughout the cortical layers II–VI (DSNN).

In the preconditioned group, infarction was localized in the middle layer of the left dorsolateral cortex. The sizes were 0.48±0.24 %, 0.11±0.04 % and 0.40±0.17 % of the ipsilateral hemisphere after 48-h, 60-h and 72-h intervals, respectively (Fig. 1); the

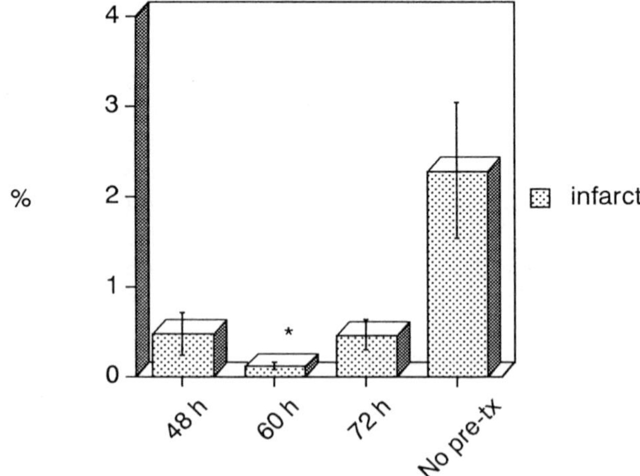

Fig. 1. Size of infarction (percentage of area of the ipsilateral hemisphere) 7 days after repeated cerebral ischemia in gerbils, with or without ischemic preconditioning. Eight minutes of ischemia (ischemic preconditioning) was experienced 48, 60 and 72 h before repeated ischemia (two 10-min occlusions of the left common carotid artery, separated by a 5-h interval). Infarction in the animals with ischemic preconditioning 60 h before repeated ischemia was significantly ($P<0.05$) smaller than that of the no-preconditioning group

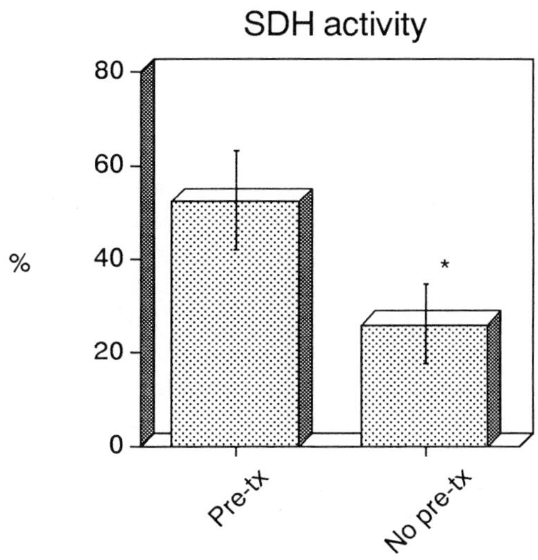

Fig. 2. Succinic dehydrogenase activity (percentage activity of the control animals) 48 h after repeated ischemia in gerbils, with or without ischemic preconditioning. The reduction was significant only in the no-preconditioning group

size after a 60-h interval was significantly ($P<0.05$) smaller than that of the no-preconditioning group. Regional SDH activity was significantly decreased in the left dorsolateral part of the cortex ($26.2\pm8.7\%$ of the control, $P<0.05$). The area of very low SDH activity (less than 20 % of the control) was observed in the cortical middle layer, which was surrounded by an area of more mild SDH reduction. In the preconditioned group, the decrease in SDH activity was less ($52.5\pm10.6\%$, n.s. compared with control) than that without preconditioning (Fig. 2). The area of very low SDH activity was smaller or not observed in the preconditioned group.

Discussion

We have observed that cortical infarction after repeated ischemia in gerbil is significantly smaller in animals with an 8-min ischemic preconditioning. An experimental model for repeated ischemic attacks has been developed, using different procedures and animal species. The effect of repetition on tissue injury has varied among different reports. Tomida et al. observed a pronounced cumulative effect on the development of edema and tissue injury in gerbils after repetitive occlusion of the bilateral common carotid artery [14]. Hanyu et al. observed that ischemic change became smaller with a longer (12 h) ischemic interval in gerbils after repetitive occlusion of the left common carotid artery [4]. Kitagawa et al. observed amelioration of CA1 injury in gerbils after bilateral common carotid-artery occlusion, when ischemic preconditioning was administered 24 h, but not 12 h before ischemia [7]. In the present study, infarction size was smaller when ischemic preconditioning was experienced 48–72 h before lethal ischemia. Therefore, the time interval between ischemic preconditioning and subsequent ischemia appears to be a crucial factor, resulting in either beneficial or harmful effects on the ischemic injury. Different mechanisms are probably triggered, depending on the interval.

Ischemic tolerance has also been observed in the heart. Brief episodes of ischemia render the myocardium more tolerant to subsequent lethal ischemia, as evidenced by reduced infarct size, delayed ultrastructural changes and improved myocardial function during reperfusion. Ischemic tolerance in the heart has been induced in multiple species between 1 min and 60 min after preconditioning and lasts for 3 h in most studies [1]. The pharmacological opening of the adenosine triphosphate (ATP)-dependent potassium (K/ATP) channel induces this tolerance [13], which is abolished by antagonists that abolish the tolerance [2]. The early window of tolerance in the heart fits with a permeability change in ionic channels. Therefore, K/ATP channels are involved in the protection of the heart by ischemic preconditioning.

The time course of the onset and duration of ischemic tolerance differs between the brain and the heart. Relatively long time intervals (24 h or more) for induction of tolerance in the brain do not fit the permeability change in ionic channels, but rather indicate the involvement of tolerance-related genes and proteins. Indeed, several studies have demonstrated the involvement of heat-shock proteins (HSPs) in the tolerance phenomenon of the brain. However, recent data indicate that the change in cellular-energy metabolism is also closely associated with the ischemic-tolerance phenomenon in the brain. Riepe et al. have observed that ischemic tolerance was induced in hippocampal slices of the brain by chemical preconditioning using an inhibitor of SDH, 3-nitropropionic acid (3-NP) [11, 12]. They noted that the application of 3-NP resulted in improved postischemic neuronal action potentials and morphological ischemic changes of neurons in rat hippocampal slices. Glibenclamide, an antagonist at K/ATP channels, partly reversed the chemical preconditioning induced by 3-NP. Benzi et al. observed that ischemic tolerance is related to a change in the activity of synaptosomal ATPases [3].

We have reported that reduction of SDH activity 48 h after repeated ischemia was milder in the preconditioned group and that the area of reduction was also smaller. These results indicate milder impairment of postischemic energy metabolism in the cortex after induction of ischemic tolerance. Since the development of infarction takes several days in the present model, the observed change may have a causative role on the infarction process.

Recently, Kuroda et al. [8] observed, in rats subjected to a transient focal cerebral ischemia, that postischemic energy impairment is a slowly developing process with a biphasic pattern of impairment. The significance of the secondary impairment on the ischemic-tissue injury was speculated in their study. We think energy impairment in the maturation of ischemic injury should be further investigated in relation to the ischemic tolerance of the brain.

References

1. Alkhulaifi AM, Pugsley WB, Yellon DM (1993) The influence of the time period between preconditioning ischemia and prolonged ischemia on myocardial protection. Cardioscience 4: 163–169
2. Auchampach JA, Gross GJ (1993) Anti-ischaemic actions of potassium channel openers in experimental myocardial ischemia/reperfusion injury in dogs. Eur Heart J 14: 10–15
3. Benzi G, Gorini A, Arnaboldi R, Ghigini B, Villa R (1993) Effect of intermittent mild hypoxia and drug treatment on synaptosomal nonmitochondrial ATPase activities. J Neurosci Res 34: 654–663
4. Hanyu S, Ito U, Hakamata Y, Yoshida M (1995) Transition from ischemic neuronal necrosis to infarction in repeated ischemia. Brain Res 686: 44–48

5. Hanyu S, Ito U, Hakamata Y, Nakano I (1997) Topographical analysis of cortical neuronal loss associated with disseminated selective neuronal necrosis and infarction after repeated ischemia. Brain Res 767: 154–157
6. Ito U, Hanyu S, Hakamata Y, Kuroiwa T, Yoshida M (1997) Maturation phenomenon in cerebral ischemia II. Springer-Verlag, Berlin Heidelberg New York, pp 115–121
7. Kitagawa K, Matsumoto M, Tagaya M, Hata R, Ueda H, Niinobe M, Handa N, Fukunaga R, Kimura K, Mikoshiba K (1990) Ischemic tolerance phenomenon found in the brain. Brain Res 528: 21–24
8. Kuroda S, Katsura K, Hillered L, Bates TE, Siesjo BK (1996) Delayed treatment with alpha-phenyl-N-tert-butyl nitrone (PBN) attenuates secondary mitochondrial dysfunction after transient focal cerebral ischemia in the rat. Neurobiol Dis 3: 149–157
9. Kuroiwa T, Terakado M, Yamaguchi T, Endo S, Ueki M, Okeda R (1996) The pyramidal cell layer of sector CA 1 shows the lowest hippocampal succinic dehydrogenase activity in normal and postischemic gerbils. Neurosci Lett 206: 1–4
10. Ohno K, Ito U, Inaba Y (1984) Regional cerebral blood flow and stroke index after left carotid artery ligation in the conscious gerbil. Brain Res 297: 151–157
11. Riepe M, Esclaire F, Kaskscheke K, Schreiber S, Nakase H, Kempski O, Ludolph AC, Dirnagl U, Hugon J (1997) Increased hypoxic tolerance by chemical inhibition of oxidative phosphorylation: "chemical preconditioning". J Cereb Blood Flow Metabol 17: 257–264
12. Riepe M, Hori N, Ludolph AC, Carpenter DO, Spencer PS, Allen CN (1992) Inhibition of energy metabolism by 3-nitropropionic acid activates ATP-sensitive potassium channels. Brain Res 586: 61–66
13. Rohmann S, Weygandt H, Schelling P, Kie Soei L, Verdouw PD, Lues I (1994) Involvement of ATP-sensitive potassium channels in preconditioning protection. Basic Res Cardiol 89: 563–576
14. Tomida S, Nowak TS Jr., Vass K, Lohr JM, Klatzo I (1987) Experimental model for repetitive ischemic attacks in the gerbil: the cumulative effect of repeated ischemic insults. J Cereb Blood Flow Metabol 7: 773–782

Upregulation of Vascular Endothelial Growth Factor Protein Levels in Global Ischemia Induced by Cardiac Arrest and Resuscitation in Rat Brain

P. Pichiule, J. C. Chávez, K. Xu, and J. C. LaManna

Summary. Cardiac arrest and resuscitation results in reperfusion injury, which produces delayed selective neuronal cell loss and, in many cases, results in delayed mortality due to cerebral edema. We have shown that, in a rat model of reversible global ischemia of 12-min duration, significant cerebral edema occurs in the brain stem after 24 h. We found that vascular endothelial growth factor (VEGF) protein levels are significantly elevated in brain after 24 h and 48 h of reperfusion. We propose that increased VEGF expression is responsible for blood–brain barrier breakdown and vasogenic edema.

Introduction

Vascular endothelial growth factor (VEGF) is a specific mitogen for endothelial cells that has the ability to induce transient vascular leakage and is a potent angiogenic factor [14]. Reduction in tissue oxygen tension in a variety of pathological processes, including tumor growth, retinal ischemia, and myocardial and cerebral infarction, often lead to a compensatory neovascularization, with VEGF considered as an important mediator of this event [2, 4, 7, 10].

Insufficiently perfused tissue is also deprived of important metabolites, such as glucose, and it has been shown that VEGF is induced in response to hypoglycemia under normoxic conditions [11]. In addition, reperfusion of ischemic tissue often involves generation of reactive oxygen intermediates, which are also known to induce VEGF expression in vitro and in vivo [5].

In regions such as the brain stem, where cardiovascular and respiratory centers are located, vasogenic edema may be a detrimental factor in the survival of an animal subjected to cardiac arrest and resuscitation. Viewing VEGF as a stress-induced protein and considering its ability to increase vascular permeability, which can lead to vasogenic edema, we investigated VEGF expression in the brain after reversible global cerebral ischemia.

Materials and Methods

Induction of Global Cerebral Ischemia

Reversible global cerebral ischemia was achieved by modification of the cardiac-arrest model of Crumrine and LaManna [3]. Male Wistar rats (250–300 g) were anesthetized with 2.5 % halothane and 70 % nitrous oxide in oxygen. A silastic catheter

Maturation Phenomenon in Cerebral Ischemia III
U. Ito et al. (Eds.)
© Springer-Verlag Berlin Heidelberg 1999

was inserted through the external jugular vein into the right atrium. The ventral tail artery was cannulated to monitor systemic arterial blood pressure and obtain samples for blood gases and pH measurements. Body temperature was monitored by means of a rectal thermoprobe and kept at 37 °C, using a feedback-controlled infrared heat lamp. The rats were allowed to recover completely from anesthesia before induction of cardiac arrest.

Cardiac arrest was induced by a rapid, sequential intra-atrial injection of D-tubocurarine (0.3 mg) and ice-cold potassium-chloride solution (0.5 M; 0.12 ml/100 g body weight). Resuscitation efforts began after 5–7 min of arrest. For this purpose, rats were orotracheally intubated for mechanical ventilation, accompanied by chest compression and intravenous saline injection. Upon return of a spontaneous heartbeat, a small variable dose of epinephrine was administered as a bolus, intravenously, to achieve a mean arterial blood pressure of at least 80 mmHg. The duration of ischemia was 11–13 min and it was defined as the period between the decrease of blood pressure to zero and its return to 80 mmHg. Ventilation was adjusted to achieve normoxia and normocapnia until the rats gained spontaneous respiration. Control animals were subjected to the whole surgical procedure, except that they did not undergo cardiac arrest and resuscitation.

Western-Blot Analysis

Animals were sacrificed 1, 24, and 48 h after cardiac arrest and resuscitation. Brains were quickly removed and cortex, brain stem and hippocampus were dissected and homogenized in ice-cold buffer (50 mM Tris/HCl, 1 mM EDTA, pH 7.4) containing protease inhibitors (1 µg/ml leupeptine, 10 µg/ml aprotinin, 100 µg/ml phenylmethylsulfonyl fluoride, 1 µg/ml pepstatin). Homogenates were centrifuged at 10,000 g for 15 min at 4 °C and the supernatants used for Western-blot analysis. Protein concentrations were determined by Bradford protein assay with bovine serum albumin as standard (Bio-Rad Inc). Samples containing 100 µg protein were electrophoresed on 12 % sodium dodecyl sulfate (SDS)-polyacrylamide gels under reducing conditions. Gels were run in sets consisting of samples from the same regions of brains from controls, after 1, 24, and 48 h of reperfusion. The proteins on the gels were transferred to polyvinylidene difluoride (PVDF) membranes that were then incubated with 10 % skim milk in Tris-buffered saline for 12 h to block nonspecific binding.

VEGF was detected by incubating the membranes with a 1: 100 dilution of polyclonal VEGF antibody (Santa Cruz Biotechnology) for 2 h at room temperature, followed by incubation with horseradish peroxidase-conjugated anti-rabbit immunoglobulin G (IgG) (1: 3000) for 2 h. The immunoreactive protein band was visualized using enhanced chemiluminescence-detection system (ECL Kit, Amersham). Autoradiographic results were quantified by means of densitometry.

Determination of Water Content by Wet/Dry Weight Ratio

The rats were allowed to recover for 1, 6, 24, and 48 h (n=5 for each group) from 12-min cardiac arrest. After in situ freeze fixation, brain samples were taken from cortical, brain stem, and hippocampal regions. The tissue samples were quickly placed into tared, dried, capped Eppendorf tubes and weighed to determine tissue wet weight. The tissues were then dried to constant weight at 100 °C to determine tissue dry weight. Water content (%) was calculated as (wet weight–dry weight)/wet weight·100.

Statistical Analysis

VEGF data were expressed as the ratio of the density of the post-resuscitation samples with respect to the control density for five different sets of brains. The data were reported as means (±1SD). The one-sample t-test was used to determine whether the ischemic:control ratio of VEGF protein density was significantly greater than one. Comparisons among VEGF ratios at various time-points were assessed by analysis of variance (ANOVA) followed by Bonferroni correction. In all cases, $P<0.05$ was considered significant.

Results

Global Cerebral Ischemia and Resuscitation

The major pathophysiological central, systemic vascular and metabolic effects of 12 min of cardiac arrest and resuscitation in the rat have been reported previously [6]. These include an initial arterial acidosis, hypertension and hemoconcentration, which returned to pre-arrest values by 30 min of reperfusion. Central changes in blood flow and metabolism are also rapidly reversed. The rats regained spontaneous respiration within 6 h after resuscitation and usually regained consciousness before 24 h. Generally, by 36 h, the resuscitated rats were able to move and feed themselves.

Western-Blot Analysis

Among the four VEGF isoforms described, $VeGF_{120}$, $VeGF_{164}$, $VeGF_{189}$ are expressed in rat brain, while $VeGF_{205}$ might be very low or not expressed in rat [1, 8]. The polyclonal VEGF antibody used in this study detected a single band at a molecular mass of ~23 kDa (Fig. 1a), which most likely corresponds to $VEGF_{164}$. This band was present in control, non-arrested rats. After 1 h of cardiac arrest and resuscitation, VEGF protein levels remained equal to the controls in the cortex, hippocampus and brain stem. However, after 24 h, VEGF protein significantly increased, about double, remaining elevated after 48 h of recovery ($n=5$). The mean increase was about the same in each region (Fig. 1b).

Wet Weight/ Dry Weight

Beginning at about 6 h of reperfusion, the rat brains exhibited signs of edema, as indicated by increased wet weight/dry weight ratios. In the cerebral cortex and hippocampus, the edema appeared to be maximum at 6 h. In the brain-stem samples, the

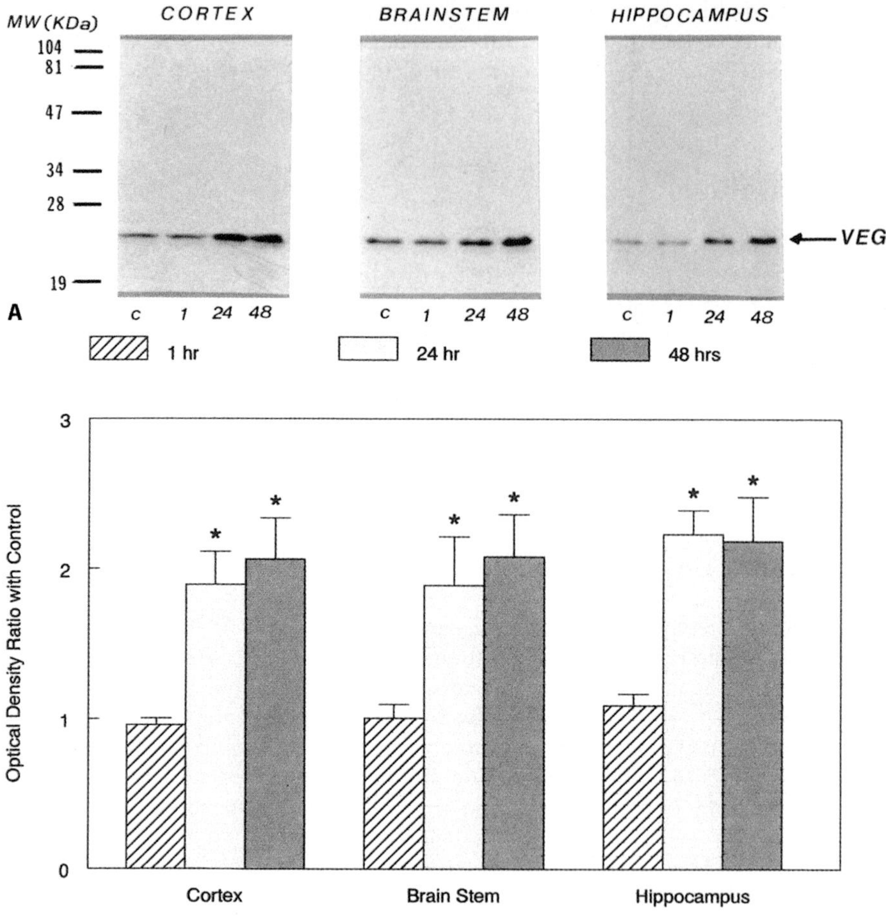

Fig. 1. A, B Increased expression of vascular endothelial growth factor (VEGF) after cardiac arrest and resuscitation. **A** An example of a Western blot of VEGF protein from cerebral cortex, hippocampus and brain-stem samples. **B** Graph of VEGF Western-blot density ratios for the three brain regions (mean±1SD, n=5, *P<0.05)

maximum effect was seen after 24 h of reperfusion. There were still signs of persistent edema after 24 h of reperfusion, although the increased wet weight/dry weight ratios did not reach statistical significance at 48 h (Fig. 2).

Discussion

Our results show an upregulation of VEGF protein levels after 24 h and 48 h of recovery from total cerebral ischemia. We were able to detect a single band that was probably associated with $VEGF_{164}$, which has been described as the predominant isoform

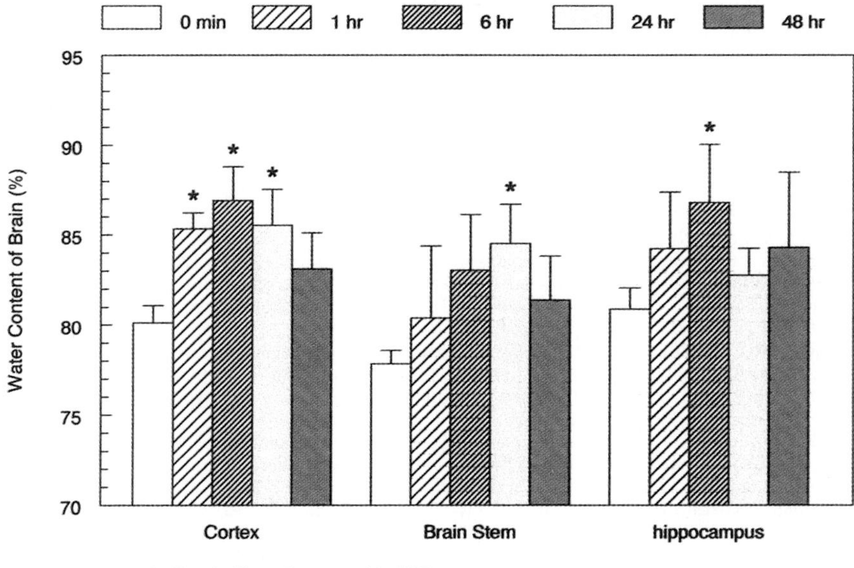

Fig. 2. Wet weight/dry weight ratios after cardiac arrest and resuscitation in cerebral cortex, hippocampus and brain stem (mean±1SD, $n=5$, *$P<0.05$)

expressed in many tissues. Immunoreactivity was observed not only in post-ischemic tissues, but also in control tissues in concordance with previous reports showing basal VEGF expression in normal brain [1, 8]. Based on our results, we cannot come to a conclusion on whether or not transient global ischemia affected the expression of the other VEGF isoforms.

Hypoxia is a strong inducer of upregulation of VEGF, which seems to be a general response, since different cultured cell types and tissues increase VEGF expression at low oxygen tensions. This upregulation is achieved, at least in vitro, by means of increasing both transcription and mRNA stability [12].

Reactive oxygen species (ROS) are also an important factor for induction of VEGF expression. In fact, it has been shown that ROS induce VEGF expression in vitro and in vivo during reperfusion of ischemic retina [5]. Our model of global cerebral ischemia induced by cardiac arrest and resuscitation includes at least two critical events: 12 min of ischemia, followed by reperfusion, during which ROS generation occurs. Both events are relevant stimuli for VEGF expression.

It is well known that VEGF plays a critical role in mediating the increase of both capillary permeability and angiogenesis. Its role in blood–brain-barrier breakdown has been proposed in tumor-associated cerebral edema and focal ischemia [4, 13]. VEGF increases permeability to $[C^{14}]$-sucrose in cultured endothelial cells derived from cerebral microvessels in a dose- and time-dependent fashion [15].

Considering its biological activity, we propose that the sustained elevation of VEGF expression after cardiac arrest and resuscitation is responsible for the increased vascular permeability and opening of the blood–brain barrier found 24 h after reversible global ischemia [9], leading to a vasogenic edema and eventually stimulation of new vessel formation. VEGF-induced brain-stem edema may be the primary cause of the increased mortality observed between 1 day and 3 days after successful resuscitation after cardiac arrest.

References

1. Bacic M, Edwards NA, Merrill MJ (1995) Differential expression of vascular endothelial growth factor (vascular permeability factor) forms in rat tissues. Growth Factors 12: 11–15
2. Banai S, Jaklitsch MT, Shou M, Lazarous DF, Scheinowitz M, Biro S, Epstein SE, Unger EF (1994) Angiogenic-induced enhancement of collateral blood flow to ischemic myocardium by vascular endothelial growth factor in dogs. Circulation 89: 2183–2189
3. Crumrine RC, LaManna JC (1991) Regional cerebral metabolites, blood flow, plasma volume and mean transit time in total cerebral ischemia in the rat. J Cereb Blood Flow Metab 11: 272–282
4. Kovács Z, Ikezaki K, Samoto K, Inamura T, Fukui M (1996) VEGF and flt expression time kinetics in rat brain infarct. Stroke 27: 1865–1873
5. Kuroki M, Voest EE, Amano S, Beerepoort LV, Takashima S, Tolentino M, Kim RY, Rohan RM, Colby KA, Yeo K-T, Adamis AP (1996) Reactive oxygen intermediates increase vascular endothelial growth factor expression in vitro and in vivo. J Clin Invest 98: 1667–1675
6. LaManna JC, Griffith JK, Cordisco BR, Bell HE, Lin C-W, Pundik S, Lust WD (1995) Rapid recovery of rat brain intracellular pH after cardiac arrest and resuscitation. Brain Res 687: 175–181
7. Miller JW, Adamis AP, Shima DT, D'Amore PA, Moulton RS, O'Reilly MS, Folkman J, Dvorak HF, Brown LF, Berse B, Yeo T-K, Yeo K-T (1994) Vascular endothelial growth factor/vascular permeability factor is temporally and spatially correlated with ocular angiogenesis in a primate model. Am J Pathol 145: 574–584
8. Monacci WT, Merrill MJ, Oldfield EH (1993) Expression of vascular permeability factor/vascular endothelial growth factor in normal rat tissues. Am J Physiol 264:C995–C1002
9. Pluta R, Lossinsky AS, Wisniewski HM, Mossakowski MJ (1994) Early blood–brain barrier changes in the rat following transient complete cerebral ischemia induced by cardiac arrest. Brain Res 633: 41–52
10. Shweiki D, Itin A, Soffer D, Keshet E (1992) Vascular endothelial growth factor induced by hypoxia may mediate hypoxia-initiated angiogenesis. Nature 359: 843–845
11. Shweiki D, Neeman M, Itin A, Keshet E (1995) Induction of vascular endothelial growth factor expression by hypoxia and by glucose deficiency in multicell spheroids: implications for tumor angiogenesis. Proc Natl Acad Sci U S A 92: 768–772
12. Stein I, Neeman M, Shweiki D, Itin A, Keshet E (1995) Stabilization of vascular endothelial growth factor mRNA by hypoxia and hypoglycemia and coregulation with other ischemia-induced genes. Mol Cell Biol 15: 5363–5368
13. Strugar J, Rothbart D, Harrington W, Criscuolo GR (1994) Vascular permeability factor in brain metastases: correlation with vasogenic brain edema and tumor angiogenesis. J Neurosurg 81: 560–566
14. Thomas KA (1996) Vascular endothelial growth factor, a potent and selective angiogenic agent. J Biol Chem 271: 603–606
15. Wang W, Merrill MJ, Borchardt RT (1996) Vascular endothelial growth factor affects permeability of brain microvessel endothelial cells in vitro. Am J Physiol 271:C1973–C1980

Neuroprotective Effect of Hepatocyte Growth Factor

T. Miyazawa, K. Matsumoto, N. Tsuzuki, H. Nakau, T. Yamashima, K. Shima, and T. Nakamura

Summary. Hepatocyte growth factor (HGF), a natural ligand for the c-Met proto-oncogene product, exhibits mitogenic, motogenic, and morphogenic activities during regeneration of the liver, kidney, and lung. Recently, HGF was clearly shown to enhance neurite outgrowth in vitro. To determine whether HGF has a neuroprotective effect, i.e., prevents the death of neurons, in vivo, we studied the effect of HGF on delayed neuronal death in the hippocampus after 5 min transient forebrain ischemia in Mongolian gerbils. Continuous postischemic intrastriatal administration of human recombinant HGF (10 µg or 30 µg) for 7 days potently prevented the delayed death of hippocampal neurons under both anesthetized and awake conditions. Even when HGF infusion started 6 h after ischemia, i.e., in a delayed manner, HGF exhibited a neuroprotective effect. We conclude that HGF, a novel neurotrophic factor, has a profound neuroprotective effect against postischemic delayed neuronal death in the hippocampus, which may have implications for the development of new therapeutic strategies for ischemic neuronal damage in humans.

Introduction

Hepatocyte growth factor (HGF) is a pleiotrophic cytokine which exhibits mitogenic, motogenic and morphogenic activities toward a wide variety of cells [16, 18, 25]. Physiologically, HGF plays an important role as an organotrophic factor, responsible for vigorous regeneration of the liver, kidney and lung [2, 16, 18, 25]. HGF and the c-Met/HGF receptor of membrane-spanning tyrosine kinase are expressed in various regions of the brain, and functional coupling of HGF and c-Met enhances the survival of hippocampal neurons in primary culture and induces neurite outgrowth during neuronal development in vitro [9, 11, 13, 24]. HGF plays a role as a chemoattractant for the projection of motor neurons to limb muscles [7], and is as potent a survival factor for motor neurons as are other survival factors, such as brain-derived neurotrophic factor (BDNF) [1, 19], ciliary neurotrophic factor (CNTF) [20], glial-cell-line-derived neurotrophic factor (GDNF) [10] and basic fibroblast growth factor (bFGF) [23]. This accumulating evidence has implied a neurotrophic function of HGF; however, there have been no reports on whether HGF exhibits a neurotrophic effect in vivo. In the present study, to determine whether HGF has a neuroprotective effect against the death of neurons in vivo, we studied the effect of HGF on delayed neuronal death following transient forebrain ischemia in gerbils [14], using continuous topical administration of HGF directly into the brain [17].

Maturation Phenomenon in Cerebral Ischemia III
U. Ito et al. (Eds.)
© Springer-Verlag Berlin Heidelberg 1999

Materials and Methods

Animal Preparation

Fifty-six male Mongolian gerbils weighing 50–70 g were divided into seven experimental groups. Anesthesia was administered with an initial concentration of 3 % halothane, then maintained with 1.5 % halothane in a mixture of 40 %O_2/60 %N_2O via a face mask. In experiments 1 and 2, a needle electrode was placed in the subscalpal space for electroencephalogram (EEG) recording to confirm electrical cessation during ischemia. Body temperature was monitored and maintained at 37 °C throughout the experiments, using a feedback-controlled heating pad.

Experiment 1:
Continuous Intrastriatal Administration of HGF Under Halothane Anesthesia

At first, an osmotic minipump (Alzet model 2001; Palo Alto, Calif., USA) containing human recombinant HGF (10 µg or 30 µg) or a physiological saline solution (PSS) was implanted. A cannula device connected to the subcutaneously implanted osmotic minipump was inserted into the right striatum from a point 1 mm anterior, 2 mm lateral, and 4 mm ventral to the bregma, and fixed with dental cement to the skull. To start infusion just after implantation, each osmotic minipump was incubated in physiological saline at 37 °C according to the instructions of Alzet. HGF was intrastriatally administered for 1 week during reperfusion. Approximately 30 min after implantation of the pump, both carotid arteries were occluded for 5 min with Sugita temporary-aneurysm clips. Complete forebrain ischemia was confirmed by the electrical cessation on EEG. The animals were divided into four groups as follows:

– Group 1 ($n=6$). Sham-operated animals. The sham operation included carotid manipulation and cannula placement in the right striatum.
– Group 2 ($n=9$). Ischemia and implantation of a minipump containing PSS.
– Group 3 ($n=9$). Ischemia and implantation of a minipump containing 10 µg HGF.
– Group 4 ($n=9$). Ischemia and implantation of a minipump containing 30 µg HGF.

Experiment 2:
Delayed Start of Continuous Intrastriatal Administration of HGF

Animals were subjected to 5 min transient forebrain ischemia similar to that described for experiment 1. After recovery from anesthesia, the animals were returned to their cages and given free access to water. Six hours after the beginning of recirculation, an osmotic minipump containing 30 µg HGF was implanted under halothane anesthesia. The osmotic minipump had been incubated in PSS at 37 °C before the experiment. Thus, the administration of HGF started 6 h after ischemia and continued for 7 days (Group 5, $n=9$). Group 2 was used as a control group.

Experiment 3:
Continuous Intrastriatal Administration of HGF Under Awake Conditions

To exclude the possibility of a secondary neuroprotective effect of halothane per se [8] and postischemic secondary hypothermia [3, 15], animals were subjected to ischemia under awake conditions. Anesthesia was initially performed and an osmotic minipump was implanted without prior incubation. To accomplish awake forebrain ischemia, the first thread was looped around both common carotid arteries, while the second thread was ligated on the loop. The ends of the first thread were led out through the nuchal muscle and back skin, and left until the start of ischemia. After closure of the wounds, halothane inhalation was discontinued, and at least 2 h were allowed for complete recovery from the anesthesia. The animals were subjected to 5 min forebrain ischemia under awake conditions, without any pain, by occlusion of both common carotid arteries; this was accomplished by pulling the ends of the first thread. The loss of the righting reflex was taken as evidence of forebrain ischemia under awake conditions. The ends of the second thread were pulled to release the carotid occlusion. In this experiment, because the osmotic minipumps were not incubated at 37 °C, the infusion usually started 3–4 h after implantation, i.e., 1–2 h after ischemia. The animals were divided into two groups as follows:

– Group 6 ($n=7$). Awake ischemia and implantation of a minipump containing PSS.
– Group 7 ($n=7$). Awake ischemia and implantation of a minipump containing 30 µg HGF.

Evaluation

Seven days after ischemia, the animals were transcardially perfused with 4 % paraformaldehyde in 0.01 M phosphate-buffered saline. Infusion of the agent into the striatum was confirmed by an empty implant pump at sacrifice. The brains were removed, immersed in the fixative for 24 h, then embedded in paraffin. Paraffin sections (3 µm) were stained with cresyl-violet. The number of intact neurons in the center of the hippocampal CA1 sector was determined, averaged, and expressed as both the neuronal density per 1 mm linear length and as a percentage of the mean value observed for the sham-operated group. The investigator performing the cell counting was blind to the treatment of each section. Statistical significance was analyzed using a one-factor analysis of variance (ANOVA), followed by Scheffé's F-test. Data are expressed as mean ± SD (Fig. 1).

Results and Discussion

The present results constitute the first hard evidence that HGF can potently protect hippocampal neurons from ischemic insult in vivo. At first, gerbils were subjected to transient forebrain ischemia under halothane anesthesia and then human recombinant HGF or saline was infused using an osmotic minipump. The absolute values per millimeter of intact neurons in a bilateral CA1 sector of the hippocampus after 7 days

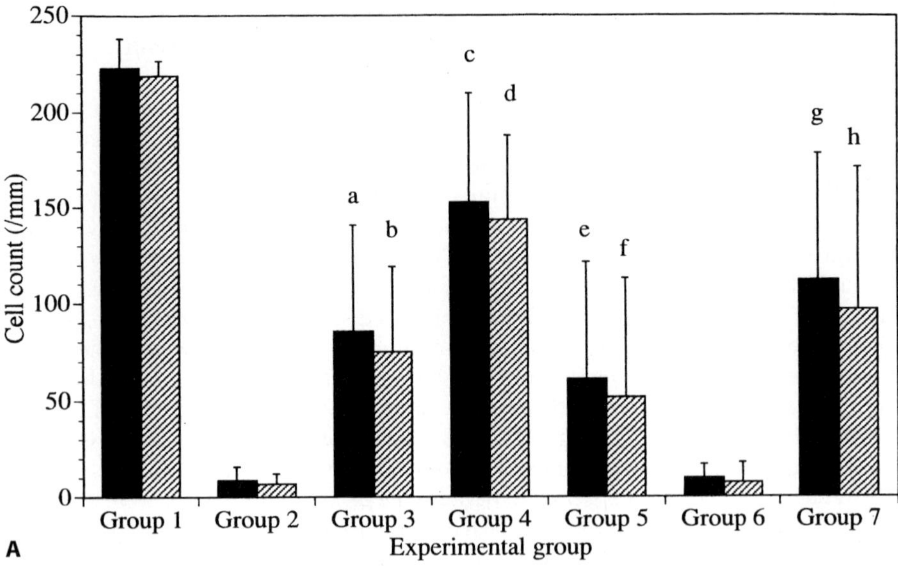

Fig. 1 A. Graphical representation of the number of viable neurons in the center of a bilateral hippo-campal CA1 sector. The number of viable neurons was determined, averaged, and expressed as the neuronal density per millimeter linear length; data is expressed as mean ± SD. *Black bars* right side; *hatched bars* left side. Group 1 ($n=6$) sham-operated animals (*right*: 222.8±15.3, *left*: 218.8±7.6); group 2 ($n=9$) ischemia and implantation of a minipump containing PSS (*right*: 8.9±6.8, *left*: 7±5.3); group 3 ($n=9$) ischemia and implantation of a minipump containing 10 µg HGF (*right*: 85.5±55.2, *left*: 75.1±44.3); group 4 ($n=9$) ischemia and implantation of a minipump containing 30 µg HGF (*right*: 152.7±57.2, *left*: 143.8±68.0); group 5 ($n=9$) delayed start of HGF-infusion 6 h after ischemia (*right*: 61.2±60.5, *left*: 51.9±61.3); group 6 ($n=7$) awake ischemia and implantation of a minipump containing PSS (*right*: 9.7±7.3, *left*: 7.6±10.4); group 7 ($n=7$) awake ischemia and implantation of a minipump containing 30 µg HGF (*right*: 112.1±66.5, *left*: 96.9±74.7). Statistical differences were evaluated by one-factor analysis of variance (ANOVA), followed by Scheffé's *F*-test. Groups 3, 4 and 5 were com-pared with group 2 on each side. Group 7 was compared with group 6 on each side. *a–d* $P<0.001$ ver-sus group 2; *e, f* $P<0.05$ versus group 2; *g, h* $P<0.01$ versus group 6

of reperfusion are shown in Fig. 1. Measured relative to sham-operated animals (group 1), control animals infused with saline (group 2) had only 3–4% of the neu-rons survive following forebrain ischemia. In contrast, continuous intrastriatal administration of HGF for 7 days during reperfusion prevented the delayed neuronal death in a dose-dependent manner (groups 3 and 4). In animals infused with 30 µg HGF (group 4), approximately two-thirds of the neurons survived relative to sham-operated animals; this number of surviving neurons is approximately 20-fold greater than that observed for PSS-infused animals.

With regard to the clinical application of neurotrophic factors, they must be neu-roprotective when administered after, not before or during, cerebral ischemia. In most studies of the neuroprotective effects in a brain ischemia model, however, the neurotrophic factors were administered before initiation of ischemia [1, 21, 22]. We, therefore, examined whether HGF had a neuroprotective effect even when HGF-infusion started 6 h after forebrain ischemia. About one-quarter of the neurons sur-vived in animals subjected to delayed HGF infusion (group 5), which was approxi-

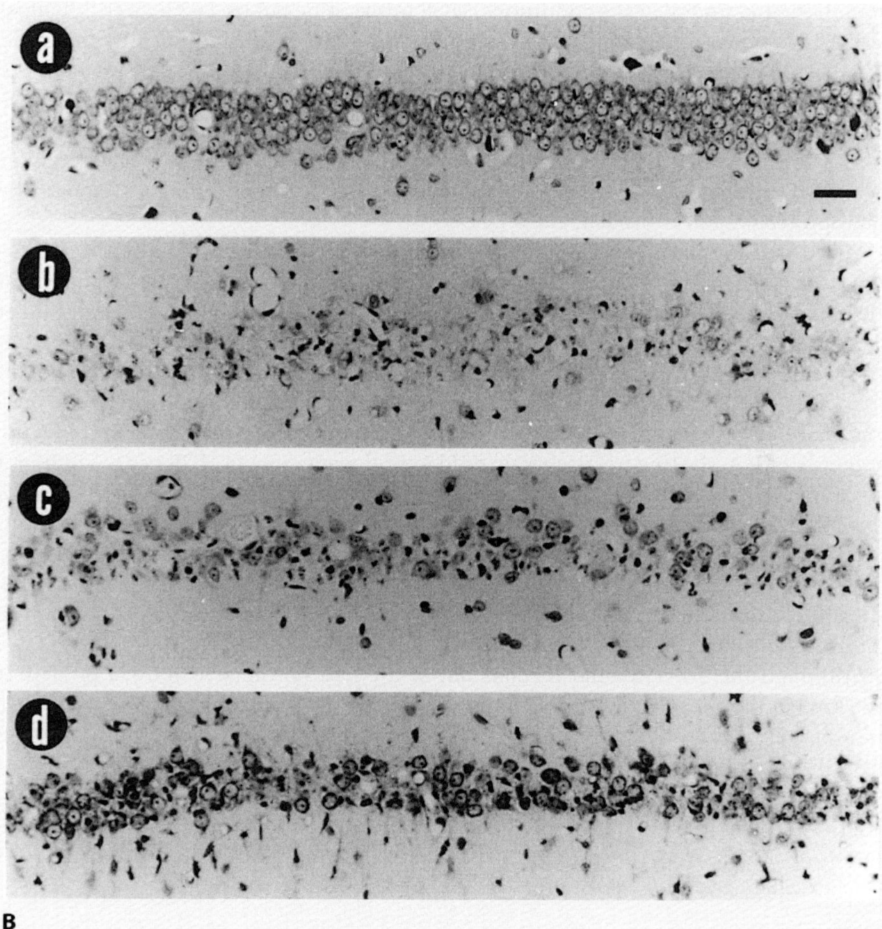

Fig. 1 B. Microphotographs of hippocampal pyramidal neurons in the CA1 sector of representative animal in each experimental group. *a* Sham-operated animal, *b* animal with PSS administration, *c* animal with 10 µg HGF administration, *d* animal with 30 µg HGF administration. *Scale bar* indicates 50 µm

mately sevenfold higher than in control PSS-infused animals. Thus, the delayed infusion of HGF significantly prevented delayed neuronal death of CA1 pyramidal neurons following forebrain ischemia. The significant neuroprotection by HGF infused in a delayed manner is encouraging for the practical application of HGF for the treatment of patients with ischemic neuronal injury.

During verification of neuroprotective agents, the neuroprotective effects of halothane per se [8] and post-anesthetic secondary hypothermia [3, 15] were found to frequently modify experimental results. To exclude the possibility of such secondary neuroprotective effects, animals were subjected to ischemia under awake conditions. At 2 h after discontinuation of anesthesia, the animals were subjected to 5 min forebrain ischemia under awake conditions. HGF infusion began by 1–2 h after ischemia. In the ischemic animals under awake conditions, 30 µg HGF significantly prevented the delayed neuronal death even after awake ischemia (group 7) compared with the data for the control group (group 6), thereby indicating that the neuroprotective effect of HGF was not due to post-anesthetic secondary hypothermia or halothane per se. Furthermore, the fact that ischemia was probably much more severe under awake conditions than under halothane anesthesia [12] rather strongly supports the neuroprotective effect of HGF.

Given that hippocampal CA1 neurons in rats express c-Met mRNA and HGF prolongs the survival of hippocampal neurons in primary culture [11], we presume that the neuroprotective effect of HGF on CA1 neurons is mediated by c-Met. Yamagata et al. [24] demonstrated selective HGF messenger ribonucleic acid (mRNA) expression in the microglia of rat brain, and c-Met mRNA expression in neurons as well as in astrocytes and microglia. This implies the possibility of interactions between neurons, astrocytes and microglia mediated by HGF and its receptor. In our study, the influence of long-lasting postischemic mild hypothermia due to HGF per se could not be completely excluded [4, 5], and we do not have data on the effects of HGF at the chronic stage (1–2 months after ischemia). Because previous studies clearly demonstrated a neurotrophic effect of HGF on neurons in primary culture under strict control of the medium temperature [11], we believe that the neurotrophic effect of HGF after forebrain ischemia persists longer, and not that HGF delays the progression of "delayed neuronal death", as seen in hypothermic animals [6].

Although the exact cellular mechanism of the neuroprotective activity of HGF is not known, our results should facilitate further studies of different modes of HGF administration as well as of the effective time window for the neuroprotective effect of HGF toward ischemic neuronal injury.

Acknowledgements. This study was partly supported by the Uehara Memorial Foundation of Japan. We wish to thank Miss Namiko Nomura and Miss Akiko Yano for their excellent technical assistance.

References

1. Beck T, Lindholm D, Castren E, Wree A (1994) Brain-derived neurotrophic factor protects against ischemic cell damage in rat hippocampus. J Cereb Blood Flow Metab 14: 689–692
2. Boros P, Miller CM (1995) Hepatocyte growth factor: a multifunctional cytokine. Lancet 345: 293–295
3. Corbett T, Evans S, Thomas C, Wang D, Jonas RA (1990) MK-801 reduced cerebral ischemic injury by inducing hypothermia. Brain Res 514: 300–304
4. Corbourne F, Corbett D (1994) Delayed and prolonged postischemic hypothermia is neuroprotective in the gerbil. Brain Res 564: 265–272
5. Dietrich WD, Busto P, Alonso O, Globus MYT, Ginsberg MD (1993) Intraischemic but not postischemic brain hypothermia protects chronically following global forebrain ischemia in rats. J Cereb Blood Flow Metab 13: 541–549
6. Dietrich WD, Lin B, Globus MYT, Green EJ, Ginsberg MD, Busto R (1995) Effect of delayed MK-801 (Dizocilpine) treatment with or without immediate postischemic hypothermia on chronic neuronal survival after global forebrain ischemia in rats. J Cereb Blood Flow Metab 15: 960–968
7. Ebens A, Brose K, Leonardo ED, Hanson MG Jr., Bladt F, Birchmeier C, Barres BA, Tessier-Lavigne M (1996) Hepatocyte growth factor/scatter factor is an axonal chemoattractant and neurotrophic factor for spinal motor neurons. Neuron 17: 1157–1172

8. Edgehouse NL, Dorman RV (1987) Ischemia-induced development of cerebral edema in awake and anesthetized gerbils. Neurochem Pathol 7: 169–179
9. Hamanoue M, Takemoto N, Matsumoto K, Nakamura T, Nakajima K (1996) Neurotrophic effect of hepatocyte growth factor on central nervous system neurons in vitro. J Neurosci Res 43: 554–564
10. Henderson CE, Phillips HS, Pollock RA, Davies AM, Lemeulle C, Armanini M, Simpson LC, Moffet B, Vandlen RA, Koliatsos VE, Rosenthal A (1994) GDNF: a potent survival factor for motoneurons present in peripheral nerve and muscle. Science 266: 1062–1064
11. Honda S, Kagoshima M, Wanaka A, Tohyama M, Matsumoto K, Nakamura T (1995) Localization and functional coupling of HGF and c-Met/HGF receptor in rat brain: implication as neurotrophic factor. Mol Brain Res 32: 197–210
12. Imon H, Mitani A, Andou Y, Arai T, Kataoka K (1991) Delayed neuronal death is induced without postischemic hyperexcitability: continuous multi-unit recording from ischemic CA1 neurons. J Cereb Blood Flow Metab 11: 819–823
13. Jung W, Castren E, Odenthal M, Van de Woude GF, Ishii T, Dienes HP, Lindholm D, Schirmacher P (1994) Expression and functional intereffect of hepatocyte growth factor-scatter factor and its receptor c-Met in mammalian brain. J Cell Biol 126: 485–494
14. Kirino T (1982) Delayed neuronal death in the gerbil hippocampus following ischemia. Brain Res 239: 57–69
15. Kuroiwa T, Bonnekoh P, Hossmann KA (1990) Prevention of postischemic hyperthermia prevents ischemic injury of CA1 neurons. J Cereb Blood Flow Metab 10: 550–556
16. Matsumoto K, Nakamura T (1996) Emerging multipotent aspects of hepatocyte growth factor. J Biochem 119: 591–600
17. Miyazawa T, Matsumoto K, Ohmichi H, Katoh H, Yamashima T, Nakamura T (1998) Protection of Hippocampal Neurons from Ischemia-Induced Delayed Neuronal Death by Hepatocyte Growth Factor: A Novel Neurotrophic Factor. J Cereb Blood Flow Metab 18: 345–348
18. Nakamura T, Nishizawa T, Hagiya M, Seki T, Shimonishi M, Shimizu S (1989) Molecular cloning and expression of human hepatocyte growth factor. Nature 342: 440–443
19. Oppenheim RW, Qin-Wei Y, Prevette D, Yan Q (1992) Brain-derived neurotrophic factor rescues developing avian motoneurons from cell death. Nature 360: 755–757
20. Sendtner M, Schmalbruch H, Stoeckli KA, Carroll P, Kreutzberg GW, Thoenen H (1992) Ciliary neurotrophic factor prevents degeneration of motor neurons in mouse mutant progressive motor neuropathy. Nature 358: 502–504
21. Shigeno T, Mima T, Takakura K, Graham DI, Kato G, Hashimoto Y (1991) Amelioration of delayed neuronal death in the hippocampus by nerve growth factor. J Neurosci 11: 2914–2919
22. Tsukahara T, Yonekawa Y, Tanaka K, Ohara O, Watanabe S, Kimura T, Nishijima T, Taniguchi T (1994) The role of brain-derived neurotrophic factor in transient forebrain ischemia in the rat brain. Neurosurgery 34: 323–331
23. Yamada K, Kinoshita A, Kohmura E, Sakaguchi T, Taguchi J, Kataoka K, Hayakawa T (1991) Basic fibroblast growth factor prevents thalamic degeneration after cortical infarction. J Cereb Blood Flow Metab 11: 472–478
24. Yamagata T, Muroya K, Mukasa T, Igarashi H, Momoi M, Tsukahara T, Arahata K, Kumagai H, Momoi T (1995) Hepatocyte growth factor specifically expressed in microglia activated Ras in the neurons, similar to the effect of neurotrophic factors. Biochem Biophys Res Commun 210: 231–237
25. Zarnegar R, Michalopoulos GK (1995) The many faces of hepatocyte growth factor: from hepatopoiesis to hematopoiesis. J Cell Biol 129: 1177–1180

III Factors Modulating Neuronal Plasticity and the Course of Maturation Phenomenon in Cerebral Ischemia (Metabolic and Inflammatory Factors)

Tumor Necrosis Factor-α-Induced Ischemic Tolerance as Manifested by Microvascular and Endothelial Cell Responses

D. Dawson, I. Ginis, J. Liu, M. Spatz, and J. M. Hallenbeck

D. Dawson and I. Ginis contributed equally to this work.

Summary. In spontaneously hypertensive rats subjected to middle-cerebral-artery occlusion, a preconditioning exposure to the cytokine-stimulating agent, lipopolysaccharide (0.9 mg/kg), 3 days prior to the focal brain ischemia conferred a state of tolerance, in which the infarct volume was smaller and the degree of microvascular-perfusion impairment was reduced, compared with control animals preconditioned with saline. In addition, brain capillary endothelial cells from Wistar–Kyoto rats could be preconditioned by a 4-h exposure to 20 ng/ml tumor necrosis factor-α (TNF-α). A second exposure to TNF-α or to hypoxia 20 h after the preconditioning stimulated significantly less expression of intercellular adhesion molecule-1 (ICAM-1) in these endothelial cell cultures compared with controls. The results indicate that protection of the microcirculation is one aspect of TNF-α-induced tolerance and that endothelial-cell activation as manifested by ICAM-1 expression can be attenuated by preconditioning exposure to TNF-α.

Introduction

The mechanisms that contribute to progressive brain damage in the penumbral region during acute focal brain ischemia are multifactorial and intricately interwoven [6]. The intricate interrelationships of these many pathogenic factors render acute stroke treatment an elusive goal. Identification of the mechanisms that regulate tolerance to ischemia could help guide investigators to more robust solutions of the stroke-treatment problem.

A variety of stressful stimuli can induce tolerance to ischemia. These would include sublethal ischemia [1, 10–12], hypothermia and oxidative stress [17]. Relative to a ligand–receptor interaction, these initiating stimuli are somewhat imprecise as starting points for the study of the intracellular signaling that regulates ischemic tolerance. The cytokines tumor necrosis factor alpha (TNF-α) and interleukin-1 (IL-1) activate intracellular signaling pathways that mediate stress responses [19] and could, therefore, function in ligand–receptor interactions that induce the tolerant state. To explore the possibility that cytokines have a role in the development of tolerance, lipopolysaccharide (LPS), which elicits the release of TNF-α and IL-1 [18], was administered to spontaneously hypertensive rats (SHRs) prior to middle-cerebral-artery occlusion (MCAO). Administration of LPS (0.9 mg/kg i.v.) 3 days before MCAO, induced a clear-cut ischemic tolerance, which could be blocked by TNF-

Maturation Phenomenon in Cerebral Ischemia III
U. Ito et al. (Eds.)
© Springer-Verlag Berlin Heidelberg 1999

binding protein, implicating TNF-α as a critical signaling factor [21]. This finding was further buttressed by the demonstration that intracisternal instillation of recombinant mouse TNF-α 0.5 g/mouse 48 h prior to MCAO-induced ischemic tolerance [3].

Tolerance to brain ischemia has generally been regarded as the consequence of factors that act upon brain parenchymal cells to induce cytoprotection. TNF-α has myriad effects on the state of the vasculature through its effects on endothelium and we have explored the possibility that ischemic tolerance induced by TNF-α involves protection of brain microcirculatory perfusion. We have also studied, in cultured brain capillary endothelial cells (BCECs), the capacity of a preconditioning exposure to hypoxia or TNF-α to suppress subsequent expression of the pro-inflammatory adhesion molecule, ICAM-1, in response to a second TNF-α exposure or hypoxia. The results show that a preconditioning exposure to LPS, which stimulates release of TNF-α, induces a state of ischemic tolerance that involves protection of the microcirculation.

Methods

Adult male SHRs were used for the in vivo experiments (*n*=5/group). Previous studies have established the most effective dose (0.9 mg/kg i.v.) and administration time point (72 h pre-MCAO) for development of LPS-induced tolerance [21]; these parameters were used in the present study.

On day 1, animals were anesthetized with halothane in nitrous oxide/oxygen (70: 30). LPS (0.9 mg/kg; from *Escherichia coli* 0111:B4 phenol extract; Sigma, St. Louis, Mo.) or an equivalent volume (1 ml/kg) of vehicle (sterile saline) was administered intravenously. Anesthetics were withdrawn and animals were returned to their home cages.

Induction of Focal Cerebral Ischemia

On day 4 (72 h post-LPS/saline injection), the rats were anesthetized again. Arterial blood pressure and blood gases were monitored and maintained at physiologic levels throughout the surgical procedure (approximately 0.5 h duration). Body temperature was maintained around 37 °C by means of a heating pad. The left MCA was exposed via a subtemporal approach and occluded between the inferior cerebral vein and lateral olfactory tract.

Following MCAO, the arterial cannula was removed, incision sites sutured and anesthetics withdrawn. The animal was kept on a heating pad until it fully regained consciousness. Rats were anesthetized 4 h post-MCAO, a tracheostomy was performed and rats were artificially respirated. The femoral vessels were recannulated. Arterial blood samples were collected as before, and blood pressure and blood gases monitored. Microvascular perfusion was measured using a double-label intravascular fluorescent-tracer technique previously described [3]. Two fluorescent tracers – Evans blue (2 % in saline; 0.2 ml/100 g body weight; Sigma) and fluorescein isothiocyanate (FITC)-dextran (10 % in saline; 0.2 ml/100 g body weight; 71,000 Da molecular weight; Sigma) – were used to obtain two measurements of microvascular perfusion within each animal. Following 4 h of MCAO, the tracers were sequentially administered into separate femoral veins 10 s (FITC-dextran) and 5 s (Evans blue) prior to decapitation. The brain was then removed, frozen in 2-methylbutane (–42 °C), and sectioned (6 μm) at –21 °C. To quantify the number of perfused microvessels (vessels containing fluorescent tracer), sections were examined by fluorescence microscopy, and images acquired and processed using the Metamorph image-processing system (Universal Imaging, West Chester, Pa.). Images were acquired from three predefined regions of cortex. The images were manually thresholded prior to automatic calculation of the number of perfused microvessels ($<$ 20 μm diameter) per field of view. Final results are expressed as the mean ($\pm$ SD) number of perfused microvessels per millimeter squared for each region of interest.

Additional cryostat sections (16 μm) were stained with hematoxylin and eosin for volumetric assessment of ischemic lesion volume. Ischemic regions were transcribed from the section onto scale drawings at eight predefined stereotactic levels [16]. Lesion areas were then measured using an image analyzer (NIH Image) and converted to total volume of ischemic damage.

BCEC Cultures

BCECs from Wistar–Kyoto (WKY) rats were isolated and cultivated by a modification of the method previously described for human BCECs [20]. Propagated ECs ($1 \cdot 10^4$ cells/100-μl well) were grown to confluency on 1 % gelatin-coated coverslips or 96-well flat-bottom microtiter plates, in a 37 °C humidified atmosphere of 5 %CO_2, in M-199 medium (25 mM Hepes buffer, Earle's salts, and L-glutamine), with 20 % heat-inactivated fetal-calf serum, 90 μg/ml heparin, 100 μg/ml streptomycin, 100 U/ml penicillin G, 0.25 μg/ml amphotericin B (all from GIBCO, Long Island, NY), and 20 μg/ml endothelial cell growth supplement (Collaborative Research, Bedford, Mass.). Endothelial cells were positively identified by both immunocytochemistry and fluorescence-activated cell sorter (FACS) analysis using endothelial-cell-specific anti-FVIII-RA (Accurate Chemical and Scientific Corp., Westbury, NY) as previously described [14].

For TNF-α preconditioning, cell cultures were incubated for 4 h with rat TNF-α 20 ng/ml (Chemicon International, Temecula, Calif.) in culture media, washed, allowed to rest in media without TNF-α for 20 h, then activated again with the same doses of TNF-α for 24 h.

Hypoxic treatment of BCECs was performed in modular incubator chambers (Billups Rothenberg); first flushed with a gas mixture of 5 %CO_2/95 %N_2 for 15 min, then sealed and incubated at 37 °C for 20 h and reoxygenated for 24 h. For preconditioning, TNF-α was incubated with BCEC cultures for 4 h at 20 ng/ml and washed out right before the beginning of hypoxic treatment.

Fluorescent cell enzyme-linked immunosorbent assay (ELISA) was performed according to Carlson et al. [2]. Cells were fixed with 1 % paraformaldehyde and the following incubations were performed at room temperature for 1 h each: first, with anti-rat ICAM-1 monoclonal antibody at 1 g/ml (Endogen, Woburn, Mass.), then with biotinylated horse anti-mouse immunoglobulin G, rat absorbed, at 10 μg/ml, then with streptavidin α-galactosidase at 10 μg/ml (Molecular Probes, Inc., Eugene, Ore.). Finally, 100 μM fluorescent substrate for α-galactosidase, fluorescein-di-α-D-galactopyranoside, was added and fluorescence was measured in a CytoFluor 4000 fluorescent plate reader at emission/excitation wavelength 485/530 nm. Background fluorescence of the cells stained without anti-ICAM-1 antibody was measured and subtracted in each experiment. Each data point was represented as the average of ten wells.

Results

Microvascular Perfusion and Ischemic Lesion Volume 4 h Post-MCAO

Microvascular perfusion 4 h post-MCAO is summarized in Table 1. The number of perfused microvessels in each region represents an average from sections cut at three levels of brain: anterior (through caudate and anterior commissure), middle (thalamus and dorsal hippocampus) and posterior (through thalamus and substantia nigra). Perfusion in region A was unaffected by MCAO and represents the normal range for the number of perfused microvessels per millimeter squared. For the saline control group, microvascular perfusion tended to be moderately reduced in region B and severely reduced in region C. In contrast, LPS pretreatment was associated with higher levels of microvascular perfusion in regions B and C, where significant differences were observed between the saline control and LPS groups after 5 s and 10 s of perfusion.

Concomitant with the preservation of microvascular perfusion, LPS pretreatment also significantly reduced ischemic lesion volume. The magnitude of the effect was similar to the previous study [21] and represented a 25 % reduction in lesion volume.

Table 1. Number of perfused brain microvessels in dorsomedial non-ischemic cortex (**A**), perifocal/penumbral region (**B**) and infarct core (**C**) 4 h after middle-cerebral-artery occlusion (mean ± SD from three coronal levels within the middle cerebral artery distribution)

	A	B	C
Saline$_{5\,s}$	408±32	85±97	16±18
LPS$_{5\,s}$	439±36	215±132	67±43
P value	0.112	0.036	0.037
Saline$_{10\,s}$	415±29	156±97	95±54
LPS$_{10\,s}$	437±33	290±99	170±60
P value	0.159	0.024	0.054

TNF-α Pretreatment Makes Cells Unresponsive to Subsequent Activation by TNF-α and Hypoxia

As expected, exposure of BCECs to TNF-α for 24 h caused an increase of surface ICAM-1 expression, which was documented by cell ELISA (Fig. 1). Inhibition of ICAM-1 induction was observed in the cells pretreated with TNF-α for 4 h, washed

TNF-α Pretreatment Attenuates TNF-α-Induced
ICAM-1 Expression in BCEC

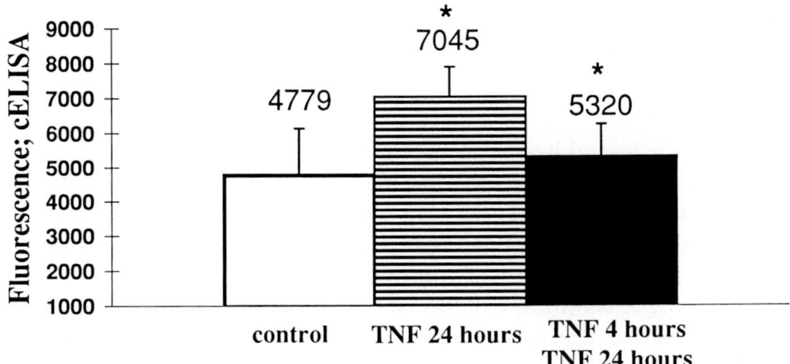

TNF-α Pretreatment Attenuates Hypoxia-Induced
ICAM-1 Expression in BCEC

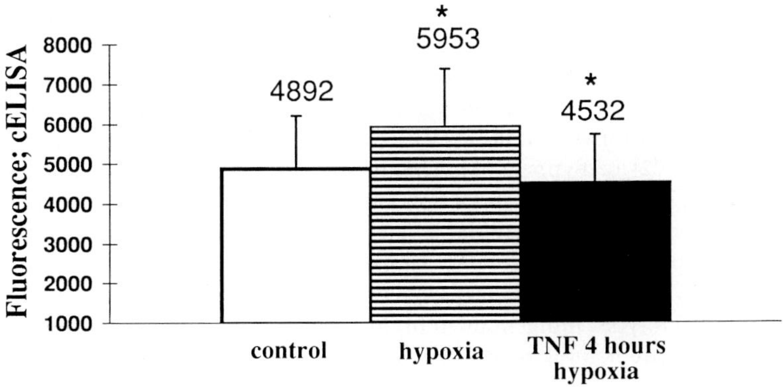

Fig. 1. Confluent cultures of brain capillary endothelial cells (BCEC) of passage 7 plated on 96-well plates have been used for the measurements of surface expression of intercellular adhesion molecule-1 (ICAM-1). Cells were treated either with 20 ng/ml tumor necrosis factor alpha (TNF-α) for 24 h (*top*) or with 20 h hypoxia/24 h reoxygenation (*bottom*). Both treatments caused a significant increase of ICAM-1 expression (*hatched bars*) over control levels (*open bars*). BCEC cultures pretreated with 20 ng/ml TNF-α for 4 h, 24 h before the TNF-α challenge (*top*) or immediately before hypoxia treatment (*bottom*) exhibited no enhancement of ICAM-1 expression (*black bars*). Each bar represents mean ± SEM of three to four experiments

and, 20 h later, activated with TNF-α. TNF-α pretreatment of BCECs for 4 h itself did not cause upregulation of ICAM-1 expression (data not shown).

We also investigated whether cell tolerance induced by short TNF-α pretreatment would attenuate ICAM-1 upregulation caused by another stimulus, which has recently been noted to cause upregulation of ICAM-1 in cultured human brain microvessels [9]. By means of cell ELISA, we have shown that in rat, BCECs subjected to 20 h of hypoxia and 24 h of reoxygenation, the amount of ICAM-1 protein on the cell surface significantly increased (Fig. 1). Incubation of BCEC with TNF-α for 4 h immediately before the beginning of the hypoxic treatment protected against hypoxia/reoxygenation-induced ICAM-1 upregulation (Fig. 1).

Discussion

The data characterize several new aspects of ischemic tolerance. The work adds evidence for a vascular component in the LPS model of tolerance to the well-studied direct effects of preconditioning stimuli on brain parenchymal elements. The evidence for a vascular component is that the secondary deficits in microvascular perfusion, which developed in non-tolerant controls, were significantly attenuated in the LPS-tolerant animals. A significant preservation of microcirculatory perfusion was noted in both the perifocal/penumbral regions and the ischemic core. This attenuation of microcirculatory-perfusion impairment was associated with a reduction of brain-infarct volume in a standardized model of MCAO in the SHR. Although the data does not permit a definite conclusion that this association is causal, the relative maintenance of microvascular perfusion in the ischemic core of animals made tolerant indicates that preservation of microcirculatory perfusion in this group cannot be fully explained by their smaller ischemic lesion volumes.

Expression of ICAM-1 protein on the membranes of BCECs was measured as the biological read-out of TNF-α-triggered cell activation in these studies. The activation of endothelial cells by TNF-α has been well studied [15, 23] and has often been used as a model for the pro-inflammatory action of TNF-α and other types of stress, such as oxidative stress [22] or hypoxia [8]. This model will permit further study of the intracellular signaling related to induction of tolerance. The sphingomyelin cycle, which leads to production of ceramide, is one candidate for study, since it has been demonstrated to play a major role in signal-transduction pathways initiated by TNF-α and other types of stress [4, 5, 7, 13]. Further study of intracellular signaling in BCECs and other cell types indigenous to brain, such as astrocytes and neurons, may lead to insights that are helpful for the development of more robust stroke therapies.

References

1. Aoki M, Abe K, Kawagoe J, Nakamura S, Kogure K (1993) Acceleration of HSP70 and HSC70 heat shock gene expression following transient ischemia in the preconditioned gerbil hippocampus. J Cereb Blood Flow Metab 13: 781–788
2. Carlson SL, Beiting DJ, Kiani CA, Abell KM, McGillis JP (1996) Catecholamines decrease lymphocyte adhesion to cytokine-activated endothelial cells. Brain Behav Immun 10: 55–67
3. Dawson DA, Ruetzler CA, Hallenbeck JM (1997) Temporal impairment of microcirculatory perfusion following focal cerebral ischemia in the spontaneously hypertensive rat. Brain Res 749: 200–208
4. Dbaibo GS, Perry DK, Gamard CJ, Platt R, Poirier GG, Obeid LM. Hannun YA (1997) Cytokine response modifier A (Crm A) inhibits ceramide formation in response to tumor necrosis factor (TNF)-alpha: CrmA and Bel-2 target distinct components in the apoptotic pathway. J Exp Med 185: 481–490
5. Ghosh S, Strum JC, Bell RM (1997) Lipid biochemistry: functions of glycerolipids and sphingolipids in cellular signaling. FASEB J 11: 45–50

6. Hallenbeck JM, Frerichs, KU, (1993) Stroke therapy. It may be time for an integrated approach. Arch Neurol 50: 768–770

7. Hannun YA (1996) Functions of ceramide in coordinating cellular responses to stress. Science 274: 1855–1859

8. Hess DC, Bhutwala T, Sheppard JC, Zhao W, Smith J (1994a) ICAM-1 expression on human brain microvascular endothelial cells. Neurosci Lett 168: 201–204

9. Hess DC, Zhao W, Carroll J, McEachin M, Buchanan K (1994b) Increased expression of ICAM-1 during reoxygenation in brain endothelial cells. Stroke 25: 1463–1468

10. Kato H, Liu Y, Araki T, Kogure K (1991) Temporal profile of the effects of pretreatment with brief cerebral ischemia on the neuronal damage following secondary ischemic insult in the gerbil. Brain Res 553: 238–242

11. Kirino T, Tsujita Y, Tamura A (1991) Induced tolerance to ischemia in gerbil hippocampal neurons. J Cereb Blood Flow Metab 11: 299–307

12. Kitagawa K, Matsumoto M, Tagaya M, Hata R, Ueda H, Ninobe M, Handa R, Kimura K, Mikoshiba K, Kameda T (1990) Ischemic tolerance phenomenon found in the brain. Brain Res 528: 21–24

13. Kolesnick R, Golde DW (1994) The sphingomyelin pathway in tumor necrosis factor and interleukin-1 signaling. Cell 77: 325–328

14. McCarron RM, Spatz M, Kempski O, Hogan RN, Muehl L, McFarlin DE (1986) Interaction between myelin basic protein-sensitized T lymphocytes and murine cerebral vascular endothelial cells. J Immunol 137: 3428–3435

15. McCarron RM, Wang L, Racke MK, McFarlin DE, Spatz M (1993) Effect of cytokines on ICAM expression and T cell adhesion to cerebrovascular endothelial cells. Adv Exp Med Biol 331: 237–242

16. Nawashiro H, Tasaki K, Ruetzler CA, Hallenbeck JM (1997) TNF-α pretreatment induces protective effects against focal cerebral ischemia in mice. J Cereb Blood Flow Metab 17: 483–490

17. Ohtsuki T, Matsumoto M, Kitagawa K, Taguchi A, Maeda Y, Hata R, Ogawa S, Ueda H, Handa N, Kamada T (1993) Induced resistance and susceptibility to cerebral ischemia in gerbil hippocampal neurons by prolonged but mild hypoperfusion. Brain Res 614: 279–284

18. Pugin J, Ulevitch RJ, Tobias PS (1995) Tumor necrosis factor-α and interleukin-1α mediate human endothelial cell activation in blood at low endotoxin concentrations. J Inflamm 45: 49–55

19. Schöbitz B, DeKloet ER, Holsboer F (1994) Gene expression and function of interleukin-1, interleukin-6 and tumor necrosis factor in the brain. Prog Neurobiol 44: 397–432

20. Spatz M, Kawai N, Merkel N, Bembry J, McCarron RM (1997) Functional properties of cultured endothelial cells derived from large microvessels of human brain. Am J Physiol 272:C231–C239

21. Tasaki K, Ruetzler CA, Ohtsuki T, Martin D, Nawashiro H, Hallenbeck JM (1997) Lipopolysaccharide pre-treatment induces resistance against subsequent focal cerebral ischemic damage in spontaneously hypertensive rats. Brain Res 748: 267–270

22. Wagener F, Feldman E, de Witte T, Abraham NG (1997) Heme induces the expression of adhesion molecules ICAM-1, VCAM-1 and E Selectin in vascular endothelial cells. Proc Soc Exp Biol Med 216: 456–463

23. Wong D, Dorovini-Zis K (1992) Upregulation of intercellular adhesion molecule-1 (ICAM-1) expression in primary cultures of human brain microvessel endothelial cells by cytokines and lipopolysaccharide. J Neuroimmunol 39: 11–21

The Role of Glial and Inflammatory Reactions in Cerebral Ischemia

H. Kato

Summary. The purpose of this study was to investigate histopathological and immunological features of the activation of glial cells and inflammatory cells in response to different degrees of cerebral ischemic insult. Transient global cerebral ischemia and focal cerebral ischemia were induced in rats, and produced sublethal injury, selective neuronal damage, and infarction within the brain. Sublethal injury induced no neuronal death but did induce transient astroglial reaction and microglial activation without any upregulation of macrophagic function. In areas with selective neuronal damage, microglial cells were rapidly activated and then transformed into macrophages when neurons were destroyed. Various immunomolecules were expressed on microglia in a time-dependent, step-wise manner. Astroglial hypertrophy was remarkable in this area of selective neuronal damage. In the ischemic core, where infarction developed later, both astroglia and microglia were destroyed in early reperfusion stages. The infarct was covered by blood-borne neutrophils and monocytes/macrophages. Perivascular cells also became positive for macrophage markers. Various immunomolecules were expressed on these blood-borne cells as well as on microglia-derived macrophages concentrated at the edge of the infarct. Thus, three classes of mononuclear phagocytes/macrophages appeared after ischemia, depending on the severity of tissue damage. The activation of microglia was strictly controlled, and their functional significance, especially before transforming into phagocytes, remains to be elucidated.

Introduction

Neuronal damage that results from cerebral ischemia is accompanied by glial reactions, both astroglial and microglial [7]. Several investigators have made histological, immunohistochemical, and biochemical analyses of glial and inflammatory reactions induced by cerebral ischemia [4, 10, 14]. However, details of the sequence of these reactions in relation to different degrees of morphological neuronal abnormalities have not been fully documented. In this study, we aimed to answer the following questions.

1. What are the morphological and immunological features of glial and inflammatory cells in tissues containing sublethal injury, selective neuronal death, and infarction?
2. What is the chronological relationship between the activation of those cells and the maturation of ischemic brain lesions?

Maturation Phenomenon in Cerebral Ischemia III
U. Ito et al. (Eds.)
© Springer-Verlag Berlin Heidelberg 1999

The information derived from these questions could be important for understanding the pathophysiological mechanisms operative in ischemic brain damage.

The brain lesions induced following global and focal cerebral ischemia grow and mature as a function of time. A brief period of global ischemia produces selective neuronal damage or delayed neuronal death in the hippocampus [8]. The lesion of the middle cerebral artery (MCA) occlusion spreads from a core (striatum) to the penumbra in the overlying cortex supplied by the MCA [9]. As such, the abnormalities evolve over time, with a spatial gradient of damage ranging from selective neuronal damage to an infarct. In this study, we investigated the characteristics of glial and inflammatory reactions in the different brain lesions of these ischemia models using histopathological and immunohistochemical methods.

Materials and Methods

Transient global ischemia was induced in male adult Wistar rats by 4-vessel occlusion for 6 min [13]. Focal cerebral ischemia was induced in Wistar rats by an intraluminal occlusion of the right MCA for 1 h [11]. The animals were sacrificed serially at 2 h to 7 days after reperfusion. Sham-operated animals were also included. Each group consisted of 4–6 animals.

The brains of the animals were perfusion fixed with 4 % paraformaldehyde in 0.1 M phosphate buffer. The brains were cryoprotected and frozen sections (20 µm) were prepared. The sections were used for histochemical visualization of microglial cells with isolectin B4 from Griffonia simplicifolia (Sigma) [15], and for immunohistochemistry with a panel of monoclonal antibodies raised against immunomolecules expressed on cells of macrophage/monocyte lineage, i.e., complement receptor type 3 (CR3, OX42; Serotec), major histocompatibility complex (MHC) class I and II antigens (OX18 and OX6; Serotec), and a monocyte/macrophage marker ED1 (Serotec). Astrocytes were immunostained with a monoclonal antibody raised against glial fibrillary acidic protein (GFAP; Chemicon). Part of the brains of the rats subjected to MCA occlusion were embedded in paraffin for better morphological observation. The paraffin sections were used for hematoxylin and eosin (HE) staining, microglial staining with isolectin, and immunostaining with the anti-GFAP antibody and the antibody ED1.

The microglial activation was classified largely into three stages according to the following criteria [6, 16]: (1) resting microglia, which are highly ramified cells present in normal adult brain; (2) activated microglia, which are cells responding to ischemia with morphological and immunophenotypic changes, as well as proliferation, but are not phagocytic. Morphological changes include enlarged cell bodies and contraction of their processes to show a stouter morphology; and (3) phagocytic microglia, which are full-blown brain macrophages with an ameboid morphology.

Results

Transient Forebrain Ischemia

The pyramidal neurons in the CA1 subfield of the hippocampus appeared preserved after 2 h and 1 day, but were destroyed after 3 days and 7 days. Many glial cells were seen at 3 days and further accumulated at 7 days. CA3 and dentate gyrus remained intact.

Two hours after ischemia, microglial cells exhibited an increase in isolectin and OX42 staining and morphological changes, such as larger cell bodies and stouter processes (activated microglia). After 1 day, these changes became more evident, and the activated microglia became OX18 positive. After 3 days, full-blown activation of microglia was seen; cell bodies were larger and the processes were stouter and shorter (ameboid). They were seen in the entire CA1 area and were most concentrated in the pyramidal cell layer; they were now ED1 positive. After 7 days, microglia further accumulated and those in the stratum radiatum had the morphology of rod cells. Ameboid cells in the pyramidal cell layer were OX6-positive. Astroglial hypertrophy started 1 day after ischemia, and became pronounced when the CA1 neurons were destroyed. Activated, but not phagocytic, microglia and reactive astrocytes were seen in the CA3 and the dentate gyrus, but to a lesser degree.

Focal Cerebral Ischemia

The MCA-supplied areas of the striatum and the cortex displayed a combination of infarction (ischemic core) and partial lesioning, with selective neuronal damage in the transitional rim surrounding the infarct (penumbra). The infarction covered the dorsolateral caudate putamen, and a variable extent of pyriform, insular, and parietal cortices. Ipsilateral cingulate and frontal cortices and medial caudate putamen remained uninjured (surrounding area).

Histology

After 4 h, almost all neurons in the striatum appeared shrunken, darkly stained, and were surrounded by perineuronal vacuolization (scalloping). In the cortex, isolated groups of neurons exhibited these changes. After 1 day, those neurons showed irreversible changes, i.e., pyknotic nuclei and cytoplasmic eosinophilia (red neurons). The extent of cortical lesions with red neurons (layers 2–6) increased. A small number of damaged neurons exhibited an apoptotic morphology; condensation of the nuclei and the formation of apoptotic bodies. After 3 days, pannecrosis developed in the striatum; the damaged neurons lost nuclear hematoxylin stainability (ghost neurons). In the cortex, infarction developed to a variable extent, together with islands of red and/or ghost neurons. After 7 days, the infarction further developed and the area was covered by macrophages that took the classical morphology of foamy macrophages. Red and/or ghost neurons were scattered in the narrow rim medial to the striatal infarct, and in the cortex that escaped infarction.

Glial Fibrillary Acidic Protein

After 4 h, astrocytes in the striatum appeared disintegrated and fragmented. After 1 day, GFAP-positive astrocytes were decreased or lost in the striatum; those in the cortex appeared slightly hypertrophic. After 3 days, no astrocytes were recognizable within the infarct, but a rim of reactive astrocytes surrounded the infarct. After 7 days, the changes became further evident. Astrocytes around the infarct were strongly hypertrophic, and those in the surrounding area were slightly hypertrophic.

Microglia

Isolectin-stained microglia decreased in the ischemic hemisphere after 4 h, especially in the striatum. OX42 immunostaining showed that microglial cells in the ischemic core were irregular in shape with fewer processes and appeared fragmented. After 1 day, microglial cells with activated morphology increased in areas peripheral to the ischemic core. Many activated microglial cells appeared to be attached to red neurons and engulfed them (neuronophagia). In the core, isolectin-positive microglia were disappearing, and a small number of round cells (monocytes/macrophages) and perivascular cells were ED1-positive. Polymorphonuclear leukocytes (PMNs) were seen within the core. After 3 days, the infarct was covered by isolectin-stained, ED1-positive round cells (monocytes/macrophages) (Fig. 1); the numbers of ED1-stained perivascular cells and the PMNs also increased. In the transitional rim, ED-1 positive phagocytic microglia were seen (Fig. 1). In the surrounding area, ED1-negative, activated microglia lay attached to normal-appearing neurons (Fig. 1). After 7 days, the

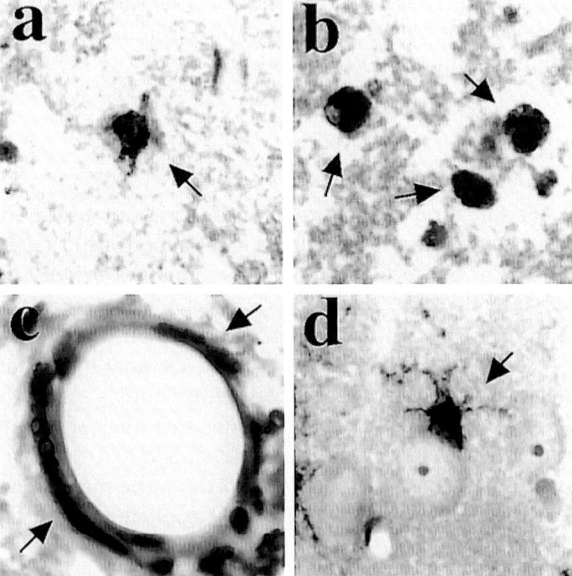

Fig. 1a–d. Three days after 1 h of middle cerebral artery occlusion in the rat. Three distinct types of cells that bear the ED1 macrophage/monocyte antigen are shown. **a** Medial striatum (the edge of the infarct). ED1-positive phagocytic microglia. **b, c** Lateral striatum (infarct). Foamy macrophages (probably monocyte origin) (**b**) and perivascular cells (**c**) are ED1 positive. **d** In the cingulate cortex (surrounding area), activated microglia (ED1 negative) are located very close to normal-appearing neurons. **a–c** Immunostaining with a pan-macrophage/monocyte marker ED1 (counterstained with hematoxylin and eosin). **d** Isolectin staining (counterstained with hematoxylin and eosin) × 400

changes in the infarct became more evident, but PMNs disappeared. Starting at 1 day, OX18, OX6 and ED1 as well as OX42 became positive in both phagocytic microglia in the peripheral rim and in the invading monocytes/macrophages in the core.

Discussion

The results of this study allow us to summarize different glial and inflammatory responses to different degrees of ischemic brain damage, ranging from sublethal injury and selective neuronal damage to infarction. The response of glial cells and the recruitment of macrophages were very different for these different brain lesions. The features of glial and inflammatory reactions are summarized in Tables 1 and 2.

Generally, three different levels of tissue damage could be classified: (1) sublethal injury in resistant areas following global ischemia (CA3 and dentate gyrus) and in the surrounding areas following MCA occlusion (cingulate and frontal cortices and medial striatum); (2) selective neuronal damage in vulnerable areas following global ischemia (CA1) and in the peripheral (penumbra) area of ischemic focus; and (3) infarction in the ischemic core following MCA occlusion (lateral striatum and part of the cortex).

Even in sublethally damaged areas, microglia were activated rapidly (within hours), and then astrocytes were activated. Microglia in these areas were morpholog-

Table 1. Activation of microglia and inflammatory cells following global and focal cerebral ischemia

Transient global ischemia
    Vulnerable area (selective neuronal damage)
        Early, transient microglial activation (activated microglia)
        Neuronal death-induced, protracted microglial (phagocytic) and astroglial activation
    Resistant area (sublethal injury)
        Early, transient microglial activation (activated microglia)
        Delayed transient astroglial activation

Focal ischemia
    Ischemic core (infarction)
        Early destruction of microglia and astroglia
        Infiltration of blood-borne neutrophils and monocytes
        Phagocytic transformation of perivascular cells
    Peripheral rim of the infarct (selective neuronal damage)
        Neuronal death-induced, protracted microglial (phagocytic) and astroglial activation
    Surrounding area (sublethal injury)
        Transient activation of microglia and astroglia

Table 2. Graded activation of microglia

Classification	Morphology	Immunomolecules
Resting microglia	Highly ramified, thin processes	CR3
Activated microglia	Enlarged cell body, stouter processes	CR3, MHC class I
Phagocytic microglia	Ameboid morphology	CR3, MHC class I and II, ED1

CR3 complement receptor type 3; *MHC* major histocompatibility complex

ically activated but did not express antigens that are observed in macrophages. These microglial cells could be seen very close to normal-appearing neurons, as if they protect the neurons from secondary injury. Because no neurons are killed in this area, it is clear that the presence of microglia does not imply neuronal death and, instead, activated microglia might act neuroprotectively [1, 6]. This issue needs to be elucidated.

Neuronal death induced strong, protracted activation of both types of glial cell. In selective neuronal damage, microglia were the sole source of brain macrophages. In the peripheral rim of an infarct, activation of microglial cells, both morphological and phenotypic, occurred, followed by astroglial hypertrophy. Microglial cells activated in the tissue with this type of neuronal death expressed the full panel of immunomolecules (OX42, OX18, OX6, ED1), suggesting that they are full-blown, phagocytic microglia. In focal ischemia, the recruitment of microglia-derived macrophages from the transitional zone into the infarct is likely.

By contrast, in the ischemic core, where infarction developed, astroglial and microglial cells, as well as neurons, were destroyed in early post-ischemic stages. Although neurons are more vulnerable to ischemia than glial cells, the development of selective neuronal damage into infarction did not take place in the maturational time course. There was a threshold at which selective neuronal damage turned into infarction. Once this threshold was reached, glial cells were damaged rapidly, leading to infarction. In this sense, glial damage is a prerequisite for the development of infarction. Because astrocytes are involved in maintaining the homeostasis of extracellular water and ion concentrations, uptake and inactivation of excitatory amino acids, and the formation of the blood–brain barrier, providing a supportive effect on neurons [3, 12, 17], it is easy to understand that a tissue with sick astrocytes cannot survive. Although several reports suggest that microglia can act neuroprotectively [1], it remains elusive whether damage to microglia contributes to the development of infarction. In the ischemic core, blood-borne neutrophils and monocytes began to infiltrate the region. This infiltration was probably facilitated by the interaction between intercellular adhesion molecule-1 (ICAM-1), expressed on endothelial cells, and a group of CD11/CD18 glycoproteins expressed on leukocytes [7]. The infarcted area was covered entirely by blood-borne monocytes/macrophages when pannecrosis was fully developed. When blood vessels in the infarct were not destroyed, perivascular cells, which are thought to derive from macrophage lineage, appeared to be a source of brain macrophages in the infarct.

Thus, three classes of mononuclear phagocytes/macrophages (microglia, perivascular cells and blood-borne monocytes) appeared after ischemia. Which source is recruited depends on the severity of damage. The relative importance of each source may also be determined by the location and route of entry. However, the absence of a marker distinguishing extrinsic macrophages from intrinsic macrophages makes the precise determination of the cell population difficult. Microglia have been known as a source of brain macrophages, which may have a neuron-killing effect [2, 5]. They have been considered intrinsic immunocompetent cells of the brain, and express a number of immunologically important surface molecules when activated, but the significance of the molecules remains enigmatic. Activated microglia may play a protective role by secreting growth factors and isolating neurons from secondary injury [1, 6]. In any ischemia paradigm and at any stage of neuronal damage, microglia/macrophages were attached to the dying or dead (necrotic) neurons engulfing them. Therefore, it is conceivable that these inflammatory cells play a pivotal role in ischemic neuronal death. However, the activational state of microglial cells varied within the brain and appeared strictly controlled in a precisely step-wise fashion. Whether the differential activation of microglia and inflammatory cells is beneficial for proper wound healing or can be a target for therapeutic intervention remains to be settled.

References

1. Banati RB, Graeber MB (1994) Surveillance, intervention and cytotoxicity: is there a protective role of microglia? Dev Neurosci 16: 114–127
2. Brierley JB, Brown AW (1982) The origin of lipid phagocytes in the central nervous system: I. the intrinsic microglia. J Comp Neurol 211: 397–406
3. Brightman M (1991) Implication of astroglia in the blood–brain barrier. Ann NY Acad Sci 633: 343–347
4. Gehrmann J, Bonnekoh P, Miyazawa T, Hossmann K-A, Kreutzberg GW (1992) Immunohistochemical study of an early microglial activation in ischemia. J Cereb Blood Flow Metab 12: 257–269
5. Giulian D (1987) Ameboid microglia as effectors of inflammation in the central nervous system. J Neurosci Res 18: 155–171
6. Kato H (1997) Microglia: inflammatory markers in stroke. In: Wood PL (ed) Neuroinflammation: mechanism and management. Humana Press, Totowa, pp 91–107
7. Kato H, Kogure K, Araki T, Itoyama Y (1994) Astroglial and microglial reactions in the gerbil hippocampus with induced ischemic tolerance. Brain Res 664: 101–107
8. Kato H, Kogure K, Araki T, Itoyama Y (1995) Graded expression of immunomolecules on activated microglia in the hippocampus following ischemia in a rat model of ischemic tolerance. Brain Res 694: 85–93
9. Kato H, Kogure K, Liu X-H, Araki T, Itoyama Y (1996) Progressive expression of immunomolecules on activated microglia and invading leukocytes following focal cerebral ischemia in the rat. Brain Res 734: 203–212
10. Morioka T, Kalehua AN, Streit WJ (1991) The microglial reaction in the rat dorsal hippocampus following transient cerebral ischemia. J Cereb Blood Flow Metab 11: 966–973.
11. Nagasawa H, Kogure K (1989) Correlation between cerebral blood flow and histologic changes in a new rat model of middle cerebral artery occlusion. Stroke 20: 1037–1043
12. Nicholls D, Attwell D (1990) The release and uptake of excitatory amino acids. Trends Pharmacol Sci 11: 462–468
13. Pulsinelli WA, Brierley JB (1979) A new model of bilateral hemispheric ischemia in the unanesthetized rat. Stroke 10: 267–272
14. Schmidt-Kastner R, Szymas J, Hossmann K-A (1989) Immunohistochemical study of glial reaction and serum protein extravasation in relation to neuronal damage in rat hippocampus after ischemia. Neuroscience 38: 527–540
15. Streit WJ (1990) An improved staining method for rat microglial cells using the lectin from Griffonia simplicifolia (GSA I-B4). J Histochem Cytochem 38: 1683–1686
16. Streit WJ, Graeber MB, Kreutzberg GW (1988) Functional plasticity of microglia: a review. Glia 1: 301–307
17. Walz W (1989) Role of glial cells in the regulation of the brain ion microenvironment. Prog Neurobiol 33: 309–333

Effect of Endothelin$_A$ Receptor Antagonist on Neuronal Injury in Global and Focal Ischemia

Y. Ohara, D. Dawson, H. Sugano, C. Ruetzler, N. Azzam, J. M. Hallenbeck, R.M. McCarron, and M. Spatz

Summary. The involvement of endogenous endothelin-1 (ET-1) was evaluated in transient global brain ischemia (8 min) with reperfusion (72 h) and in focal permanent ischemia (4 h) of spontaneously hypertensive rats (SHR). In gerbils, postischemic treatment with an ET$_A$ receptor antagonist, Ro 61-1790, reversed the ischemia-induced hypoperfusion and preserved 64–74 % of hippocampal CA1 neurons, compared with controls (20–44 %). The pretreatment of SHR with Ro 61-1790 significantly increased cerebral microvascular perfusion, which was associated with a significant decrease (27 %) in the volume of the ischemic lesion. These findings support the hypothesis that endogenously released ET-1 is an important mediator of ischemic injury.

Introduction

In general, it is a well-accepted notion that the mechanisms involved in the development and progression of cerebral ischemia are multifactorial in nature. There is also little doubt that a severely compromised blood flow to the brain results in energy failure, cessation of glucose metabolism and anoxia. This, in turn, leads to disturbances of other metabolic pathways affecting the functional integrity of the cellular constituents of the brain. The evolving degree of tissue injury depends on the duration, site and severity of the primary insult, as well as the predisposing vascular factors. Therefore, our renewed attention has been drawn to endogenous mediators derived from the vascular and microvascular beds of the brain.

In particular, we have been interested in endothelin-1 (ET-1), the most potent vasoconstrictive peptide, which is predominantly produced by the endothelium [3, 17, 24]. Reports indicate that the potential vasoconstrictive effect of ET-1 is opposed by nitric oxide (NO), which is a powerful vasodilatory gas also produced (among other vasoactive substances) by the endothelium [3, 7, 9]. It has been thought that these two substances create a balanced system implicated in the regulation of vascular tone and blood flow [7]. However, impaired endothelial vasodilatory responses noted in hypertensive patients and animals (ineffectiveness of acetylcholine to induce NO) implicate disturbances in the balance between ET-1 and NO in cerebrovascular-disease processes [14]. In addition, an elevated ET-1 level has been reported in circulating plasma and/or cerebrospinal fluid (CSF) of patients with vasospasm, ischemia and essential hypertension, among other disease processes [6, 21]. These observations, strengthened by similar findings described in experimental global and focal brain ischemia, validate a role for ET-1 in the pathogenic mechanisms of brain ischemia [1, 2, 12, 18, 19, 23].

Maturation Phenomenon in Cerebral Ischemia III
U. Ito et al. (Eds.)
© Springer-Verlag Berlin Heidelberg 1999

Recent experimental results also suggested an association of early (induced by inhibition of NO synthase) and late postischemic hypoperfusion, with an increased content of ET-1 in the CSF [18]. Based on these data, our working hypothesis embraced the possibility that ischemia-induced and endogenously released ET-1 is responsible for the noted postischemic hypoperfusion. This concept was substantiated by the observed reversal of postischemic hypoperfusion in the same model of transient global brain ischemia (15 min) in gerbils treated with selective ET_A receptor antagonists (BQ123 or Ro 61-1790). Therefore, it is important to examine whether the ET_A receptor-mediated improvement of postischemic or ischemic cerebral circulation is associated with modulation of ischemic injury. For this purpose, we used two different models: transient global cerebral ischemia (8 min) with reperfusion (72 h) in gerbils, and focal brain ischemia (4 h) in spontaneously hypertensive rats (SHR), a strain known to develop the largest and most reproducible neocortical infarct after middle cerebral artery (MCA) occlusion [10]. This report summarizes data demonstrating the effect of ET_A receptor antagonists on: (1) postischemic hypoperfusion and neuronal survival in the CA1 region of the hippocampus after transient global brain ischemia, and (2) the microvascular perfusion and volume of the lesion in focal ischemia in SHR.

Materials and Methods

Global Cerebral Ischemia/Reperfusion

Separate groups (9–14) of 3-month-old female Mongolian gerbils under pentobarbital (20 mg/kg) anesthesia and spontaneous ventilation were used for induction of ischemia by bilateral carotid-artery occlusion (8 min) and release (72 h). Mean arterial pressure (MAP) [using Universal Harvard Oscillograph (Kent, UK) and blood-pressure transducer], cerebral blood flow (CBF), and head (temporal muscle) and rectal temperature were continuously monitored and maintained at 37–38 °C with a thermostatic heating lamp (Model 73, Yellow Spring Instruments Co., Inc.) during the entire experiment. The severity of the ischemic insult and the pattern of the CBF were assessed by measuring CBF using laser Doppler flowmetry (Laserflo Model BPM 403 A, TSI; St. Paul, Minn.). The probe was placed in the temporoparietal area of the brain, as previously described [18].

The treatment consisted of intravenously (i.v.) injecting (12.5 min after release of MCA occlusion) the selective ET_A receptor antagonist Ro 61-1790 (1 mg/kg/ml saline); saline-treated (1 ml/kg) animals served as controls. Ro 61-1790 was a generous gift from Drs. M. Clozel and S. Roux (F. Hoffmann-La Roche Ltd., Basel, Switzerland).

Focal Cerebral Ischemia

Adult male SHR, under halothane in nitrous oxide and oxygen (70: 30) anesthesia, were artificially respirated via a tracheotomy. Cannulated femoral vessels served for monitoring mean arterial blood pressure (MAP) and blood gases; a heating pad was used to maintain body temperature at 37 °C. The left MCA was occluded by electro-coagulation midway between the inferior cerebral vein and lateral olfactory tract (using the subtemporal approach). The selective ET_A receptor antagonist (10 mg/kg) or saline (1 ml/kg) was administered i.v. 5 min prior to MCA occlusion. Microvascular perfusion was assessed using the double-labeled fluorescent tracers Evans' blue and fluorescein isothiocyanate (FITC)-dextrose (71,000 Da), both purchased from Sigma, St. Louis, Mo., according to a previously described technique by Dawson et al. [4, 5]. Briefly, the tracers were administered sequentially into separate femoral veins, 10 s (FITC-dextran) and 5 s (Evans' blue) prior to termination of the experiment (4 h). All animal procedures were in strict accordance with the National Institutes of Health (NIH) Guide for the Care and Use of Laboratory Animals.

Gerbils were perfused with formaldehyde prior to removal of the brain and freezing, whereas the removed SHR brains were in 2-methylbutane. Hematoxylin-eosin (H&E) or terminal deoxynucleotidyltransferase-mediated dUTP-biotin nick-end labeling (TUNEL)-stained cryostat sections (20 μm) were used to evaluate neuronal integrity in the CA1 region of the hippocampus. H&E-stained cryostat sections were also used for light microscopy to assess ischemic injury in the SHR brain. Ischemic regions were transcribed from the sections onto scale drawings at eight predefined stereotactic levels. Lesion areas were then measured using an image analyzer (NIH

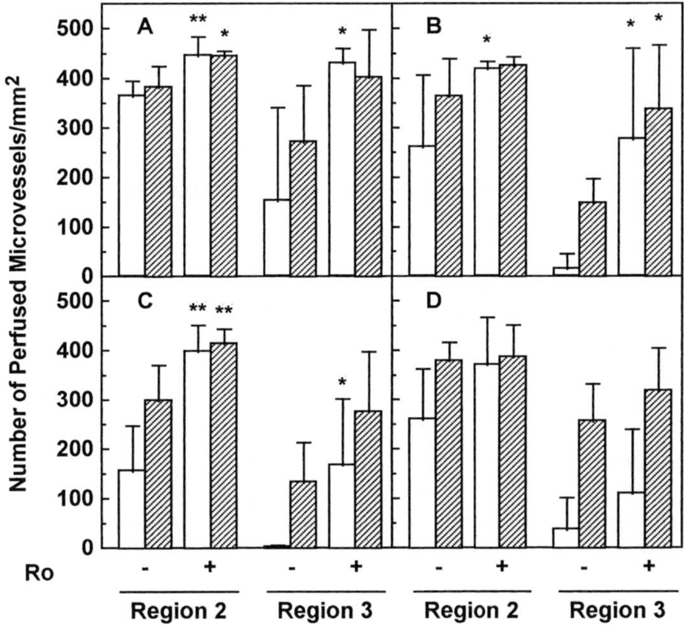

Fig. 1 A–D. Microvascular perfusion measured 4 h post-middle cerebral artery (MCA) occlusion in rats pretreated with Ro61-1790 or saline. The mean (±SD) number of microvessels perfused within a 5-s or 10-s time period were measured in five cortical regions at four levels of brain tissue. Ro61-1790 (10 mg/kg, i.v., 5 min pre-MCA occlusion) resulted in significant increases in the number of perfused microvessels, particularly in penumbral-peri-ischemic regions 2 and 3, compared with the same control group ($P^*<0.05$, $^{**}P<0.01$; unpaired t-tests)

Image) and converted to total volume of ischemic damage. The use of scale drawings circumvents the confounding influence of edema on lesion measurement and negates the use of an edema correction factor [13].

Microvessels (vessels containing fluorescent tracer) in frozen cryostat sections (6 µm) of SHR brains at four coronal levels (Fig. 1) were examined by means of fluorescence microscopy. Images acquired from five cortical regions at each of four coronal levels were processed using the Metamorph Image Processing System (Universal Imaging, West Chester, Pa.) and used to quantify the number of perfused microvessels. The chosen coronal levels (1–3) represent the territory of the MCA, whereas level 4 exhibits the area near the border of the MCA. The images were manually thresholded prior to automatic calculation of the number of perfused microvessels (< 20 µm diameter) per field of view. Region 1 depicts the normal (control) range of microvascular perfusion; regions 2 and 3 depict the number of perfused microvessels in the penumbra; and regions 4 and 5 exhibit the number of perfused microvessels in the ischemic core. Final results are expressed as the mean number of perfused microvessels per millimeter squared for each region of interest.

Statistical Analysis

Unpaired *t*-tests were used to compare data regarding the number of perfused microvessels and the significance of differences in ischemic lesion volume between Ro 61-1790-pretreated and control (saline) rats.

Results

Global Cerebral Ischemia/Reperfusion General Physiological Parameters

Temperature

There were no significant differences in rectal and temporal muscle temperature observed between the saline- and Ro 61-1790-treated gerbils during the entire experimental period.

Arterial Blood Pressure

Values (mean ± SD) for saline-injected gerbils were not significantly different from those treated with Ro 61-1790 in either preischemia (87.9±6.7 mmHg and 84.9±8 mmHg, respectively) or postischemia (87.8±7.2 mmHg and 93.0±11 mmHg, respectively). The level of MAP increased (31–42 %) during ischemia.

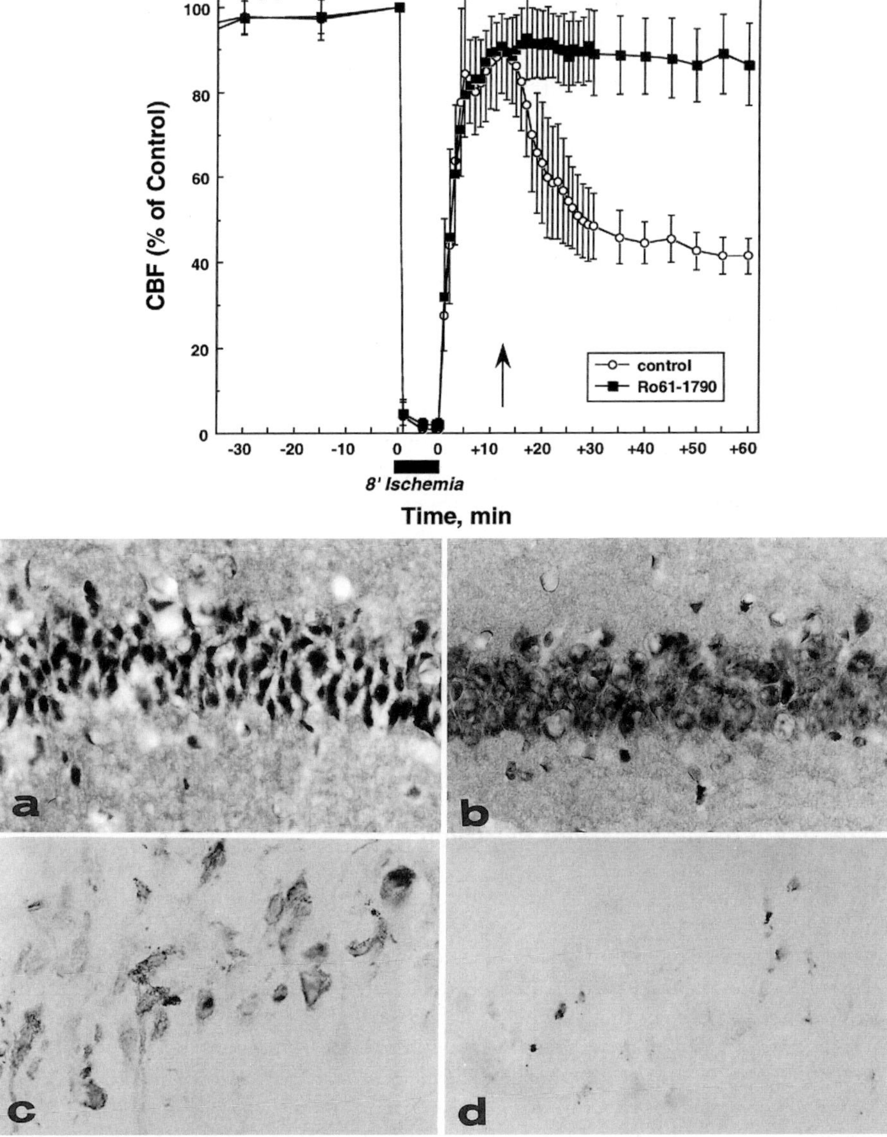

Fig. 2. A Effect of ET$_A$ receptor antagonist Ro61-1790 on changes in cerebral blood flow (CBF). Ro61-1790 (1 mg/kg/ml) was administered i.v. 12.5 min after release of bilateral carotid artery occlusion (8 min); saline-treated animals served as controls. The data are presented as means ± SD of 12 gerbils in each group injected either with Ro61-1790 or saline. **B** Effect of bilateral carotid artery occlusion (8 min) with release (72 h) on hippocampal CA1 neurons. The representative photomicrographs of brain sections were obtained from gerbils treated with saline (*a, c*) or Ro 16-1790 (*b, d*) and stained with H&E (*a, b*) or TUNEL (*c, d*)

Cerebral Blood Flow

The release of bilateral carotid occlusion transiently recovered CBF, which gradually declined starting at approximately 15 min after release of occlusion (Fig. 2A). The ET_A receptor antagonist completely reversed the postischemic hypoperfusion (Fig. 2A).

Light Microscopy

A bilateral loss of viable neurons (56–80 %) was observed in the CA1 region of the hippocampus following ischemia and reperfusion, compared with sham-operated controls (Fig. 2Ba). Most of these cells were shrunken and were represented by pyknotic and pigmented nuclei in H&E-stained sections. These changes were accompanied by increased TUNEL staining, which was observed in many of the shriveled cells (Fig. 2Bc). In contrast, the Ro 61-1790-treated animals showed either no, or significantly less (26–36 %), reduction in the number of viable neurons (Fig. 2Bb), compared with sham controls; no detectable levels of TUNEL staining (except slight staining of occasional cells) was observed in these animals Fig. 1Bd).

Focal Cerebral Ischemia

The blood gases ($PaCO_2$ 35±2 mmHg to 38±2 mmHg and PaO_2 128.4±7 mmHg to 132±10 mmHg) and MBP (125±1 mmHg and 132±1 mmHg) were within physiological limits and not significantly different between saline- and Ro 61-1790-pretreated groups at either the time of MCA occlusion or 4 h post-MCA occlusion.

Assessment of Microvascular Perfusion

Microvascular perfusion was not compromised in region 1 at 4 h after MCA occlusion in either saline- or Ro 61-1790-pretreated SHR. The number of perfused microvessels in region 1 saline- and Ro 61-1790-treated was: 410.29±3.9 and 429.7±24.04 (5 s); 420.57±25.75 and 442.29±25.75 (10 s), respectively. As illustrated in Fig. 1B, a moderately reduced microvascular perfusion was observed in region 2 in the saline control group. The reduced microvascular perfusion was more accentuated in regions 3–5 (except for level 4, close to the border of the MCA territory, where the decreased perfusion was less severe). Overall, Ro 61-1790 pretreatment was associated with higher levels of microvascular perfusion. Particularly significant differences between the microvascular perfusion in saline controls and Ro 61-1790 groups were seen in region 2 (levels 1–3). In the ischemic core (regions 4 and 5, levels 1–3; data not shown), perfusion was higher with Ro 61-1790 pretreatment than in controls, but did not reach the same degree of improvement seen in regions 1 and 2. The selective ET_A receptor antagonist Ro 61-1790 also significantly (unpaired t-test, $P<0.02$) decreased the volume of the ischemic lesion by 27 % [saline, 120±3 mm^3 ($n=5$); Ro 61-1790, 87±10 mm^3 ($n=6$)].

Discussion

The findings of this study indicate that the selective ET$_A$-antagonist, Ro 61-1790, treatment reversed the postischemic hypoperfusion following transient global ischemia (8 min) in gerbils, and improved the observed impaired microcirculatory perfusion seen in focal brain ischemia (4 h) of SHR. Recently, ET$_A$-receptor-mediated amelioration of postischemic hypoperfusion was also reported in rats, cats and rabbits [2, 11, 15]. Therefore, the results presented here confirm not only the use of ET$_A$-receptor antagonists to improve the postischemic perfusion in gerbils, but also in other species.

The noted effect of the postischemic Ro 61-1790 administration also modified the ischemic neuronal injury seen in the CA1 region of the gerbil hippocampus, since the animals treated with this agent showed a greater number of viable cells in the same area (Fig. 2Bb). The absence of TUNEL-positive cells in adjacent tissue sections (Fig. 2Bd) supports this conclusion. In addition, the significantly reduced volume of ischemic injury accompanying the enhanced microcirculatory perfusion seen in MCA occlusion of SHR, pretreated with Ro 61–1790, deserves special attention in order to assess the contribution of improved microcirculatory perfusion to the reduction of ischemic injury. Both the use of this model of ischemia and the method to evaluate microcirculatory perfusion have been disputed, since 4 h of MCA occlusion might not reflect a maximally developed ischemic lesion. Therefore, we wish to reiterate that previous reports including the present and previous observations from our laboratory demonstrated that 4 h of MCA occlusion in SHR induces a reproducible topographic volume of neocortical ischemic lesion suitable for the measurement of ischemic impairment of cerebral microcirculatory perfusion [10]. It has also been shown, in this study, that the use of intravascular fluorescent tracers to determine brain-capillary perfusion, originally developed by Kuschinsky and his associates, is more reliable than other techniques, e.g., carbon black, to assess the ischemia-induced deficit in microvascular perfusion [4, 5, 8, 22].

The modulatory effect of the ET$_A$-receptor antagonist on ischemic microvascular perfusion and lesion strongly suggests that preventing ischemic deterioration of microvascular perfusion is beneficial. This conclusion is particularly supported by the observed Ro 61-1790-induced amelioration of ischemic microvascular perfusion in regions 2 and 3, i.e., peri-ischemic/penumbral tissue, an area considered important for potential pharmacological intervention and rescue.

In conclusion, the effect of Ro 61-1790, the competitive ET-1 inhibitor, (with ~1000 times greater selectivity for ET$_A$ than ET$_B$ receptors) further supports the involvement of ET$_A$-mediated hypoperfusion in the development of cerebral injury [16]. This substance and other selective ET$_A$-receptor antagonists have been useful in preventing or treating other vascular disorders, e.g., vasospasm, hypertension [16, 20]. Therefore, based on the data presented here, as well as in previous studies, further exploration of the relationship between CBF and tissue injury is warranted. These findings will hopefully provide an impetus for continued studies of this phenomenon through the use of ET$_A$ antagonists alone or as part of a treatment regimen for multifactorial pathogenic processes such as stroke.

References

1. Barone FC, Globus MY-T, Price WJ, et al. (1994) Endothelin levels increase in rat and focal global ischemia. J Cereb Blood Flow Metab 14: 337–342
2. Bian L-G, Zhang T-X, Zhao WG, et al. (1994) Increased endothelin-1 in the rabbit model of middle cerebral artery occlusion. Neurosci Lett 174: 47–50
3. Boulanger C, Luscher T (1990) Release of endothelin from the porcine aorta; inhibition by endothelin-derived nitric oxide. J Clin Invest 85: 587–590
4. Dawson DA, Ruetzler CA, Carlos TM (1996) Polymorphonuclear leukocytes and microcirculatory perfusion in acute stroke in the SHR. Keio J Med 45: 248–253
5. Dawson DA, Ruetzler CA, Hallenbeck JM (1997) Temporal impairment of microcirculatory perfusion following focal cerebral ischemia in the spontaneously hypertensive rat. Brain Res 749: 200–208
6. Ehrenreich H, Lange M, Near KA, et al. (1992) Long-term monitoring of immunoreactive endothelin-1 and endothelin-3 in ventricular cerebrospinal fluid, plasma, and 24 hr urine of patients with subarachnoid hemorrhage. Res Exp Med 192: 257–268
7. Ehrenreich H, Schilling L (1995) New developments in the understanding of cerebral vasoregulation and vasospasm: the endothelin-nitric oxide network. Cleveland J Med 62: 105–116
8. Gobel U, Theilen H, Kuschinsky W (1990) Congruence of total and perfused capillary network in rat brains. Circ Res 66: 271–281
9. Hunley TE, Iwasaki S, Homma T, et al. (1995) Nitric oxide and endothelin in pathophysiological settings. Pediatr Nephrol 9: 235–244.
10. Kaplan B, Brint S, Tanabe J, et al. (1991) Temporal thresholds for neocortical infarction in rats subjected to reversible focal ischemia. Stroke 22: 1032–1039
11. Kelly PAT, Edvinsson L, Ritchie IM (1995) The endothelin antagonist FR139317 attenuates the cerebrovascular effects of N^Gnitro-L-arginine methyl ester in vivo. J Cereb Blood Flow Metab 15[Suppl 1]:S458
12. Macrae IM, Robinson MJ, Graham DI, et al. (1993) Endothelin-1 induced reduction in cerebral blood flow: dose dependency, time course and neuropathological consequences. J Cereb Blood Flow Metab 13: 276–284
13. Osborne KA, Shigeno T, Balarsky AM, et al. (1987) Quantitative assessment of early brain damage in a rat model of focal cerebral ischaemia. J Neurol Neurosurg Psychiatry 50: 402–410
14. Panza JA, Quyyumi AA, Brush JE, Jr., et al. (1990) Abnormal endothelin-dependent vascular relaxation in patients with essential hypertension. N Engl J Med 323: 22–27
15. Patel TR, Galbraith S, Graham DI, et al. (1996) Endothelin receptor antagonist increases cerebral perfusion and reduces ischaemic damage in feline focal cerebral ischaemia. J Cereb Blood Flow Metab 16: 95–958
16. Roux S, Breu V, Giller T, et al. (1997) Ro 61-1790, a new hydrosoluble endothelin antagonist: general pharmacology and effects on experimental cerebral vasospasm. J Pharmacol Exp Ther 283: 1110–1118
17. Rubanyi GM, Polokoff MA (1994) Endothelins: molecular biology, biochemistry, pharmacology, physiology and pathophysiology. Pharmacol Rev 46: 325–415
18. Spatz M, Stanimirovic D, Strasser A, et al. (1995) Nitro-L-arginine augments the endothelin-1 content of cerebrospinal fluid induced by cerebral ischemia. Brain Res 684: 99–103
19. Spatz M, Yasuma Y, Strasser A, et al. (1996) Cerebral postischemic hypoperfusion is mediated by ET_A receptors. Brain Res 726: 242–246
20. Stasch J-P, Hirth-Dietrich C, Frobel K, et al. (1995) Prolonged endothelin blockade prevents hypertension and cardiac hypertrophy in stroke-prone spontaneously hypertensive rats. Am J Hyperten 11: 1128–1134
21. Suzuki R, Masaoka H, Hirata Y, et al. (1992) The role of endothelin-1 in the original of cerebral vasospasm in patients with aneurysmal subarachnoid hemorrhage. J Neurosurg 77: 96–100
22. Theilen H, Schrock H, Kuschinsky W (1993) Capillary perfusion during incomplete forebrain ischemia and reperfusion in rat brain. Am J Physiol 265: H642–H648
23. Willette RN, Sauermelch C, Ezekiel M, et al. (1990) Effect of endothelin on cortical microvascular perfusion in rats. Stroke 21: 451–458
24. Yanagisawa M, Kurihara H, Kimura S, et al. (1988) A novel potent vasoconstrictive peptide produced by endothelial cells. Nature 332: 411–415

Lowering of Ameboid Microglial Resistance to Hydrogen Peroxide by Propentofylline

M. Tomita, Y. Fukuuchi, N. Tanahashi, M. Kobari,
H. Takeda, and M. Yokoyama

Summary. Employing video-enhanced contrast/differential-interference contrast (VEC–DIC) microscopy, we examined the effects of 10^{-5} M propentofylline on the hydrogen peroxide (H_2O_2)-enhanced cellular activity of ameboid microglia. The 20-min survival rate of ameboid microglia after H_2O_2 exposure in the control was two of two at 10^{-4} M, five of six at 10^{-3} M, one of two at 10^{-2} M, and none of four at 10^{-1} M. The value of TC_{50} (toxic concentration for 50 % survival) was $10^{-2.5}$ M. When ameboid microglia were pretreated with propentofylline, their resistance to H_2O_2 was greatly decreased. Upon exposure to millimolar H_2O_2, the microglia exhibited drastic changes, with the immediate commencement of a large ruffling wave at the peripheral part of the lamellipodia, formation of giant phagocytic vesicles containing H_2O_2, rapid transportation of a phagosome to the nucleus, evacuation of its contents onto the nucleus, immediate fragmentation of the lamellipodia, and shrinkage of the nucleus with condensation of chromatin. These changes usually occurred within a few minutes after exposure to H_2O_2. The survival rate of ameboid microglia pretreated with propentofylline was one of one at 10^{-7} M, three of six at 10^{-5} M, none of one at 10^{-4} M, and none of six at 10^{-3} M. The value of the TC_{50} was 10^{-5} M. At 10^{-3} M, five control cells survived, whereas all six cells pretreated with propentofylline died ($P<$ 0.05). It was concluded, therefore, that propentofylline lowered the resistance of ameboid microglia to H_2O_2.

Introduction

Microglia modify the maturation process of cerebral ischemia through their ability to differentiate into brain macrophages, releasing several secretory products, e.g., proteinases, cytokines, reactive oxygen intermediates, and reactive nitrogen intermediates [5]. Banati et al. [1] observed that propentofylline, a xanthine derivative, could completely inhibit the Ca^{2+}-dependent concanavalin A (Con A)-induced increase in production of reactive oxygen intermediates by a respiratory burst, whereas it did not affect the phorbol 12-myristate-13-acetate (PMA)-induced rise in respiratory burst activity. According to them, propentofylline can suppress reduced nicotinamide adenine dinucleotide phosphate (NADPH)-dependent production of reactive oxygen intermediates released from microglia/macrophages, so that its effect is, in large part, neuroprotective.

When analyzing the morphological changes of cultured microglia by video-enhanced contrast/differential-interference contrast (VEC–DIC) microscopy [8], we observed that nanomolar hydrogen peroxide (H_2O_2) activated ramified microglia,

Maturation Phenomenon in Cerebral Ischemia III
U. Ito et al. (Eds.)
© Springer-Verlag Berlin Heidelberg 1999

transforming them into rod-type microglia [9]. Micromolar concentrations of H_2O_2 appeared to facilitate transformation into the reactive form, which displayed strong phagocytic activity. Such hyperactivity sometimes led the microglia to undergo aggregation and cell death through coagulation necrosis. With or without H_2O_2, the reactive forms of microglia immediately transformed themselves into an ameboid morphology with spreading lamellipodia, as soon as the tip of the filopodia of floating villous microglia (reactive form) touched a coverslip surface [8]. Ameboid microglia became tolerant to millimolar H_2O_2, which apparently enhanced their phagocytic activity with ruffling movements of the lamellipodia and phagosome formation [6]. These observations suggest that microglia are a source of H_2O_2 and, at the same time, a target for it.

In the present study, we examined the effects of propentofylline, a microglial suppressor, on the morphological changes of ameboid microglia following exposure to millimolar H_2O_2.

Materials and Methods

We employed our recently developed technique of VEC–DIC microscopy to observe the detailed morphological changes of living ameboid microglia at an electron-microscopic level of magnification, as reported elsewhere [7]. Briefly, the VEC–DIC microscope consisted of an inverted Nomarski microscope (Axiovert 135, Carl Zeiss), which was equipped with a differential-interference-contrast (DIC) objective lens. Optical images were obtained using a charge-coupled device (CCD) camera (C3077, Hamamatsu Photonics) in digitized signal form. Video signals from the small detection area (7 mm×9 mm) of the camera were fed into an image processor (Argus-10, Hamamatsu Photonics) linked to a personal computer, which enhanced the contrast and increased the electrical magnification of the video images. The total magnification so reached was 20,000·. All images obtained were recorded on videotape (30 frames/s) for storage. To analyze the motions of the microglia at a high spatial and temporal resolution, selected parts of the videotape of specific interest were played back and fed into an image analyzer (Avio Excel, Nippon Avionics) coupled to the above computer.

Microglia were obtained from the brains of embryonic SD rats employing the technique reported by Nakajima et al. [4]. Cells were grown routinely, being co-cultured with astroglia in a bottle containing Dulbecco's modified Eagle medium (DMEM, GIBCO) supplemented with 10 % fetal bovine serum plus penicillin–streptomycin, and incubated in a humidified 5 %CO_2/95 %O_2 atmosphere at 37 °C. At 7–20 days after seeding, numbers of round and flattened cells were observed on the surface of the astroglial cell layer. The bottle was shaken gently by hand for 2–3 min and the cells floating in the medium were collected as a source of microglia. The isolated microglia displayed a strong phagocytic activity for latex beads, were positive for ED 1 and negative for anti-GFAP [4]. The collection rate of microglia achieved by the present technique amounted to 97 % purity [4]. Observations of the microglia were made on a coverslip which was mounted on the objective glass of the inverted microscope with oil. The microglia were superfused continuously with DMEM, employing a double-pump system (infusion- and suction-pumps). As reported previously, the microglia exhibited four distinct forms in terms of their phenotype: (1) process-bearing ramified microglia paved onto or buried in the co-cultured astroglial cell layer; (2) rod-type microglia characterized by ever-moving filopodia and lamellipodia; (3) reactive microglia of two types, with abundant fine filopodia or with a skirt of wide, thin, undulating lamellipodia, both of which displayed swift locomotion and strong phagocytotic activity; and (4) ameboid microglia, which were used for the present study ($n=28$). As a control, 14 ameboid microglia were observed before, during, and after exposure to H_2O_2 at concentrations ranging widely between 10^{-9} M and 10^{-1} M, prepared by diluting 3 % H_2O_2 with saline. Another 14 ameboid microglia were pretreated with propentofylline (supplied by Hoechst Japan) at a final concentration of 10^{-6} M, and the cells were then exposed to H_2O_2 at different concentrations, as in the control group. We monitored the cells for more than 20 min and compared the survival rates of the microglia, which were expressed in terms of half-maximal toxicity concentration (TC_{50}).

Results

Ameboid Microglia and H_2O_2

When reactive microglia were flowing or drifting in the medium, their shape was spherical and, in most cases, they had filopodia on their surface (villous form) which moved violently. On coming into contact with the glass surface of the coverslip at their filopodia, the floating reactive microglia immediately spread themselves out and transformed into the ameboid form. Thin, transparent, sheet-like structures (lamellipodia) extended from the cell bodies toward the outside so as to form a peripheral band on the cell body. The ameboid microglia remained at the same place, just moving and waving their lamellipodia. If any directional movement was observed, it was extremely slow. H_2O_2 at concentrations of 10^{-7} M, 10^{-6} M, 10^{-5} M, and 10^{-4} M, to which both ramified and reactive microglia had reacted strongly, now produced no appreciable changes in the ameboid microglia. With H_2O_2 at 10^{-3} M, the control microglia ($n=6$) became gradually activated, exhibiting an enhanced ruffling motion of their lamellipodia and formation of large vesicles (phagosomes). Subsequently, five of the six cells continued to be active for 30 min, while one died. Unlike in the reactive form of microglia, we observed little ameboid locomotion of these microglia within a period of 60 min, even under such hyperactivated conditions. With H_2O_2 at 10^{-2} M ($n=2$) and 10^{-1} M ($n=4$), the microglia began to show signs of degeneration; their granular activity slowed down, and they became quiet, with no movements of the lamellipodia. The cell membrane underwent gradual fragmentation, and the nucleus shrank with spotty chromatin condensation within 2 min. All the cells ($n=6$) ultimately died. The cell death resembled the state of apoptosis. A summary of the control changes is presented in Table 1. As shown, the 20-min survival rate of the ameboid microglia after exposure to H_2O_2 in the control group was two of two (100 %) at 10^{-4} M, five of six (83 %) at 10^{-3} M, one of two (50 %) at 10^{-2} M, and none of four (0 %) at 10^{-1} M. The value of the TC_{50} was $10^{-2.5}$ M.

Table 1. Control Microglia exposed to H_2O_2 (10^{-1}–10^{-4} M)

No	Concn.	Observed changes	Final outcome
1	10^{-1}	Coagulated and Immobile	XCell death
2	10^{-1}	Coagulated	XCell death
3	10^{-1}	Plasma membrane fragmented and chromatin condensed	XCell death
4	10^{-1}	Vacuolization, degeneration	XCell death
5	10^{-2}	Coagulated, degeneration, membrane ballooning	XCell death
6	10^{-2}	Activated with ruffling, phagosome formation	O
7	10^{-3}	Activated, ruffling	O
8	10^{-3}	Activated, ruffling	O
9	10^{-3}	Activated, ruffling, granular agitation	O
10	10^{-3}	Activated, abundant phagosome formation, ruffling	O
11	10^{-3}	Coagulation necrosis (5 min), ballooning (15 min)	XCell death
12	10^{-3}	Ruffling, ballooning, cell body swelling (60 min)	O
13	10^{-4}	Abundant phagosome formation, ruffling, stunned condition	O
14	10^{-4}	Activated, phagosome formation, bleb formation	O

Propentofylline-Pretreated Ameboid Microglia and H_2O_2

The same procedure was repeated with propentofylline (10^{-5} M)-pretreated ameboid microglia (n=14). In contrast to the control group, drastic changes were observed in the propentofylline-pretreated ameboid microglia, as illustrated in Fig. 1. Upon administration of 10^{-3} M H_2O_2 (n=6), part of the lamellipodia reacted (Fig. 1A), became inflated, folded back (Fig. 1B, C) and internalized H_2O_2-containing fluid to form a giant phagosome (Fig. 1D), which was rapidly transported to the nucleus (Fig. 1E). As soon as the phagosome had reached the nucleus and emptied itself by sprinkling the H_2O_2-containing fluid onto the nucleus (Fig. 1F), chromatin underwent immediate condensation, and the peripheral lamellipodia fragmented. The nucleus shrank and became swollen with spotty chromatin aggregations (Fig. 1F–H). Such

Table 2. Propentofyline-pretreated microglia exposed to H_2O_2 (10^{-3}–10^{-7} M)

No	Concn.	Observed changes	Final outcome
1	10^{-3}	Degenration (13 min), nucleus coagulation, granule Brownian motion	XCell death
2	10^{-3}	Lamellipodia abrasion, necrosis	XCell death
3	10^{-3}	Homogenized nucleus, ruffling, giant phagosome, granule Brownian motion	XCell death
4	10^{-3}	Ruffling, giant phagosome, granule Brownian motion (5 min)	XCell death
5	10^{-3}	Ruffling, giant phagosome, granule Brownian motion, nucleus shrinkage	XCell death
6	10^{-3}	10^{-5} H_2O_2 no change; 10^{-3} add. ruffling, coagulation (5 min)	XCell death
7	10^{-4}	Coagulation necrosis	XCell death
8	10^{-5}	Ruffling, 3–4 phagosomes on & off; rapid degeneration (7 min)	XCell death
9	10^{-5}	With 10^{-5} ruffling enhanced, 7 phagosomes, coagulation	XCell death
10	10^{-5}	Ruffling slightly activated	O
11	10^{-5}	Ruffling activated	O
12	10^{-5}	Chromatin condensation, vesicle formation in nucleus	XCell death
13	10^{-5}	Ruffling activated and then subsiding	O
14	10^{-7}	Giant wrinkling, star-like shape, transformation to ameboid form	O

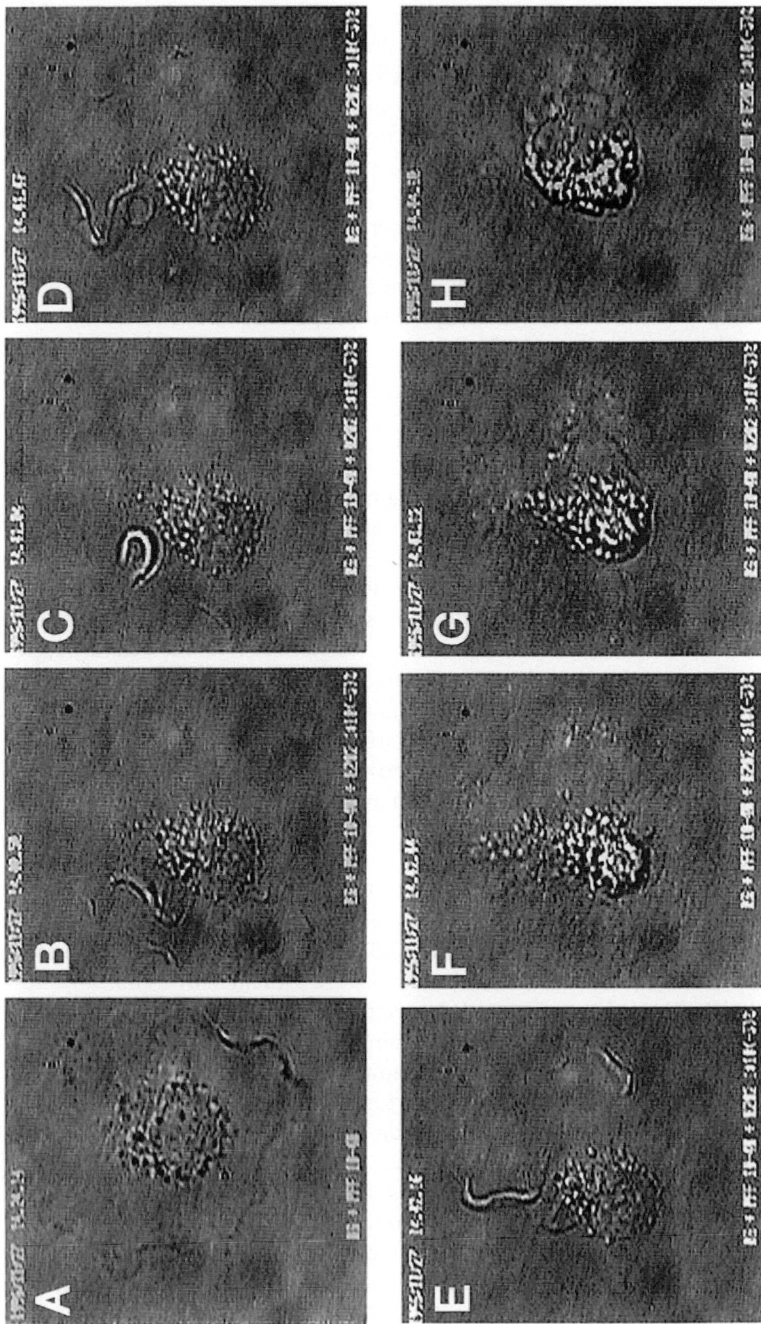

Fig. 1A–H. Sequential morphological changes of propentofylline-pretreated ameboid microglia after exposure to 10^{-3} M H_2O_2. **A** Control. **B**, Immediately; **C** 10 s; **D** 20 s; **E** 30 s; **F** 40 s; **G** 50 s; and **H** 3 min after H_2O_2

changes were completed within 1 min after the application of 10^{-3} M H_2O_2, leading to cell death, which resembled apoptosis in four of the six cells, while the remainder suffered necrotic cell death with swelling of the cell membrane and randomly moving particles in the inner solution. As summarized in Table 2, the survival rate of ameboid microglia in the propentofylline group was one of one (100 %) at 10^{-7} M, three of six (50 %) at 10^{-5} M, none of one (0 %) at 10^{-4} M, and none of six (0 %) at 10^{-3} M. The value of the TC_{50} was 10^{-5} M.

As described above, the TC_{50} in the control was $10^{-2.5}$ M, and that in the propentofylline group was 10^{-5} M. Comparing the two groups at 10^{-3} M H_2O_2, it can be seen that one of six cells died in the control group, whereas all of the cells died in the propentofylline group ($P<0.05$). These data imply that propentofylline lowered the resistance of the ameboid microglia to H_2O_2.

Comments and Conclusion

In a previous communication, we reported that nanomolar concentrations of H_2O_2 activated ramified microglia into the rod-type, then the reactive form [7]. Such a reaction appeared to be non-specific for ramified microglia, since similar activation was induced by several other stimuli, e.g., application of lipopolysaccharide, supernatant of zymosan-A solution, supernatant of dead neurons, shear stress imposed on the cell surface, etc. We also observed that micromolar concentrations of H_2O_2 enhanced the migration and phagocytosis of reactive microglia. In the present experiments, we found that ameboid microglia were not affected by nanomolar, micromolar, or even millimolar concentrations of H_2O_2, but became affected only when the concentration was increased to values higher than 10^{-3} M. The microglial sensitivity to H_2O_2 appeared to be differentiation dependent. This suggests that microglia may regulate protection from H_2O_2. As mentioned above, microglia are a source of reactive oxygen species through activation of NADPH oxidase, including free radicals and H_2O_2. However, microglia have also been reported to be a target for H_2O_2. Hastie et al. [3] observed that H_2O_2 (100 μM)-induced filamin translocation from the membrane to cytosol occurred after 1 min of H_2O_2 treatment. H_2O_2 exposure rapidly lowered the intracellular cyclic adenosine monophosphate (cAMP) levels, while H_2O_2-induced cAMP decreases were prevented by inhibiting phospholipase D (PLD). Their data indicate that metabolites produced downstream from H_2O_2-induced PLD activation could mediate filamin redistribution and F-actin rearrangement. They also reported that the H_2O_2-induced filamin redistribution resulted from inhibition of the cAMP-dependent protein kinase pathway [2].

The effect of propentofylline on the activation of microglia in lowering the resistance or, in other words, increasing the sensitivity to H_2O_2 was diametrically opposed to our expectations. One possible explanation is that propentofylline not only halted free-radical production by inhibiting the respiratory burst, but also stopped induction of the defense mechanisms against free radicals/H_2O_2. There must be a mechanism of coupled regulation between the rate of production of reactive microglia and induction of self-protection from H_2O_2 so that the cells are not killed by their own toxic substances. It is feasible that microglia may regulate protection from H_2O_2.

Acknowledgement. The research reported here was supported by Hoechst Japan.

References

1. Banati RB, Schubert P, Rothe G, Gehrmann J, Rudolphi K, Valet G, Kreutzberg GW (1994) Modulation of intracellular formation of reactive oxygen intermediates in peritoneal macrophages and microglia/brain macrophages by pentofylline. J Cereb Blood Flow Metab 14: 145–149
2. Hastie LE, Patton WF, Hechtman HB, Shepro DJ (1997) H_2O_2-induced filamin redistribution in endothelial cells is modulated by the cyclic AMP-dependent protein kinase pathway. J Cell Physiol 172: 373–381
3. Hastie LE, Patton WF, Hechtman HB, Shepro D (1998) Metabolites of the phospholipase D pathway regulate H_2O_2-induced filamin redistribution in endothelial cells. J Cell Biochem 68: 511–524
4. Nakajima K, Hamanoue M, Shimojo M (1989) Characterization of microglia isolated from a primary culture of embryonic rat brain by a simplified method. Biomed Res 10[Suppl 3]:411–423
5. Raivich G, Bluethmann H, Kreutzberg GW (1996) Signaling molecules and neuroglial activation in the injured central nervous system. Keio J Med 45: 239–247
6. Takeda H, Fukuuchi Y, Tomita M, Tanahashi N, Kobari M, Yokoyama M, Takao M, Ito D (1998) Hydrogen peroxide enhances phagocytic activity of ameboid microglia. Neurosci Lett 240: 5–8
7. Tomita M, Fukuuchi Y, Tanahashi N, Kobari M, Takeda H, Yokoyama M, Ito D, Terakawa S (1996) Swift transformation and locomotion of PMNL and microglia as observed by VEC-DIC microscopy (video microscopy). Keio J Med 45: 213–224
8. Tomita M, Fukuuchi Y, Tanahashi N, Kobari M, Takeda H, Yokoyama M, Tomita Y, Ito D (1997) Rapid transformation of ramified microglia by nanomolar hydrogen peroxide into reactive form (abstract). Jpn J Cereb Blood Flow Metab 45: 73
9. Tomita M, Fukuuchi Y, Tanahashi N, Takeda H (1998) Changes in resistance of cultured microglia to hydrogen peroxide with differentiation. Microcirculation Annu 14: 17–18

Combination Therapy:
A Promising Treatment Strategy for Cerebral Ischemia

E. Hungerhuber, S. Zausinger, A. Baethmann,
H.-J. Reulen, and R. Schmid-Elsaesser

Introduction

Investigations of the mechanisms of cerebral ischemia have revealed that cell death is mediated, among other things, by a massive release of excitatory amino acids [9], generation of free radicals [50] and, as a final step, calcium influx into cells [49]. This understanding has led to a search for pharmacologic agents that protect the brain against these mechanisms. Although the molecular processes of the postischemic events are still only partially understood, numerous experimental neuroprotective drugs have been developed. Many of them are currently under clinical evaluation for the treatment of ischemic stroke, subarachnoid hemorrhage (SAH), or head injury. Yet, encouraging results from clinical trials are still rare. No trial has shown any single agent to be effective so far [57]. As a multitude of mechanisms is involved in ischemic brain injury, it is conceivable that a single pharmacotherapeutic agent aimed at just one process of ischemic damage is unlikely to be sufficient, and that a combination of treatment procedures would be more promising.

Pharmacological Neuroprotection

Excitatory Amino Acid Antagonism

Ischemia leads to a massive release and accumulation of glutamate in the extracellular space, followed by an interaction with several classes of receptors [29]. The N-methyl-D-aspartate (NMDA)-, the alpha-amino-3-hydroxy-5-methyl-4-isoxazole propionic acid (AMPA)-, and the kainate-receptors are ion-channel-coupled receptors. Glutamate binding, particularly at the NMDA receptor, leads to calcium influx, with the known deleterious consequences of an increased intracellular calcium concentration. Furthermore, influx of sodium ions, predominantly via non-NMDA receptors (AMPA, kainate) facilitates depolarization and may eventually result in neuronal as well as glial swelling [47].

The most extensively studied NMDA antagonist MK-801 (dizocilpine) binds noncompetitively with the ionophore. This drug exhibits a marked therapeutic efficacy, particularly in focal ischemia, when administered within the first 2 h after artery occlusion [40], but severe psychomimetic and neurotoxic side effects prevent its administration in humans. Competitive NMDA antagonists such as selfotel, 2-(2-carboxypiperazine-4-yl)-1-propenyl-1-phosphonic acid (d-CPP-ene) and eliprodil have shown a reduction of infarct formation by more than 70 % when their adminis-

Maturation Phenomenon in Cerebral Ischemia III
U. Ito et al. (Eds.)
© Springer-Verlag Berlin Heidelberg 1999

tration was started before middle cerebral artery occlusion (MCAO) [51]. Despite these promising results, most NMDA antagonists have intolerable side effects [34]; therefore, clinical trials with, e.g., selfotel, cerestat and eliprodil have been suspended [7].

The noncompetitive NMDA antagonist and widely used antitussive dextromethorphan is metabolized to dextrorphan. Both compounds bind inside the NMDA-receptor-associated channel, thereby attenuating glutamate neurotoxicity in cultured neurons as well as in animals in vivo [53]. A safety and tolerance study on dextromethorphan in neurosurgical patients has already been completed. Side effects proved to be acceptable, as these were reversible [52].

In animal models of global and focal ischemia, AMPA antagonists such as 6-nitro-7-sulfamoylbenzo(f)quinoxaline-2,3-dione (NBQX) have marked neuroprotective properties with an unusual time window of effectiveness [18]. Recently, however, evidence is accumulating on adverse effects of NBQX, causing clinical trials to be terminated [15].

Calcium Antagonism

Calcium plays a pivotal role in the regulation of many physiological cell functions. Under regular conditions, the cytosolic calcium concentration is maintained at a much lower level than in the extracellular space; this is attributable to specific cellular control mechanisms involving consumption of metabolic energy. Ca^{2+} ions enter the intracellular compartment through different classes of gates, such as the voltage-sensitive calcium channels (VSCC) or receptor-operated calcium channels (ROCC). Neuronal ischemia causing membrane depolarization eventually leads to a progressive derangement of the cellular calcium homeostasis [21]. The intracellular calcium-ion accumulation may promote numerous secondary processes, leading to neuronal damage, such as activation of proteolytic enzymes, phospholipases, and generation of free radicals [6].

In contrast to many other calcium antagonists, nimodipine – an inhibitor of VSCC – penetrates the intact blood–brain barrier. It has been extensively investigated in a number of randomized, placebo-controlled trials and has been shown to improve outcome following SAH [39]. However, in acute ischemic stroke there is a lack of convincing results; to the contrary, even worsening of outcome and increased mortality have been described [25]. This may be due to arterial hypotension after nimodipine administration.

Magnesium is a naturally occurring calcium antagonist inducing dilatation of cerebral arteries. The mechanisms of magnesium ions are numerous and not completely understood. Magnesium ions participate in a voltage-sensitive blockade of ion channels, resulting in a noncompetitive antagonism of NMDA receptors [38]. They compete with extracellular calcium ions, thereby reducing entry of calcium ions into the cell [2]. Finally, Mg^{2+} ions inhibit the release of intracellular calcium and of excitatory amino acids [14]. In animals, administration of magnesium has been observed to decrease morbidity from cerebral ischemia, trauma, and SAH. According to the results of a pilot study, magnesium has been found to be safe and well-tolerated by patients with acute stroke [35].

Free Radical Scavengers

Oxygen free radicals are highly reactive due to their unpaired electron. During cerebral ischemia, the electron transport chain in the mitochondria is highly reduced, which may result in oxygen-radical formation as soon as oxygen is re-supplied. Such conditions prevail during incomplete ischemia as well as in the penumbra zone of focal ischemia. Free radicals predominantly attack membrane phospholipids and induce lipid peroxidation, resulting in irreversible damage of cell membranes and release of free fatty acids [54]. The autoxidation of arachidonic acid results in an increase of the formation of superoxide radicals, thromboxanes and prostaglandins which affect the vascular reactivity post ischemia. Moreover, free radicals were found to attack DNA and oxidize proteins. They may thereby adversely affect the structure and function of membranes, receptors, ion channels, and enzymes [50].

Native superoxide dismutase (SOD) has a short half-life and is unable to cross the blood–brain barrier. Neuroprotection by SOD was demonstrated only at very high doses [33]. Conjugation of the antioxidant SOD with polyethylene glycol (PEG) prolongs its half-life in the plasma. PEG-SOD exhibits neuroprotective properties predominantly in experimental focal ischemia. Although results of a phase-II trial in head injury with PEG-SOD have been encouraging [36], it was not found to be effective in subsequent phase-III trials [58].

The 21-aminosteroid tirilazad mesylate is a potent inhibitor of the free-radical-induced lipid peroxidation; however, due to its low barrier permeability, its efficacy is largely restricted to the vascular endothelium. Tirilazad has been proven to exert neuroprotective effects under numerous pathophysiological conditions studied in vitro and in vivo. It has recently become clinically available [24]. In a SAH trial, evidence was obtained for an improved outcome in male but not female patients. Women may metabolize the drug more rapidly than men. Moreover, a clinical trial on ischemic stroke was suspended because interim analyses indicated a lack of clinical efficacy. As both trials on tirilazad were producing inconclusive results, further studies with administration of higher doses are currently under way [26].

Evidence is accumulating that lipophilic antioxidants which penetrate the intact blood–brain barrier may be more effective than agents with a limited permeability. Some are integrated into neuronal and other cell membranes and may thereby inhibit the process of lipid peroxidation more effectively [54]. In addition, these drugs may also penetrate the mitochondrial membrane and afford protection against free-radical damage to components of the respiratory chain [37]. The recently discovered group of pyrrolopyrimidines [19], which are antioxidants with an improved blood-brain barrier permeability, have more powerful neuroprotective properties than 21-aminosteroids [45], which must enter the brain parenchyma via the vascular endothelium.

Combination Pharmacotherapy

Regarding the complexity of pathophysiological mechanisms operating in cerebral ischemia, many neuroprotective drug combinations are conceivable. An overview of studies that have evaluated combination pharmacotherapies is given in Table 1.

Table 1. Combination pharmacotherapies

Treatment	Ischemia/animal	Results	Reference
MK-801 + NBQX	Focal/rat	MK-801 alone more effective than combination	Gill and Lodge [16],
	Focal/mice	Over-additive protection by combination therapy	Lippert et al. [28]
MK-801 + kynurenic acid	Global/gerbil	Reduced hippocampal neurodegeneration by drug combination	Gill and Woodruff [17]
MK-801 + PBN	In vitro	Improved efficacy, prolonged time window of protection	Barth et al. [5]
MK-801 + tirilazad + insulin + diazepam	Global/rat	Less damage of neocortex by combination therapy	Auer [3]
MK-801 + nicardipine	Global/gerbil	Additive protective effects against CA1 neuronal loss	Hewitt and Corbett [22]
MK-801 + nimodipine	Focal/cat	Improved histological outcome with combination therapy	Uematsu et al. [55]
Magnesium + tirilazad	Focal/rat	Reduced infarct volume. Improved functional outcome	Schmid-Elsaesser et al. [42]
Dextrorphan + cycloheximide	Focal/rat	Additive protective effects. Reduced infarct volume	Du et al. [11]
Dextromethorphan + tirilazad	Focal/rat	Combination annihilates effects afforded by single therapies	Schmid-Elsaesser et al. [44]
MK-801 + muscimol	Focal/rat	Combination therapy prolongs therapeutic window	Lyden and Lonzo [30]
U-101033 E + U-74389G	Focal/rat	Combination results in more rapid functional recovery	Schmid-Elsaesser et al. [46]

Experiments with the NMDA antagonist MK-801 and the AMPA antagonist NBQX have provided conflicting results [12, 28]. Gill and Woodruff combined MK-801 and kynurenic acid, a noncompetitive antagonist at the glycine binding site of the NMDA receptor. The combination therapy attenuated hippocampal neurodegeneration by 86 %, which is more effective than each drug alone [17]. Uematsu et al. demonstrated enhanced neuroprotection by combined administration of a NMDA antagonist and a calcium-channel antagonist. These authors found an inhibition of the increase of the intracellular calcium concentration in cerebral cortex during middle cerebral artery occlusion (MCAO) as well as an improved histological outcome of animals receiving MK-801 plus nimodipine [55].

Another promising approach is the concurrent administration of calcium-channel or NMDA-receptor antagonists together with radical scavengers. Treatment with α-phenyl-tert-butyl nitrone (PBN) and MK-801 afforded an increase of both the efficacy and the time window of protection after global ischemia [5]. Surprisingly, in focal ischemia, the combination of tirilazad and dextromethorphan was observed to abolish the beneficial effects obtained by each therapy alone [44]. The combination of these drugs might have led to mutual inhibition or intensified adverse effects. Recently, we have observed enhanced neuroprotection by the combination therapy of tirilazad and magnesium [42]. In another study, rats subjected to transient forebrain ischemia suffered less damage of the neocortex when administered with MK-801 in addition to tirilazad than with tirilazad alone. Even greater neuroprotection of neocortex was achieved with tirilazad in combination with MK-801 plus insulin and diazepam [3].

Damage of both the vascular endothelium and brain parenchyma may be involved in the radical-mediated injury. It is therefore conceivable that administration of a combination of drugs exerting antioxidative properties in blood vessels and brain parenchyma might protect the brain against free-radical-mediated damage more effectively [46].

Another possibility is the use of a single drug that simultaneously acts at different targets. Lubeluzole, for example, prevents the release of glutamate and inhibits glutamate-induced nitric-oxide-related neurotoxicity. In a phase-II trial, lubeluzole was found to reduce mortality [10], and phase-III trials on ischemic stroke have recently been completed. Preliminary results also appear to be promising, since lubeluzole is well tolerated [57].

Hypothermia

Hypothermia has already been shown to exert protective effects if brain temperature is lowered by only $2-3\,^{\circ}\mathrm{C}$ [8]. Brain cooling reduces metabolism and delays depletion of ATP stores. Maintenance of the blood–brain barrier function, suppression of glutamate release, and decreased generation of oxygen free radicals and of NO were reported to be involved in the neuroprotective mechanisms of hypothermia. In view of the multitude of pathomechanisms of ischemia, it is not surprising that hypothermia currently represents the most effective monotherapy to prevent ischemic brain damage [4]. Although administration of deep hypothermia ($<25\,^{\circ}\mathrm{C}$) is well established for cardio- or neurovascular procedures, it is associated with severe side effects. In contrast, mild to moderate hypothermia ($30-35\,^{\circ}\mathrm{C}$) appears to be well tolerated. A variety of centers utilize mild hypothermia for neuroprotection during aneurysm surgery. Recent clinical investigations of the treatment of traumatic brain injury by moderate hypothermia indicate a tendency toward an improved outcome [31].

Only a few experiments on hypothermia in combination with pharmacotherapy have been reported (Table 2). We have recently investigated protective properties of tirilazad plus magnesium in combination with mild hypothermia ($33\,^{\circ}\mathrm{C}$) in transient focal ischemia of rats. The results of this study suggest that the neuroprotective properties of hypothermia can be enhanced by using this combination of therapies. Hypothermia alone significantly reduced infarct formation in the cortex but not in the basal ganglia, whereas the combination with tirilazad and magnesium significantly inhibited infarction in both cortex and the basal ganglia. The multimodal treatment with tirilazad, magnesium, and hypothermia afforded almost complete suppression of infarct formation in the cortex and major reduction in the basal ganglia. Furthermore, the animals subjected to this treatment had fewer neurological deficits and enjoyed enhanced electrophysiological recovery [43].

Table 2. Combination therapies with mild to moderate hypothermia

Treatment	Ischemia/ animal	Results	Reference
Hypothermia (34 °C) + magnesium	Spinal cord/ rabbit	Enhanced tolerance against duration of ischemia	Vacanti and Ames [56]
Hypothermia (33 °C) + U-74389G	Trauma/rats	Combination no more protective than single therapies	Marion and White [32]
Hypothermia (35 °C) + selfotel	Global/gerbil	Combination protective against repetitive ischemia	Shuaib et al. [48]
Hypothermia + MK-801	Global/rat focal/rat	Chronic protection only by combination therapy (30 °C). Treatments had similar, but no additive effects (33 °C)	Lin et al. [27], Frazzini et al. [13]
Hypothermia (33 °C) + mannitol	Focal/rat	Combination no more protective than hypothermia alone	Karibe et al. [23]
Hypothermia (33 °C) + magnesium + tirilazad	Focal/rat	Combination therapy inhibits infarct formation, affords improved functional outcome and electrophysiological recovery	Schmid-Elsaesser et al. [43]

Conclusions

Although many drugs exert potent neuroprotective properties in animal experiments, no single agent has been found to be effective in clinical trials on stroke patients so far. An ideal treatment should provide neuroprotection on a broad basis, aiming at: (1) reduction of cerebral metabolism, (2) antagonism of glutamate neurotoxicity, (3) scavenging of free radicals, (4) inhibition of the cellular calcium overload, and (5) amelioration of reperfusion. As no single compound currently meets all of these requirements, the need for clinical trials using a combination of drugs may be emphasized [1, 7, 20, 41]. Before clinical trials are initiated, however, the efficacy and safety of promising drug combinations should be investigated in animal models also suitable for identifying the interactions of given drugs. Nevertheless, interventions by hypothermia or by pharmacological agents interfering with different mechanisms of neuronal cell damage, possibly in combination, promise to achieve an improved neuroprotection.

References

1. Akins PT, Hsu CY (1998) Future directions in research and development of new treatments for ischemic stroke. In: Hsu CY (ed) Ischemic stroke: from basic mechanisms to new drug development. Karger, Basel, pp 151–162
2. Altura BT, Altura BM (1984) Interactions of Mg and K on cerebral vessels – aspects in view of stroke. Review of present status and new findings. Magnesium 3: 195–211
3. Auer RN (1995) Combination therapy with U74006F (tirilazad mesylate), MK- 801, insulin and diazepam in transient forebrain ischaemia. Neurol Res 17: 132–136
4. Barone FC, Feuerstein GZ, White RF (1997) Brain cooling during transient focal ischemia provides complete neuroprotection. Neurosci Biobehav Rev 21: 31–44

5. Barth A, Barth L, Newell DW (1996) Combination therapy with MK-801 and alpha-phenyl-tert-butyl-nitrone enhances protection against ischemic neuronal damage in organotypic hippocampal slice cultures. Exp Neurol 141: 330–336

6. Belch JJF (1992) Free radicals and their scavenging in stroke. Scott Med J 37: 67–68

7. Bogousslavsky J, De Keyser J, Diener HC, Fieschi C, Hacke W, Kaste M, Orgogozo JM, Pulsinelli W, Wahlgren NG (1998) Neuroprotection as initial therapy in acute stroke. Third report of an ad hoc consensus group meeting. Cerebrovasc Dis 8: 59–72

8. Busto R, Dietrich WD, Globus MY, Valdes I, Scheinberg P, Ginsberg MD (1987) Small differences in intraischemic brain temperature critically determine the extent of ischemic neuronal injury. J Cereb Blood Flow Metab 7: 729–738

9. Choi DW (1992) Excitotoxic cell death. J Neurobiol 23: 1261–1276

10. Diener HC, Hacke W, Hennerici M, Radberg J, Hantson L, Dekeyser J (1996) Lubeluzole in acute ischemic stroke: a double-blind, placebo-controlled phase II trial. Stroke 27: 76–81

11. Du C, Hu R, Csernansky CA, Liu XZ, Hsu CY, Choi DW (1996) Additive neuroprotective effects of dextrorphan and cycloheximide in rats subjected to transient focal cerebral ischemia. Brain Res 718: 233–236

12. Foutz AS, Pierrefiche O, Denavit Saubie M (1994) Combined blockade of NMDA and non-NMDA receptors produces respiratory arrest in the adult cat. Neuroreport 5: 481–484

13. Frazzini VI, Winfree CJ, Choudhri HF, Prestigiacomo CJ, Solomon RA (1994) Mild hypothermia and MK-801 have similar but not additive degrees of cerebroprotection in the rat permanent focal ischemia model. Neurosurgery 34: 1040–1045

14. Ghribi O, Callebert J, Verrecchia C, Plotkine M, Boulu RG (1995) Blockers of NMDA-operated channels decrease glutamate and aspartate extracellular accumulation in striatum during forebrain ischaemia in rats. Fundam Clin Pharmacol 9: 141–146

15. Gill R (1994) The pharmacology of a-amino-3-hydroxy-5-methyl-4-isoxazole propionate (AMPA)/kainate antagonists and their role in cerebral ischemia. Cerebrovasc Brain Metab Rev 6: 225–256

16. Gill R, Lodge D (1993) The neuroprotective effects of a combination of MK-801 and NBQX in focal ischaemia (abstract). J Cereb Blood Flow Metab 13:S668

17. Gill R, Woodruff GN (1990) The neuroprotective actions of kynurenic acid and MK-801 in gerbils are synergistic and not related to hypothermia. Eur J Pharmacol 176: 143–149

18. Graham SH, Chen J, Lan JQ, Simon RP (1996) A dose-response study of neuroprotection using the AMPA antagonist NBQX in rat focal cerebral ischemia. J Pharmacol Exp Ther 276: 1–4

19. Hall ED, Andrus PK, Smith SL, Oostveen JA, Scherch HM, Lutzke BS, Raub TJ, Sawada GA, Palmer JR, Banitt LS, Tustin JS, Belonga KL, Ayer DE, Bundy GL (1996) Neuroprotective efficacy of microvascularly-localized versus brain-penetrating antioxidants. Acta Neurochir Suppl (Wien) 66: 107–113

20. Hallenbeck JM, Frerichs KU (1993) Stroke therapy – it may be time for an integrated approach. Arch Neurol 50: 768–770

21. Harris RJ, Symon L (1984) Extracellular pH, potassium, and calcium activities in progressive ischemia of rat cortex. J Cereb Blood Flow Metab 4: 178–186

22. Hewitt K, Corbett D (1992) Combined treatment with MK-801 and nicardipine reduces global ischemic damage in the gerbil. Stroke 23: 82–86

23. Karibe H, Zarow GJ, Weinstein PR (1995) Use of mild intraischemic hypothermia versus mannitol to reduce infarct size after temporary middle cerebral artery occlusion in rats. J Neurosurg 83: 93–98

24. Kassell NF, Haley EC, Appersonhansen C, Stat M, Alves WM, Dorsch NW, Fabinyi G, Matheson J, Reilly P, Siu K, Stokes B, Stuart G, Koos W, Calliauw L, Selosse P, Astrup J, Gjerris F, Mendelow AD, Castel JP, Christiaens JL, Cophignon J, Keravel Y, Lagarrigue J, Mourier K, Philippon J, Brandt L, Vonessen C, Persson L, Brock M, Fahlbusch P, Gilsbach J, Hassler W, Perneczky A, Samii M, Schmiedek P, Mee E, Arista A, Cantore G, Carteri A, Collice M, Dapian R, Marini G, Menonna P, Baena RRY, Matteo PS, Testa PC, Villani R, Antunes JL (1996) Randomized, double-blind, vehicle-controlled trial of tirilazad mesylate in patients with aneurysmal subarachnoid hemorrhage: a cooperative study in Europe, Australia, and New Zealand. J Neurosurg 84: 221–228

25. Kaste M, Fogelholm R, Erila T, Palomaki H, Murros K, Rissanen A, Sarna S (1994) A randomized, double-blind, placebo-controlled trial of nimodipine in acute ischemic hemispheric stroke. Stroke 25: 1348–1353

26. Koroshetz WJ, Moskowitz MA (1996) Emerging treatments for stroke in humans. Trends Pharmacol Sci 17: 227–233

27. Lin B, Dietrich WD, Busto R, Kraydieh S, Globus MYT, Ginsberg MD (1994) Postischemic brain hypothermia combined with delayed MK-801 treatment protects chronically after global ischemia in rats. Stroke 25: 254

28. Lippert K, Welsch M, Krieglstein J (1993) Overadditive effect of dizocilpine and NBQX against neuronal damage (abstract). J Cereb Blood Flow Metab 13:S672

29. Lipton SA, Rosenberg PA (1994) Excitatory amino acids as a final common pathway for neurologic disorders. N Engl J Med 330: 613–622
30. Lyden PD, Lonzo L, Nunez S (1995) Combination therapy extends the therapeutic window to 60 minutes after stroke. J Neurotrauma 12: 223–230
31. Marion DW, Penrod LE, Kelsey SF, Obrist WD, Kochanek PM, Palmer AM, Wisniewski SR, DeKosky ST (1997) Treatment of traumatic brain injury with moderate hypothermia. N Engl J Med 336: 540–546
32. Marion DW, White MJ (1996) Treatment of experimental brain injury with moderate hypothermia and 21-aminosteroids. J Neurotrauma 13: 139–147
33. Matsumiya N, Koehler RC, Kirsch JR, Traystman RJ (1991) Conjugated superoxide dismutase reduces extent of caudate injury after transient focal ischemia in cats. Stroke 22: 1193–1200
34. Muir KW, Lees KR (1995) Clinical experience with excitatory amino acid antagonist drugs. Stroke 26: 503–513
35. Muir KW, Lees KR (1995) A randomized, double-blind, placebo-controlled pilot trial of intravenous magnesium sulfate in acute stroke. Stroke 26: 1183–1188
36. Muizelaar JP, Marmarou A, Young HF, Choi SC, Wolf A, Schneider RL, Kontos HA (1993) Improving the outcome of severe head injury with the oxygen radical scavenger polyethylene glycol-conjugated superoxide dismutase: a phase II trial. J Neurosurg 78: 375–382
37. Nakai A, Kuroda S, Kristian A, Siesjö BK (1997) The immunosuppressant drug FK506 ameliorates secondary mitochondrial dysfunction following transient focal cerebral ischemia in the rat. Neurobiol Dis 4: 288–300
38. Nowak L, Bregestovski P, Ascher P, Herbet A, Prochiantz A (1984) Magnesium gates glutamate-activated channels in mouse central neurones. Nature 307: 462–465
39. Ohman J, Heiskanen O (1988) Effect of nimodipine on the outcome of patients after aneurysmal subarachnoid hemorrhage and surgery. J Neurosurg 69: 683–686
40. Park CK, Nehls DG, Graham DI, Teasdale GM, McCulloch J (1988) The glutamate antagonist MK-801 reduces focal ischemic brain damage in the rat. Ann Neurol 24: 543–551
41. Sacchetti ML, Toni D, Fiorelli M, Argentino C, Fieschi C (1997) The concept of combination therapy in acute ischemic stroke. Neurology 49:S70-S74
42. Schmid-Elsaesser R, Zausinger S, Hungerhuber E, Baethmann A, Reulen HJ (1999) Neuroprotective effects of combination therapy with tirilazad and magnesium in rats subjected to reversible focal cerebral ischemia. Neurosurgery 44: 163–172
43. Schmidt-Elsaesser R, Zausinger S, Hungerhuber E, Baethmann A, Reulen HJ (1998) Optimal cerebroprotection by mild hypothermia plus combination pharmacotherapy during temporary middle cerebral artery occlusion in rats (abstract). Zentralbl Neurochir [Suppl 98]:89–89
44. Schmid-Elsaesser R, Zausinger S, Hungerhuber E, Baethmann A, Reulen HJ (1998) Monotherapy with dextromethorphan or tirilazad – but not a combination of both – improves outcome after transient focal cerebral ischemia in rats. Exp Brain Res 122: 121–127
45. Schmid-Elsaesser R, Zausinger S, Hungerhuber E, Plesnila N, Baethmann A, Reulen HJ (1997) Superior neuroprotective efficacy of a novel antioxidant (U-101033E) with improved blood–brain barrier permeability in focal cerebral ischemia. Stroke 28: 2018–2024
46. Schmid-Elsaesser R, Hungerhuber E, Zausinger S, Baethmann A, Reulen HJ (1999) Neuroprotective efficacy of combination therapy with two different antioxidants in rats subjected to transient focal ischemia. Brain Res 816: 471–479
47. Schneider GH, Baethmann A, Kempski O (1992) Mechanisms of glial swelling by glutamate. Can J Physiol Pharmacol 70: 334–343
48. Shuaib A, Ijaz S, Mazagri R, Senthilsevlvan A (1993) CGS-19755 is neuroprotective during repetitive ischemia – this effect is significantly enhanced when combined with hypothermia. Neuroscience 56: 915–920
49. Siesjö BK (1992) Pathophysiology and treatment of focal cerebral ischemia. Part II: mechanisms of damage and treatment. J Neurosurg 77: 337–354
50. Siesjö BK, Agardh CD, Bengtsson F (1989) Free radicals and brain damage. Cerebrovasc Brain Metab Rev 1: 165–211
51. Simon R, Shiraishi K (1990) N-methyl-D-aspartate antagonist reduces stroke size and regional glucose metabolism. Ann Neurol 27: 606–611
52. Steinberg GK, Bell TE, Yenari MA (1996) Dose escalation safety and tolerance study of the N-methyl-D-aspartate antagonist dextromethorphan in neurosurgery patients. J Neurosurg 84: 860–866
53. Steinberg GK, Kunis D, DeLaPaz R, Poljak A (1993) Neuroprotection following focal cerebral ischaemia with the NMDA antagonist dextromethorphan, has a favourable dose response profile. Neurol Res 15: 174–180
54. Traystman RJ, Kirsch JR, Koehler RC (1991) Oxygen radical mechanisms of brain injury following ischemia and reperfusion. J Appl Physiol 71: 1185–1195

55. Uematsu D, Araki N, Greenberg JH, Sladky J, Reivich M (1991) Combined therapy with MK-801 and nimodipine for protection of ischemic brain damage. Neurology 41: 88–94
56. Vacanti FX, Ames A, 3rd (1984) Mild hypothermia and Mg++ protect against irreversible damage during CNS ischemia. Stroke 15: 695–698
57. Wahlgren NG (1997) Neuroprotectants in late clinical development: a status report. Cerebrovasc Dis 7[Suppl]:13–17
58. Young B, Runge JW, Waxman KS, Harrington T, Wilberger J, Muizelaar JP, Boddy A, Kupiec JW (1996) Effects of pegorgotein on neurologic outcome of patients with severe head injury. A multicenter, randomized controlled trial (comments). JAMA 276: 538–543

Another Facet of Nitric Oxide: Reduction of Toxic Zinc Influx Through Voltage-Gated Channels

B. J. Snider, J.-Y. Choi, D. M. Turetsky, L. M. T. Canzoniero, S. L. Sensi, C. T. Sheline, and D. W. Choi

Summary. The neurotoxicity of zinc, released from nerve terminals during global ischemia, may contribute to the delayed death of certain selectively vulnerable neuronal populations. A likely first event in zinc-induced neuronal death appears to be its permeation across the plasma membrane, largely through voltage- and agonist-gated calcium channels. Considering the possibility that cellular Zn^{2+} overload might be lethal for reasons similar to cellular calcium overload, we tested the hypothesis that Zn^{2+} neurotoxicity might be mediated by activation of neuronal nitric oxide synthase (NOS), an event implicated in the pathogenesis of excitotoxic neuronal death. However, physiologically relevant concentrations of zinc (30–100 nM) had no effect on NOS activity, while 100–300 µM Zn^{2+} actually inhibited NOS activity in solution. The addition of extracellular Zn^{2+} did not affect NOS activity in cultured murine neocortical neurons, assessed by measuring cyclic guanosine 5'-monophosphate (cGMP) levels, and the concurrent addition of NOS inhibitors did not alter Zn^{2+}-induced neuronal death (cultures were exposed to 300–500 µM Zn^{2+} for 5 min under depolarizing conditions; neuronal degeneration was assessed 24 h later). Rather, addition of the nitric oxide (NO) precursor, L-arginine, or the diazeniumdiolate (NONOate) NO donors (DEA/NO) or 1-propanamine,3-(2-hydroxy-2-nitroso-1-propylhydrazino) NONOate (PAPA/NO) markedly reduced Zn^{2+}-induced neuronal death and produced a dose-dependent block of high K^+-stimulated cellular $^{45}Ca^{2+}$ uptake. The oxidizing agents thimerosal and 2,2'-dithiodipyridine (DTDP) also reduced K^+-stimulated cellular $^{45}Ca^{2+}$ uptake, while alkylation of thiols by pretreatment with N-ethylmaleimide (NEM) blocked the reduction of $^{45}Ca^{2+}$ uptake by NO donors. These results suggest that Zn^{2+}-induced neuronal death is not mediated by the activation of NOS; rather, any available NO may attenuate Zn^{2+} neurotoxicity, in part through a down-modulation of Zn^{2+} entry through voltage-gated Ca^{2+} channels.

Introduction

Zn^{2+} is present at high concentrations in the central nervous system and is localized in synaptic boutons, usually of glutamatergic neurons [3, 8, 10]. It is released with nerve cell activity; extracellular concentrations may reach the 100-µM range in regions such as the mossy fiber terminals in the CA3 region of the hippocampus [5, 7, 16, 17]. The basis of Zn^{2+} neurotoxicity has not been established, but likely involves Zn^{2+} entry into neurons through both agonist and voltage-gated Ca^{2+} channels. Several types of evidence suggest that voltage-gated Ca^{2+} channels are the major route by which excessive Zn^{2+} can enter neurons under depolarizing conditions. Depolariza-

Maturation Phenomenon in Cerebral Ischemia III
U. Ito et al. (Eds.)
© Springer-Verlag Berlin Heidelberg 1999

tion enhances accumulation of $^{65}Zn^{2+}$ in cultured neurons (H.S Ying et al., unpublished results), as well as $[Zn^{2+}]_i$ [11] and neuronal vulnerability to Zn^{2+}-induced death [18]. Zn^{2+} entry and Zn^{2+}-induced neuronal death can be attenuated by the application of voltage-gated Ca^{2+}-channel antagonists, particularly the L type (H.S Ying et al., unpublished results) [4, 11, 18].

Because Zn^{2+} probably enters neurons through many of the same routes as Ca^{2+}, it is possible that the neuronal death induced by cellular Zn^{2+} overload might result from some of the same mechanisms responsible for Ca^{2+}-overload-induced neuronal death, such as occurs following glutamate-receptor over-stimulation. A prominent mechanism in the latter category is the over-activation of nitric oxide synthase (NOS) leading to the production of toxic levels of nitric oxide (NO). While extremely high (100 μM) concentrations of Zn^{2+} have been reported to inhibit brain-tissue NOS in crude enzyme preparations [1, 15], activation of NOS by the 1–100 nM Zn^{2+} concentrations that may be relevant to physiological or even pathophysiological conditions [11] can be considered.

We exposed primary cultures of murine neocortical neurons to Zn^{2+} under depolarizing conditions to test the hypothesis that Zn^{2+} neurotoxicity, like excitotoxic neuronal death, is substantially mediated by the activation of neuronal NOS (nNOS).

Materials and Methods

Cell Culture and Exposure to Drugs

Mixed neocortical cultures were prepared from mouse cortices as previously described [9]. Cultures were maintained in a 37 °C, humidified incubator in a 5 % CO_2 atmosphere. All experiments were performed after 14 days in vitro.

Mixed cultures of neocortical neurons and glia were exposed to Zn^{2+} (300–500 μM $ZnCl_2$) for 6 min in room air in the presence of 45 mM KCl. The exposure was performed in *N*-2-hydroxyethylpiperazine-*N*'-2-ethanesulfonic acid (HEPES)-buffered control salt solution (HCSS: 120 mM NaCl, 5.4 mM KCl, 0.8 mM $MgCl_2$,1.8 mM $CaCl_2$, 10 mM NaOH, 10 μM glycine, 20 mM HEPES, 5.5 mM glucose, pH 7.4). HCSS with increased potassium was made by substituting KCl for NaCl. Since exposure to high potassium could be expected to induce secondary glutamate release, we included the competitive *N*-methyl-D-aspartate (NMDA) antagonist D-4-(3-phosphopropyl)piperazine-2-carboxylic acid (D-CPP) (100 μM) in the exposure medium to block NMDA receptor-mediated toxicity. The NO donors diethylamine NONOate (DEA/NO) or 1-propanamine,3-(2-hydroxy-2-nitroso-1-propylhydrazino) NONOate (PAPA/NO) were made up at 100–300 mM in 10 mM NaOH, stored at 4 °C and used the same day. The stock solution was diluted into neutral pH buffer immediately before use. Cell death was estimated 20–24 h after exposure to drugs by phase-contrast microscopy and quantified by measuring lactate dehydrogenase (LDH) present in the bathing medium [13]. To determine the percentage of neurons dying, LDH efflux from treatment conditions was divided by LDH efflux from sister cultures treated for 24 h with 300 μM NMDA, a treatment that kills virtually all the neurons.

Measurement of Radiolabeled $^{45}Ca^{2+}$ Uptake

$^{45}Ca^{2+}$ uptake was measured in cultures over a 5-min epoch in HCSS identical to that described above, but nominally Ca^{2+} free, with 2 μCi/ml $^{45}Ca^{2+}$ (2 μM Ca^{2+}). Cultures were washed three times in Ca^{2+}-free HCSS and exposed to drugs and $^{45}Ca^{2+}$ for 5 min. After 5 min, the cultures were washed four times in the same buffer (lacking radiolabeled Ca^{2+}), solubilized in warm 0.2 % sodium dodecyl sulfate, mixed with scintillant, and counted in a liquid-scintillation counter.

Results

Mixed cultures of neocortical neurons and glia exposed to 300 μM Zn^{2+} in the presence of 45 mM KCl and 100 μM CPP (to block activation of NMDA receptors induced by secondary glutamate release) developed widespread neuronal damage over the next 24 h. Inhibition of NOS with N^G-nitro-L-arginine methyl ester, HCl (L-NAME, HCl) or 7-nitroindazole, a more specific inhibitor of nNOS [2, 14], did not alter this process of Zn^{2+}-induced neuronal necrosis, or the release of LDH into the bathing media (Fig. 1). Similar lack of neuroprotection was observed with two other NOS inhibitors: N^G-nitro-L-arginine (N-Arg) and L-thiocitrulline (both at 0.1–1 mM; data not shown).

Surprisingly, administration of the NOS substrate L-arginine (data not shown), or the NO donors DEA/NO or PAPA/NO attenuated the neurotoxic effects of Zn^{2+} plus KCl in a NO-donor-concentration-dependent manner (Table 1 and data not shown). DEA/NO that had decayed at neutral pH for over 24 h did not alter Zn^{2+} toxicity (data not shown).

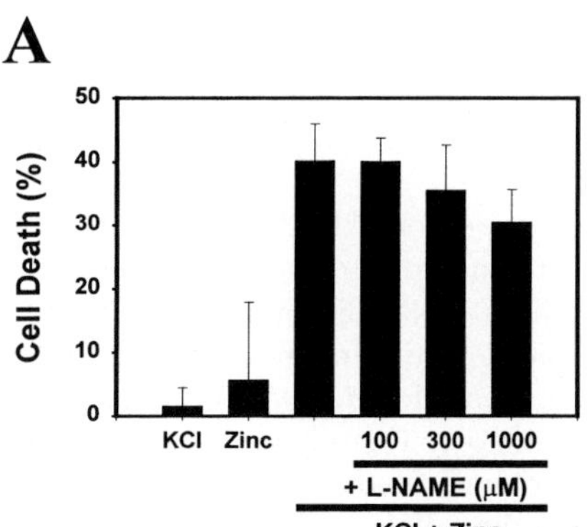
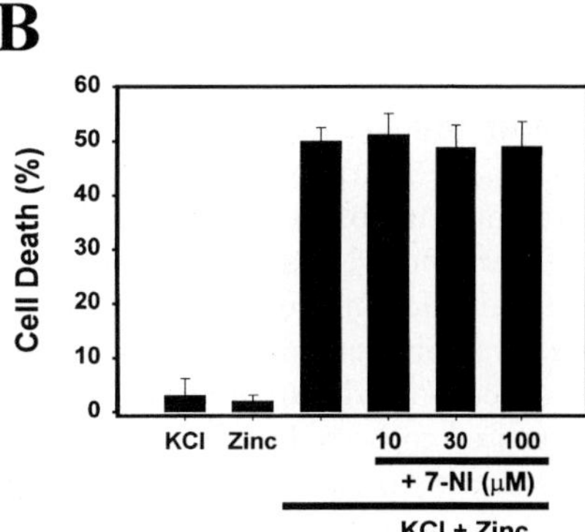

Fig. 1A, B. Toxicity of Zn^{2+} and high potassium in cultured cortical neurons. Mixed cortical cultures were exposed to 45 mM KCl and 300 μM $ZnCl_2$ separately (*first two bars*), or together (*last four bars*), for 5 min in the presence of 100 μM D-4-(3-phosphonopropyl)piperazine-2-carboxylic acid as well as the indicated concentration of N^G-nitro-L-arginine methyl ester, HCl (L-NAME) (**A**), or 7-nitroindazole (*7 NI*) (**B**). Each value represents the mean (± the standard error of the mean) lactate dehydrogenase efflux into the bathing media sampled 24 h after exposure to Zn^{2+}, n=12 sister cultures per condition

Table 1. NO donors reduce zinc neurotoxicity. Mixed cortical cultures were exposed to 45 mM KCl and 500 µM ZnCl$_2$ for 5 min in the presence of 100 µM D-4-(3-phosphonopropyl)piperazine-2-carboxylic acid and the NO donors diethylamine NONOate (DEA/NO), or 1-propanamine-3-(2-hydroxy-2-nitroso-1-propylhydrazino) NONOate (PAPA/NO). Each value represents the mean (± standard error of the mean) lactate dehydrogenase efflux into the bathing media sampled 24 h after exposure to Zn^{2+}. * indicates significant difference from K+Zn condition. Significance ($P<0.001$) analyzed by student's t test. $n=4$ cultures per condition

Condition	Cell death (%)
Experiment 1:	
KCl 45 mM	3.1±3.2
Zinc 500 µM	1.9±1.7
KCl + zinc	71.6±3.6
KCl + zinc + 300 µM DEA/NO	31.1±1.4 *
Experiment 2:	
KCl + zinc	85.0±5.4
KCl + zinc + 1 mM PAPA/NO	22.3±2.5 *

Reduction of Zn^{2+} influx through voltage-gated Ca^{2+} channels is one plausible mechanism through which NO might reduce Zn^{2+} neurotoxicity. ^{45}Ca^{2+} accumulation induced by exposure to 60 mM K$^+$ in the presence of 10 µM MK-801 was mediated by nimodipine-sensitive Ca^{2+} channels (unpublished results). The NO donors DEA/NO and PAPA/NO inhibited this K$^+$-stimulated ^{45}Ca^{2+} uptake, with DEA/NO again more potent than PAPA/NO (data not shown).

NO mediates its biologic effects through several pathways, the best-characterized of which is mediated by the interaction of NO with the heme component of guanylate cyclase, with enhancement of the enzyme's activity and subsequent increases in cellular cGMP levels [6]. However, even with a 24-h pretreatment with the cGMP analogue dibutryl-cGMP (1 mM), there was no reduction in Zn^{2+} neurotoxicity (data not shown).

Discussion

Present data do not support the hypothesis that the neuronal death induced by intracellular zinc overload occurs for reasons identical to neuronal death induced by intracellular calcium overload. Neither the NOS inhibitor L-NAME nor the more specific nNOS inhibitor 7-nitroindazole altered zinc-induced cortical neuronal death. Rather, the neuronal death induced by exposure to Zn^{2+} under depolarizing conditions appeared to be reduced by the addition of NO donors. This neuroprotective effect, presumably mediated by NO itself, was associated with a reduction in K$^+$-stimulated ^{45}Ca^{2+} accumulation, a parameter likely reflecting the cellular influx of Ca^{2+} [12] and, thus, may be due to modulation of voltage-gated Ca^{2+} channels. Calcium-channel antagonists block both depolarization-induced neuronal death and increases in [Zn^{2+}]$_i$ in cultured cortical neurons [11, 18]. Further study will be necessary to determine whether the neuroprotective effect of NO on Zn^{2+}-induced neuronal death observed here reflects a direct effect of NO (upon Ca^{2+}channels) or an indirect effect mediated by second-messenger cascades.

References

1. Persechini A, McMillan K, Masters BSS (1995) Inhibition of nitric oxide synthase activity by Zn^{2+} ion. Biochemistry 34: 15091–15095
2. Moore PK, Wallace P, Gaffen Z, Hart SL, Babbedge RC (1993) Characterization of the novel nitric oxide synthase inhibitor 7-nitro indazole and related indazoles: antinociceptive and cardiovascular effects. Br J Pharmacol 110: 219–224
3. Perez-Clausell J, Danscher G (1985) Intravesicular localization of zinc in rat telencephalic boutons. A histochemical study. Brain Res 337: 91–98
4. Freund W-D, Reddig S (1994) AMPA/Zn^{2+}-induced neurotoxicity in rat primary cortical cultures:involvement of L-type calcium channels. Brain Res 654: 257–264
5. Perez-Clausell J, Danscher G (1986) Release of zinc sulphide accumulations into synaptic clefts after in vivo injection of sodium sulphide. Brain Res 362: 358–361
6. Ignarro LJ, Byrns RE, Buga GM, Wood KS (1987) Endothelium-derived relaxing factor from pulmonary artery and vein possesses pharmacologic and chemical properties identical to those of nitric oxide radical. Circ Res 61: 866–879
7. Charton G, Rovira C, Ben-Ari Y, Leviel V (1985) Spontaneous and evoked release of endogenous Zn^{2+} in the hippocampal mossy fiber zone of the rat in situ. Exp Brain Res 58: 202–205
8. Haug F-MS (1967) Electron microscopical localization of the zinc in hippocampal mossy fibre synapses by a modified sulfide silver procedure. Histochemie 8: 355–368
9. Rose K, Choi DW, Goldberg MP (1993) Cytotoxicity in murine neocortical cell culture. In: Tyson C, Frazier J (eds) In vitro biological methods. Academic, San Diego, pp 46–60
10. Frederickson CJ (1989) Neurobiology of zinc and zinc-containing neurons. Int Rev Neurobiol 31: 145–238
11. Sensi SL, Canzoniero LMT, Yu SP, Ying HS, Koh J-Y, Kerchner GA, Choi DW (1997) Measurement of intracellular free zinc in living cortical neurons: routes of entry. J Neurosci 17: 9554–9564
12. Hartley DM, Kurth MC, Bjerkness L, Weiss JH, Choi DW (1993) Glutamate receptor-induced 45Ca2+ accumulation in cortical cell culture correlates with subsequent neuronal degeneration. J Neurosci 13: 1993–2000
13. Koh J-Y, Choi DW (1987) Quantitative determination of glutamate mediated cortical neuronal injury in cell culture by lactate dehydrogenase efflux assay. J Neurosci Methods 20: 83–90
14. Moore PK, Bland-Ward PA (1996) 7-nitroindazole: an inhibitor of nitric oxide synthase. Methods Enzymol 268: 393–398
15. Mittal CK, Harrell WB, Mehta CS (1995) Interaction of heavy metal toxicants with brain constitutive nitric oxide synthase. Mol Cell Biochem 149/150: 263–265
16. Howell GA, Welch MG, Frederickson CJ (1984) Stimulation-induced uptake and release of zinc in hippocampal slices. Nature 308: 736–738
17. Assaf SY, Chung SH (1984) Release of endogenous Zn^{2+} from brain tissue during activity. Nature 308: 734–736
18. Weiss JH, Hartley DM, Koh J-Y, Choi DW (1993) AMPA receptor activation potentiates zinc neurotoxicity. Neuron 10: 43–49

Slowly Progressive Neuronal Degeneration in Remote Areas After Focal Cerebral Ischemia

A. Tamura, M. Nakane, T. Kuroiwa, T. Nagaoka, H. Nakanishi, T. Nakagomi, T. Matsui, and K. Sano

Summary. Recently, it has become clear that focal cerebral ischemia causes slowly progressive neuropathological changes in certain distant nonischemic areas, such as the ipsilateral thalamus and ipsilateral substantia nigra (SN), remote from the original infarct. In rats, neuronal loss and atrophy were observed in these areas a few weeks after occlusion of the middle cerebral artery (MCA), and an in vitro electrophysiological slice study showed hyperexcitation in the SN neurons. In clinical studies, we have detected secondary changes in the SN using magnetic resonance imaging (MRI) as a high-signal-intensity spot and in the thalamus using computed tomography (CT). However, the mechanism giving rise to these changes is still not clear. For the purpose of interpreting the signal changes on MRI, we attempted to analyze (1) the nigral change by means of MRI and electron microscopy and (2) the changes in water content and capillary permeability in the SN after MCA occlusion in the rat. In the rat, proton density-, T2-, and T1-weighted images were obtained at 1, 4, 7, 14 and 28 days after occlusion of the MCA using a 4.7-T superconductive magnetic resonance (MR) unit. T2-weighted images revealed an area of high signal intensity in the ipsilateral SN at 4 days after occlusion. A low-signal-intensity lesion appeared in the ipsilateral thalamus 7 days after occlusion in proton density- and/or T2-weighted images. Diffusion-weighted images at 4 days after occlusion revealed a high-signal-intensity lesion in the ipsilateral SN. Neuropathological examination showed swelling of perineuronal and perivascular end-feet of astrocytes and also swelling of dendrites. In the ipsilateral SN, no significant change in specific gravity and no demonstrable change in capillary permeability was detected. In the ipsilateral thalamus, there were slight increases in specific gravity, although no change in capillary permeability was demonstrated. In conclusion, we identified two types of secondary neuronal degeneration based on MRI findings, suggesting that secondary degeneration may occur through various mechanisms.

Introduction

Focal cerebral ischemia leads to slowly progressive degeneration of neurons in remote areas having fiber connections with the ischemic area. In the rat, neuronal loss and atrophy were observed in such remote areas as the ipsilateral thalamus and the ipsilateral substantia nigra (SN) a few weeks after occlusion of the middle cerebral artery (MCA) [2, 13]. In clinical studies, we have detected secondary changes in SN using magnetic resonance imaging (MRI) as a high-signal-intensity spot and in the thalamus using computed tomography (CT) [6, 14]. However, the mechanism giving rise

Maturation Phenomenon in Cerebral Ischemia III
U. Ito et al. (Eds.)
© Springer-Verlag Berlin Heidelberg 1999

to these changes is still not clear. For the purpose of interpreting the signal changes on MRI, we attempted to analyze the nigral change by MRI and electron microscopy (EM) and the changes in water content and capillary permeability in SN after MCA occlusion in the rat.

Materials and Methods

Animal Model

Male Sprague-Dawley rats, 9–10 weeks of age, weighing 320–350 g, were anesthetized with 2 % halothane. The proximal part of the left MCA was exposed and permanently cauterized [11]. After the surgery, the animals were transferred to observation cages and permitted free access to food and water until the time of experiments.

MR Imaging

The rats were re-anesthetized with ketamine and this anesthesia was maintained with 1 % isoflurane via a face mask. Animals were fixed by a hand-made folder with a coil. Body temperature was maintained between 36 °C and 37 °C. MRI was performed in each animal only once.

All examinations were performed using a 4.7-T imager/spectrometer system (Unity plus SIS 200/330, Varian, Palo Alto, Calif., USA) equipped with a 33-cm-horizontal-bore magnet (Oxford Instruments, England) with a gradient strength of 50 mT/m. To achieve reproducible images, a T1-weighted midsagittal scout view was taken, and nine consecutive coronal sections were selected. The section thickness was 2 mm, with a 128·128 matrix zero-field to 512·512 over a field of view of 4·4 cm. We obtained T1-weighted [T1-W; repetition time (TR) 600 ms; echo time (TE) 20 ms], T2-weighted (T2-W; TR 2500 ms; TE 100 ms), and proton density-weighted (PD-W; TR 1800 ms; TE 25 ms) spin-echo images at 1, 4, 7, 14 and 28 days after MCA occlusion ($n=3$ at each time point). The sham-operated rats were also subjected to the same MRI protocol as outlined above ($n=2$ at each time point).

T2-W (TR 2500 ms; TE 100 ms) spin-echo images were obtained 4 days after MCA occlusion ($n=3$). Thereafter, diffusion-weighted images (DWI) were obtained using a modified spin-echo pulse sequence (TR 1500 ms; TE 70 ms) with unipolar diffusion gradients before and after the refocusing pulse at the slice which included the SN. The slice thickness was 2 mm with a 64·64 matrix zero-field to 256·256 over a field of view of 4·4 cm. B values of 531 seconds/mm^2 were used and the times between the rising edges of the two diffusion gradients, D and d, were 40 ms and 10 ms, respectively. The diffusion-encoding gradient was irradiated along one axis (Z-axis). Apparent diffusion coefficient (ADC) values were calculated, and the quantitative ADC values were obtained using a Sun Spark 10 workstation.

Electron Microscopy

Four rats were perfusion-fixed 4 days after MCA occlusion. The fixative contained 2.5 % glutaraldehyde and 2 % paraformaldehyde in 0.1 M cacodylate buffer (pH 7.3). Perfusion was carried out at a pressure of 130 cm H_2O; 500 ml of fixative was used for each animal. The brains were left in situ at 4 °C overnight, then removed, and cut coronally to obtain sections of the SN. These sections were postfixed in 1 % OsO_4, mordanted in 1.5 % aqueous solution of uranyl acetate, dehydrated in graded ethanol, and embedded in Araldite CY-212. One-micrometer sections were prepared and stained with toluidine blue. Thin sections of the SN were cut with a diamond knife, contrasted with uranyl acetate and lead citrate, and observed under a Philips 300 or a JEOL 100 U electron microscope.

Cerebrovascular Permeability

Microvascular permeability was studied using alpha-aminoisobutyric acid labeled with carbon-14 (^{14}C-AIB) as described previously. Briefly, 50 mCi ^{14}C-AIB was injected intravenously 4 days after MCA occlusion ($n=4$). The blood–tissue transfer ratio (Ki) values were determined by autoradiography.

Measurement of Specific Gravity

Animals were killed to measure the specific gravity in the thalamus and SN at 4, 7 and 14 days after MCA occlusion ($n=5$ at each time point). A tissue sample, weighing approximately 10 mg, was carefully resected from the SN on each side. The specific gravity was determined 2 min after immersion into a bromobenzene/kerosene gradient column, which was prepared according to the method reported by Marmarou et al. [4]. The sham-operated rats and normal rats were also subjected to the same protocol as outlined above ($n=5$ at each time point).

Results

MR Imaging

T1-W, T2-W, and PDW Images

Ischemia developed in all operated rats and was observed on T2-WI as a high signal intensity in the left caudate putamen and cortex, suggestive of cerebral infarction. The area of infarction was observed as a slightly high signal intensity on PD-WI and as an iso-signal intensity on T1-WI at 1 day after occlusion of the MCA. A small cortical high signal intensity, observed on T2-WI in some sham-operated rats, was considered to be due to cerebral contusion during the sham operation.

T2-WI at 4 days after MCA occlusion revealed a high signal intensity in the ipsilateral SN in all animals. However, the lesion was not observed at 1, 7, 14 or 28 days after

MCA occlusion. The lesion in the SN was observed as a slight high signal intensity on PD-WI, and as an iso-signal intensity on T1-WI. The signal intensity on PD-WI and/or T2-WI decreased in the ipsilateral thalamus as early as 7 days after MCA occlusion. The low signal intensity was located in the ventral thalamus, and was observed even at 28 days after MCA occlusion. T1-WI revealed no signal abnormality in the thalamus.

In sham-operated rats, no significant abnormality was observed in the SN or in the thalamus at 1, 4, 7, 14 and 28 days after MCA occlusion.

Diffusion-Weighted Image

The area of infarction was manifested as a slightly high signal intensity on DWI and as an iso-signal intensity on T1-WI at 1 day after occlusion. T2-WI and DWI at 4 days after MCA occlusion revealed a high signal intensity in the ipsilateral SN in all animals (Fig. 1). The lesion in the SN was observed as a slightly high signal intensity on PD-WI, and as an iso-signal intensity on T1-WI.

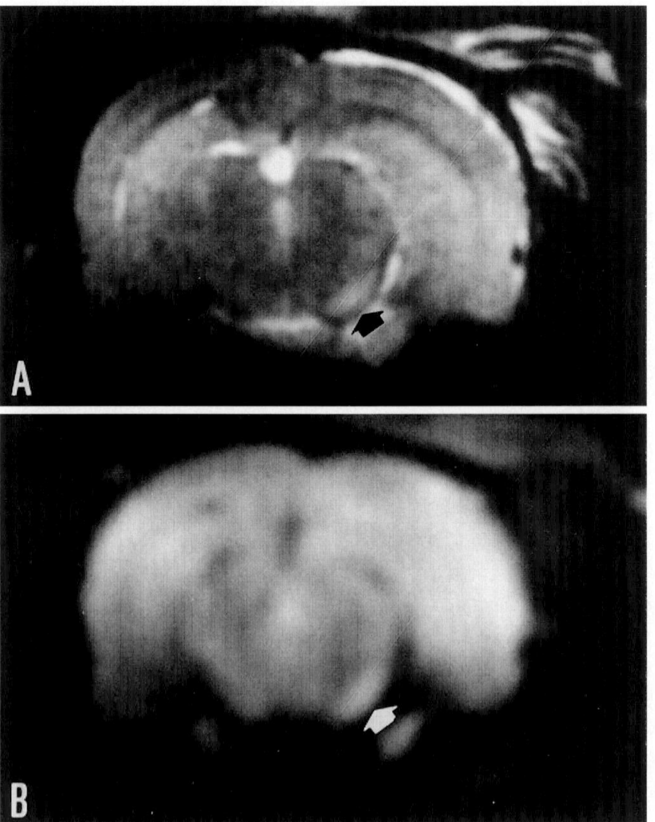

Fig. 1A, B. T2-weighted (A) and diffusion-weighted (B) images at 4 days after the middle cerebral artery occlusion in the rat reveal high signal intensity in the ipsilateral substantia nigra (*arrows*)

Observations by Electron Microscopy

Neuropathological examination by EM in the ipsilateral SN showed swelling of peri-neuronal and perivascular end-feet of astrocytes and also swelling of dendrites. Some neurons showed slight hydropic swelling.

Cerebrovascular Permeability

The mean ($\pm$SD) nigral blood-to-brain transfer constant in the ipsilateral side was 1.103$\pm$0.243 ml/g/min·100 and that in the contralateral side was 0.9875$\pm$0.1072 ml/g/min·100. There was no statistically significant difference in cerebrovascular permeability between the ipsilateral and contralateral SN.

Measurement of Specific Gravity

The mean specific gravities in the SN and the thalamus on each side after MCA occlusion are shown in Table 1. There was no statistically significant difference in specific gravity between the ipsilateral and contralateral SN.

Table 1. Specific gravity (mean $\pm$ SD)

Structure	Left (ipsilateral)	Right (contralateral)
Substantia nigra		
MCAO		
Day 4	1.043$\pm$0.002	1.044$\pm$0.001
Day 7	1.044$\pm$0.002	1.043$\pm$0.002
Day 14	1.044$\pm$0.002	1.043$\pm$0.002
Sham		
Day 4	1.045$\pm$0.001	1.044$\pm$0.001
Day 7	1.044$\pm$0.001	1.045$\pm$0.001
Day 14	1.044$\pm$0.001	1.044$\pm$0.001
Normal	1.045$\pm$0.001	1.045$\pm$0.001
Thalamus		
MCAO		
Day 4	1.044$\pm$0.001	1.047$\pm$0.002
Day 7	1.045$\pm$0.002	1.047$\pm$0.002
Day 14	1.046$\pm$0.002	1.048$\pm$0.001
Sham		
Day 4	1.046$\pm$0.001	1.046$\pm$0.001
Day 7	1.047$\pm$0.001	1.048$\pm$0.001
Day 14	1.046$\pm$0.002	1.046$\pm$0.002
Normal	1.047$\pm$0.001	1.046$\pm$0.003

Discussion

Following MCA occlusion in rats, we noted a marked reduction in cerebral blood flow (CBF) in the territory of the occluded artery, an absolute increase in CBF in the ipsilateral globus pallidus and SN, and a slight decrease in CBF in the ipsilateral thalamus [12]. Subsequently, in the chronic phase, we detected a similar pattern of increase in CBF and a marked increase in local cerebral glucose utilization (CGU) in the SN and decreases in CBF and CGU in the thalamus [15]. In this model, both SN and thalamus lie outside the ischemic area, but have neuronal connections with the ischemic foci, such as the caudate nucleus and cortex. Therefore, we believe that changes in CBF and CGU in these remote areas may be explained as being a reflection of altered neuronal function in these areas.

The caudate nucleus of the rat contains high concentrations of several neurotransmitters, such as acetylcholine, dopamine, glutamate and gamma-aminobutyric acid (GABA). The inhibitory neurotransmitter plays an important functional role in the striato-nigral pathway. Nakayama et al. reported that the long-lasting decrease in GABA and aspartate in the ipsilateral SN after MCA occlusion was due to ischemic damage of afferent tracts and subsequent degeneration of the synaptic terminals in SN [9]. Therefore, it is probable that the decrease in the level of GABA, a potent inhibitor of neuronal discharge, renders the SN neurons liable to fire spontaneously, leading to coupled increase in CBF and CGU. We reported detection of neuronal degeneration, gliosis, and marked atrophy of this area after MCA occlusion and concluded that the nigral degeneration may be explained by trans-synaptic, neurotransmitter-mediated disinhibition as a result of infarction of the striatum [13].

This hypothesis is supported by the results of a study by Saji and Reis who reported anterograde trans-synaptic degeneration of neurons in the SN after destruction of the caudate nucleus by administration of an excitotoxin, ibotenic acid [10]. Furthermore, they found that neuronal death was prevented by long-term intraventricular infusion of the GABA agonist muscimol. We also reported that intraventricular muscimol infusion prevented neuronal death in the SN after MCA occlusion [15]. Recently, Nakanishi et al. reported sequential changes in the electrophysiological profiles of the ipsilateral SN neurons in an in vitro slice preparation obtained from MCA-occluded rats [8]. They showed marked atrophy and neuronal degeneration in the ipsilateral SN pars reticulata at 14 days after MCA occlusion and a significant increase in the input resistance and spontaneous firing rate of the neurons in the SN pars compacta at 13–16 days after MCA occlusion. However, there were no significant changes in the electrical membrane properties and synaptic responses of SN pars reticulata neurons. Their results strongly suggest that changes in electrophysiological responses observed in the neurons of the SN pars compacta are caused by degeneration of GABAergic afferents from the SN pars reticulata following MCA occlusion.

Focal brain lesions induce decreases in CBF and CGU in areas remote from the original lesion, an effect called diaschisis. This phenomenon is believed to be secondary to interruption of neuronal connections and the consequent metabolic suppression. Because rich nerve-fiber connections exist between the thalamus and the cerebral cortex, diaschisis can occur in the thalamus following infarction of the cerebral cortex. The concept of diaschisis does not imply irreversible morphologic change. However, it has been reported that the ipsilateral half of the thalamus progressively shrinks several months following MCA occlusion in the rat [2]. The thalamic degeneration after cortical infarction might be secondary and, judging from the results of several experimental studies, may primarily result from retrograde degeneration [3, 5]. In this study, we attempted to detect secondary changes in these remote areas after MCA occlusion in rats using high-resolution MRI. It was shown that MRI can be used to detect secondary changes in the ipsilateral thalamus and SN after MCA occlusion [7]. Although both regions were similar with respect to their sequential morphological alterations, MRI findings in the two regions were different. Secondary thalamic change was observed as a low signal intensity on PD-WI and/or T2-WI. However, secondary change in the SN was observed as a high signal intensity on T2-WI. The differences in the MRI findings between these areas may be explained by the occurrence of different types of neuronal degeneration, predominantly retrograde degeneration in the thalamic neurons and anterograde trans-synaptic degeneration in the SN.

For the purpose of interpreting the signal changes on MRI, we attempted to analyze the nigral change in DWI, on which changes in the self-diffusion of water molecules that associated with early cytotoxic edema can be detected. The signal abnormalities in the ipsilateral SN seen in DWI in this study seem to be caused by reduced diffusion of interstitial water, owing to a relative decrease in the interstitial space, which suggests cell swelling, i.e., cytotoxic edema. This interpretation is supported by the results of EM and changes in specific gravity and cerebrovascular permeability obtained in our study.

Nigral degeneration after striatal destruction, and thalamic degeneration after cortical damage are well known in the domain of anatomy. However, neuronal death in

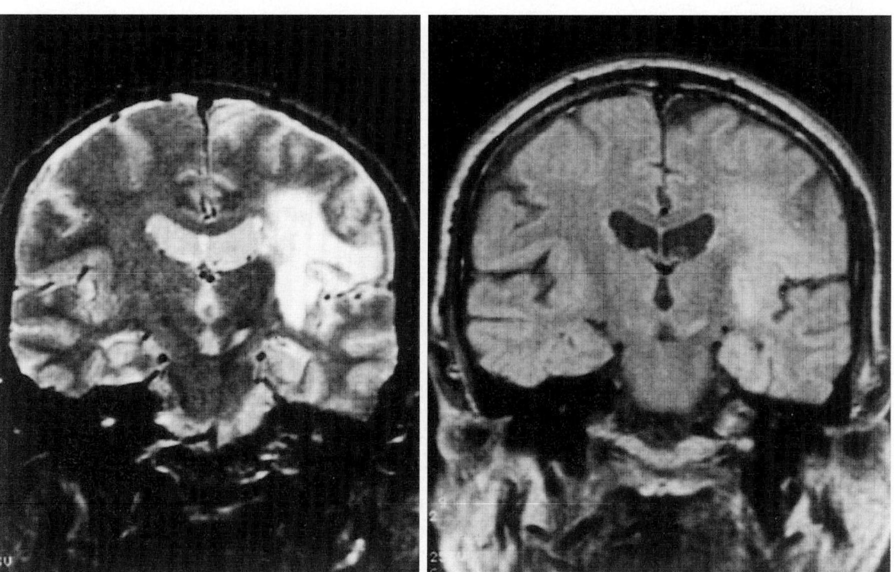

Fig. 2. T2-weighted (*left*) and proton density-weighted (*right*) images at 4 weeks after the onset of infarction. T2-weighted and proton density-weighted images reveal a markedly high signal intensity spot in the ipsilateral substantia nigra. However, the ipsilateral thalamus was visualized as a slightly low-signal-intensity region on T2-weighted and proton density-weighted images

remote areas following focal cerebral ischemia has not been investigated systematically, particularly in humans. There are only a few autopsy reports of neuropathological changes in the SN following massive basal ganglia infarction. Forno reported a slight to moderate nerve-cell loss in the ipsilateral SN from 6 months to 10 years after massive infarction of the basal ganglia [1]. Nakane et al. investigated changes in the SN following striatal infarction by means of MRI [6]. Consequently, they demonstrated a high-signal-intensity spot in T2-WI in this area a few weeks after the striatal infarction. This change became obscure a few months later because of decreased signal intensity of the lesion and/or wallerian degeneration and atrophy in the adjacent cerebral peduncle. However, the ipsilateral thalamus was visualized as a slightly low signal intensity region on PD-WI and/or T2-WI at about 2 weeks after the onset of cortical infarction (Fig. 2). In conclusion, we identified two types of secondary neuronal degeneration based on MRI findings. The thalamic changes observed on MRI were quite different from those observed in the SN, suggesting that secondary degeneration may occur through various mechanisms.

References

1. Forno LS (1983) Reaction of the substantia nigra to massive basal ganglia infarction. Acta Neuropathol (Berl) 62: 96–102
2. Fujie W, Kirino T, Tomukai N, Iwasawa T, Tamura A (1990) Progressive shrinkage of the thalamus following middle cerebral artery occlusion in rats. Stroke 21: 1485–1488
3. Iizuka H, Sakatani K, Young W (1990) Neural damage in the rat thalamus after cortical infarctions. Stroke 21: 790–794
4. Marmarou A, Tanaka K, Shulman K (1982) An improved gravimetric measure of cerebral edema. J Neurosurg 56: 246–253
5. Matthews MA (1973) Death of the central neuron: an electron microscopic study of thalamic retrograde degeneration following cortical ablation. J Neurocytol 2: 265–288
6. Nakane M, Teraoka A, Asato R, Tamura A (1992) Degeneration of the ipsilateral substantia nigra following cerebral infarction in the striatum. Stroke 23: 328–332
7. Nakane M, Tamura A, Nagaoka T, Hirakawa K (1997) MR detection of secondary changes remote from ischemia: preliminary observations after occlusion of the middle cerebral artery in rats. AJNR Am J Neuroradiol 18: 945–950
8. Nakanishi H, Tamura A, Kawai K, Yamamoto K (1997) Electrophysiological studies of rat substantia nigra neurons in an in vitro slice preparation after middle cerebral artery occlusion. Neuroscience 77: 1021–1028
9. Nakayama H, Tamura A, Kanazawa I, Sano K (1990) Time-sequential change of amino acid neurotransmitters -GABA, aspartate and glutamate- in the rat basal ganglia following middle cerebral artery occlusion. Neurol Res 12: 231–234
10. Saji M, Reis DJ (1987) Delayed transneuronal death of substantia nigra neurons prevented by gamma-aminobutyric acid agonist. Science 235: 66–69
11. Tamura A, Graham DI, McCulloch J, Teasdale GM (1981) Focal cerebral ischemia in the rat. 1. Description of technique and early neuropathological consequences following middle cerebral artery occlusion. J Cereb Blood Flow Metab 1: 53–60
12. Tamura A, Graham DI, McCulloch J, Teasdale GM (1981) Focal cerebral ischemia in the rat. 2. Regional cerebral blood flow determined by [14C]iodoantipyrine autoradiography following middle cerebral artery occlusion. J Cereb Blood Flow Metab 1: 61–69
13. Tamura A, Kirino T, Sano K, Takagi K, Oka H (1990) Atrophy of the ipsilateral substantia nigra following middle cerebral artery occlusion in the rat. Brain Res 510: 154–157
14. Tamura A, Tahira Y, Nagashima H, Kirino T, Gotoh O, Hojo S, Sano K (1991) Thalamic atrophy following cerebral infarction in the territory of the middle cerebral artery. Stroke 22: 615–618.
15. Tamura A, Kirino T, Fujie W, Nakane M, Teraoka A, Tahira Y, Narita K, Nagashima H, Sano K (1992) Neuropathological changes in remote areas after focal cerebral ischemia. In: Ito U, Kirino T, Kuroiwa T, Klatzo I (eds) Maturation phenomenon in cerebral ischemia. Springer, Berlin Heidelberg New York, pp 57–63

Metabolic Disturbances and Gene Responses Following Cortical Injury in Rats: Relationship to Spreading Depression

D. M. Hermann, G. Mies, and K.-A. Hossmann

Summary. The effects of a cortex lesion on alterations in cortical direct-current (DC) potential, cerebral metabolism and gene expression were examined in rats at 1–6 h after transcranial cold injury. In 14 of 21 injured rats, spreading depression (SD)-like depolarizations were recorded, which were accompanied by a transient decrease in electroencephalogram activity and a parallel increase in perfusion. Metabolic disturbances did not differ between injured animals with and without SD. The lesion surrounding was characterized by increased glucose and lactate contents without major disturbances of protein synthesis or energy state. A transient peri-focal decrease in tissue pH by 0.4 units was noticed after 1 h, followed by tissue alkalosis 3 h post-injury. In injured animals without SD, a short-lasting expression of immediate-early gene (IEG) mRNAs was found in piriform cortex, in the dentate gyrus and hippocampal CA3/CA4 subfields at 1 h after lesioning. In injured animals with SDs, a strong elevation of IEGs was seen additionally in layers II–IV and VI of the injury-remote ipsilateral cerebral cortex, which persisted for as long as 6 h. The mRNA levels for c-fos, junB and mitogen-activated protein kinase phosphatase (MKP)-1 were closely related to the time interval between the last DC deflection and the termination of the experiment, yielding a post-depolarization decline with half-lives of 48, 75, and 58 min for c-fos, junB and MKP-1, respectively. The results of the present study demonstrate that SD is a prominent factor influencing trauma-related gene responses in the lesion-remote cerebral cortex. In contrast to focal cerebral ischemia, however, SDs do not aggravate the metabolic dysfunction in the area surrounding the lesion.

Introduction

Spreading depression (SD) waves, characterized by transient negative shifts of the cortical direct-current (DC) potential, have been associated with various pathologies of the human brain, such as migraine, chronic subdural hematoma, or head injury [1–4]. In fact, SD-like DC shifts have been recorded in a patient following brain trauma [5], but it has not been established whether such depolarizations contribute to the severity of injury. Elicitation of SD waves in intact cortex does not lead to lasting disturbances [6], because the increased energy demand required for cell repolarization is coupled to a proportional increase of blood flow that covers the elevated glucose and oxygen utilization [7, 8]. SDs in the normal cortex may even induce tolerance to subsequent ischemia by activating a protective gene-response program [9]. In focal ischemia, however, SD waves are thought to contribute to infarct growth into the

Maturation Phenomenon in Cerebral Ischemia III
U. Ito et al. (Eds.)
© Springer-Verlag Berlin Heidelberg 1999

oligemic surrounding of the ischemic lesion [10] because they aggravate the mismatch between substrate delivery and energy demand [8]. There are indications that secondary hemodynamic and metabolic alterations also occur in the area surrounding traumatic brain lesions, as reflected by cerebral hypoperfusion [11], increased glucose consumption [12] and, as a consequence of both, activation of anaerobic glycolysis [13]. Besides these metabolic disturbances, immediate-early genes (IEGs) are activated after the onset of experimental brain trauma [14–16]. It remains to be shown, however, whether these alterations are caused by SDs. We, therefore, examined the relationship between transient depolarizations, metabolic alterations and gene responses in the peri-lesion and lesion-remote tissue following traumatic injury of rat brain cortex.

Materials and Methods

Experimental Protocol

Male Sprague-Dawley rats (180–300 g) were anesthetized with 0.8 % halothane (30 % O_2, remainder N_2O). Catheters were inserted into both femoral arteries and veins for arterial blood-pressure recording, arterial blood sampling and intravenous infusions of drugs and tracers. Animals were tracheotomized, immobilized with tubocurarine chloride (1.5 mg/kg) and mechanically ventilated. Rectal temperature was maintained between 36.5 °C and 37.0 °C. The cortical DC potential and electroencephalogram (EEG) were recorded with miniature calomel electrodes positioned on the right parietal skull (5 mm caudal to bregma) and 15 mm further rostrally above the olfactory bulb. A laser Doppler-flowmetry (LDF) probe was placed 5 mm rostral to the bregma. Prior to cortex injury, arterial blood gases were measured and controlled repeatedly during the experiment. Cortical lesions were produced using a liquid-nitrogen-cooled thermal probe (tip diameter 2 mm), which was applied to the intact skull over the right parietal cortex at the level of bregma. For measurement of cerebral protein synthesis (CPS), L-[4,5-^{3}H]-leucine (1 mCi/animal; specific activity 151 Ci/mmol) was administered for 45 min by programmed intravenous infusion to achieve a constant level of specific activity of arterial plasma leucine [17]. Arterial blood samples were collected at 5-min intervals for the analysis of plasma-leucine specific activity. Experiments were terminated by in-situ freezing of the animals' heads in liquid nitrogen.

Following cold injury of the right sensorimotor cortex, animals were allowed to survive for 1, 3 or 6 h ($n=7$ in each group). Control animals were subjected only to sham surgery ($n=7$).

Multiparametric Imaging

Brains were removed in a cold box at –20 °C, cut into 20-µm coronal sections at –20 °C using a cryostat and placed either on poly-lysine-coated object slides or on coverslips. Cortical tissue samples were taken for enzymatic analysis of tissue adenosine triphosphate (ATP), glucose and lactate contents [18]. For measurement of regional pH and tissue ATP, glucose and lactate content, cryostat sections were processed using the umbelliferone method [19] or substrate-specific bioluminescence imaging [20–22]. Images were digitized and calibrated with graded pH standards and with the ATP, glucose or lactate values measured enzymatically in tissue samples taken from the cryostat block. High-performance liquid chromatography (HPLC) determinations of free-tissue-leucine and plasma-leucine specific activity were carried out as described earlier [17]. For the quantitative determination of regional CPS, sections were incubated in 10 % trichloroacetic acid to remove labeled free leucine and metabolites other than those incorporated into proteins. Sections were exposed for 2 weeks to Hyperfilm ^{3}H together with calibrated [^{3}H]-standards to perform quantitative ^{3}H-autoradiography [23]. Autoradiograms were digitized and converted to tissue isotope radioactivity, and the CPS rate was calculated as described previously [17].

In-Situ Hybridization and Immunohistochemistry

The probes and the in situ hybridization protocol for the detection of c-fos, junB, c-jun and mitogen-activated protein kinase phosphatase-1 (MKP-1) mRNAs have previously been described in detail [24, 25]. Briefly, sections were fixed in 4 % paraformaldehyde and treated with 0.25 % acetic anhydride in 0.1 M triethanolamine, before overnight hybridization with 5 pg/μl of a [^{35}S]-labeled oligoprobes at 42 °C. The following day, sections were washed for 1 h at 42 °C in 2·sodium saline citrate (SSC)/ 50 % formamide/5 mM dithiothreitol (DTT), dehydrated, dried and exposed to Amersham βmax Hyperfilm.

Immunocytochemistry was carried out on acetone-fixed sections, which were immersed in 0.1 % H_2O_2/phosphate-buffered saline (PBS) and PBS containing 1 % bovine serum albumin (PBS-BSA/normal goat serum; 1 : 50). Sections were subsequently incubated overnight at 4 °C with a polyclonal rabbit c-Fos antibody (PC05, Oncogene Science; 1 μg/ml) and for 2 h at room temperature with biotinylated goat anti-rabbit antibody (IgG, Vector Labs; 1 : 200), then immersed in an avidin biotin peroxidase complex (ABC) mix. The staining was developed with diaminobenzidine tetrahydrochloride and 0.01 % H_2O_2.

Statistics

Tissue ATP, glucose, lactate and pH values were analyzed using one-way analysis of variance (ANOVA) followed by the Scheffé test. In situ-hybridization data were fitted to a mono-exponential function to estimate the half-life of mRNA decay. Differences between groups are considered significant for a P value < 0.05.

Results

Physiological Variables

Systemic parameters remained within physiologic limits throughout the duration of the experiment and did not differ between the control and experimental groups (pH 7.3–7.4; pCO_2 37.7–38.6 mmHg; pO_2 196–213 mmHg; mean arterial blood pressure 112–127 mmHg).

Electrophysiology and Laser-Doppler Flowmetry

After cortex lesioning, SD-like depolarizations occurred in 14 of 21 injured animals. Recordings from SD-positive animals of cortical EEG, DC potential and perfusion as assessed by LDF revealed that during the first hour after cold injury several spontaneous depolarizations of the cortical DC potential were elicited, followed by transient SDs at more irregular intervals at later times of the experiment. The cortical DC deflections were accompanied by a transient decrease in EEG amplitude and by a 20–40 % increase in perfusion [26].

Metabolic Imaging

In Fig. 1, the development of metabolic changes after generation of a cortex lesion is demonstrated in a control and in a SD-positive animal, each surviving for 6 h post-injury. As is evident from the ATP and CPS images, lesions were sharply demarcated and affected 60–95 % of the cortical depth. The lesion size was the same in animals with and without SDs. In the injury-remote cortical tissue, no differences in tissue ATP, glucose, lactate or regional pH were found, irrespective of the occurrence of SDs. A minor reduction in cortical CPS by 10–15 % was noticed only in a few animals, in which transient depolarizations occurred during the 45 min [^{3}H]-leucine infusion.

In the rim around the lesion, at 1 h post-injury, tissue pH was significantly reduced by 0.4±0.3 units ($P<0.05$). However, tissue acidosis resolved within 3 h following trauma, and tissue alkalosis developed in the lesion border, which became significant 6 h after lesioning (0.3±0.2 units above the contralateral value; $P<0.05$). At 3 h post-injury, tissue lactate content was elevated not only within, but also in a small zone around the lesion (4.2±2.0 vs 1.8±0.4 µmol/g on the contralateral side; $P<0.05$). Moreover, a significant increase of tissue glucose content was observed at 6 h in the tissue around the lesion (7.2±2.7 vs 4.5±2.1 µmol/g; $P<0.05$), probably reflecting the widening of the glucose-rich extracellular space by vasogenic edema.

In Situ Hybridization and Immunohistochemistry

In sham-operated controls, expression of c-fos, junB, c-jun, and MKP-1 mRNAs was absent or weak. In injured animals, in which no SD waves were detected, a weak elevation of c-fos, junB, c-jun and MKP-1 mRNA levels was observed in the ipsilateral cortex at 1 h post-injury (Fig. 2). At the same time, a marked rise in mRNA

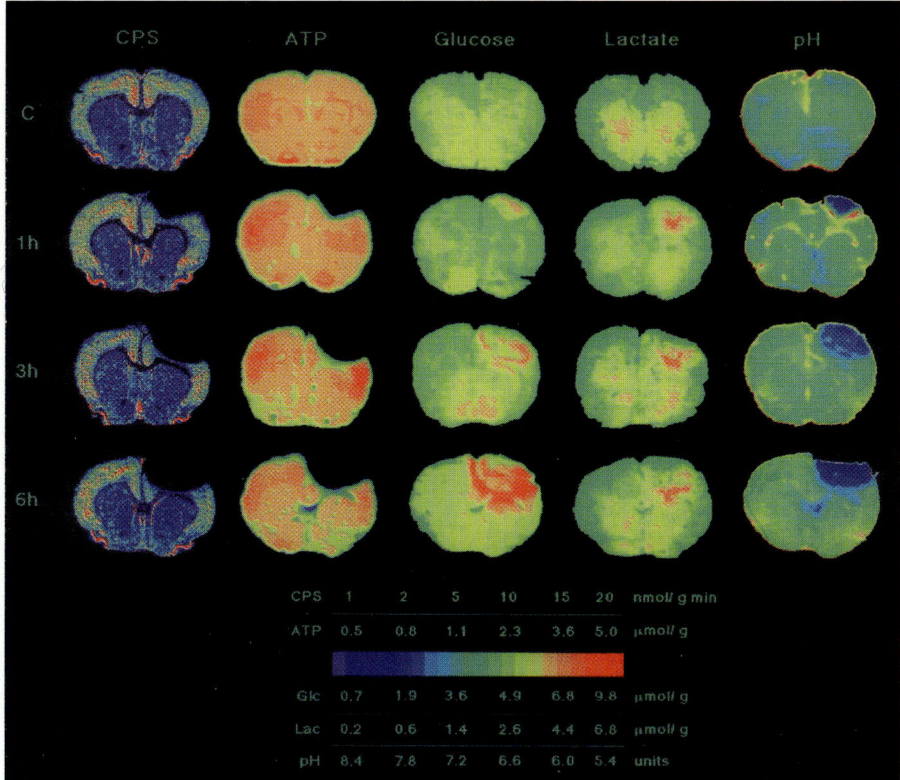

Fig. 1. Cerebral protein synthesis, tissue adenosine triphosphate, glucose, lactate, and pH images from a sham-operated rat and from rats submitted to cortical injury followed by 1, 3, and 6 h survival. Cortical lesions were surrounded by a narrow rim with a mild inhibition of overall protein synthesis and increase in tissue glucose and lactate content. Note a transient decrease in tissue pH (acidosis) in the lesion rim at 1 h followed by alkalosis at 3 h and 6 h post-injury in the peri-lesion cortex and underlying white matter, which is probably related to vasogenic edema

levels was bilaterally seen in the piriform cortex and – with ipsilateral dominance – in dentate gyrus and hippocampal CA3/4 subfields. The mRNA response, however, completely subsided at later survival times, i.e. at 3 h and 6 h post-injury.

Additionally, in lesioned animals with transient depolarizations, strong hybridization signals for c-fos, junB, c-jun and MKP-1 mRNAs were found in layers II–IV and VI throughout the ipsilateral lesion-distant cerebral cortex, which lasted until 6 h post-injury (Fig. 2). Interestingly, a close relationship was noticed between mRNA levels for c-fos, junB and MKP-1 and the time interval between the last DC deflection and the termination of experiment. mRNA levels were highest in animals that experienced SD shortly before sacrifice, but decreased mono-exponentially with increasing time delay. Kinetic analysis revealed half-lives of 48, 75 and 58 min for c-fos, junB and MKP-1 mRNAs, respectively. In the peri-lesion surrounding of SD-positive animals, c-fos mRNA was elevated at 1 h post-injury but was deficient at 3 h and 6 h, although energy metabolism and protein synthesis were not disturbed.

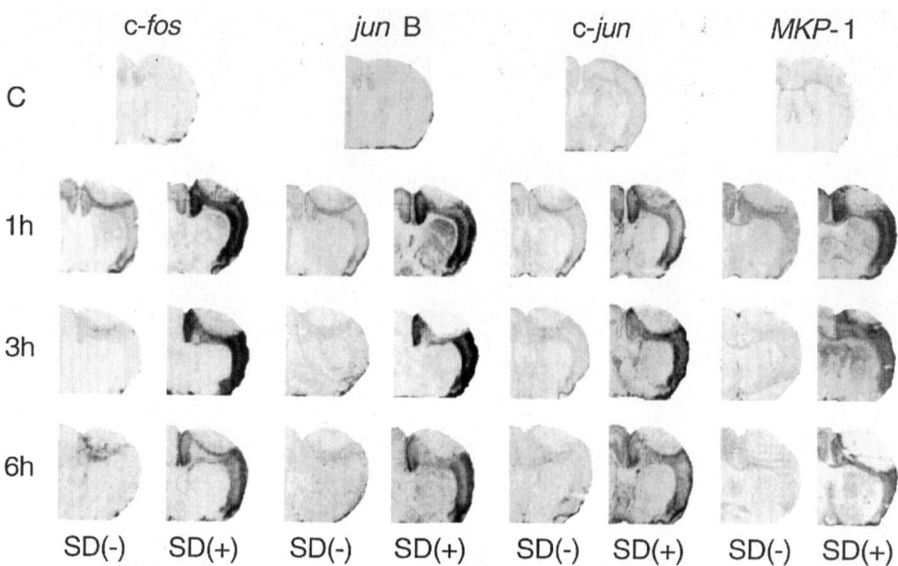

Fig. 2. In situ hybridization autoradiograms of c-fos, junB, c-jun, and MKP-1 mRNAs from a sham-operated rat and from rats submitted to cortical injury followed by 1, 3, and 6 h survival. In the *left column*, mRNA expression is shown in animals without spreading depressions (SDs), and in the *right column* in animals with SDs. Note the marked induction of immediate-early genes in lesion-remote ipsilateral cortex of animals with SDs at 1 h post-injury, and circumscribed c-fos deficits in the peri-lesion surrounding with normal cerebral protein synthesis, at 3 and 6 h post-injury

Discussion

In order to evaluate the role of SD in the pathophysiology of brain trauma, we compared the metabolic disturbances and the changes of gene expression between animals with and without transient cortical depolarizations after cold injury. We found metabolic disturbances in the lesion rim, i.e. an increase in tissue lactate and transient acidosis, which most likely reflect stimulation of anaerobic glycolysis and which are in line with similar studies that have been carried out before [27–32]. However, in contrast to focal cerebral ischemia, where peri-infarct SDs contribute to the evolution of brain infarction [8, 33–35], lesion-related SDs did not aggravate the metabolic disturbances. The fact that tissue acidosis develops only transiently after cortical injury could be of importance for the timing of head-injury treatment. Clinical trials with drugs that reduce tissue acidosis did not improve the outcome in head-trauma patients [36, 37], but this could have been due to the fact that treatment started too late.

In contrast to the metabolic disturbances in the lesion rim, IEG responses in the injury-remote brain tissue could be clearly differentiated into SD-dependent and -independent changes. Expression of AP-1 family genes (c-fos, junB, c-jun) or of MKP-1 are of particular interest because they encode for transcription factors that activate promoters of target genes involved in the regulation of neuronal function, adaptive processes or apoptotic cell death [38] or for second messengers implicated in the induction of such genes [25]. C-fos, junB, c-jun and MKP-1 mRNAs were strongly expressed in the injury-remote cerebral cortex of animals with transient DC depolarizations. This confirms previous studies which suggested that SD is responsible for the cortical induction of AP-1 genes after traumatic brain lesions [15, 16]. Since DC-potentials and the gene response after cortical injury were measured in the same experiment, it was possible to investigate the interrelationship between mRNA responses and SD more precisely. We found that the intensity of IEG mRNA expression was inversely related to the time interval between the last SD and the termination of the experiment, and that it did not depend on the survival time of animals after cortex injury or the total number of preceding DC shifts. The kinetic analysis revealed that the decline of SD-induced levels of c-fos, junB and MKP-1 mRNAs occurred at decay rates with half-lives of 48, 75 and 58 min, respectively. Our in-vivo results are in line with data previously obtained in cell culture after transient serum stimulation with soluble growth factors. In these studies, c-fos mRNA levels sharply increased after stimulation, followed by a gradual decline over 1–2 h [39, 40].

In injured animals, tissue adjacent to the lesion revealed a circumscribed region in which c-fos and junB mRNA were induced at 1 h post-injury, but not at 3 h and 6 h after cortex injury, although energy metabolism and protein synthesis were not disturbed. This could be due to the fact that SDs did not propagate into the border adjacent to the lesion. In focal ischemia, c-fos-mRNA antisense application prior to brain injury exacerbates tissue damage [41]. It is, therefore, conceivable that disturbances of c-fos transcription and translation in the rim of traumatic brain lesions are responsible for the previously shown lesion growth that occurs during the first day after cold injury [42].

In conclusion, cortical SDs, generated in the area surrounding cortical lesions, upregulate the expression of IEGs but do not aggravate the metabolic injury. However, the lack of c-fos expression in the lesion's immediate surroundings, in combination with the observed metabolic disturbances, may be involved in the peri-focal maturation of secondary tissue damage.

Acknowledgements. This study was supported by the grant 01K09508/0 of the BMBF, Germany.

References

1. Oka H, Kako M, Matsushima M, Ando K (1977) Traumatic spreading depression syndrome. Review of a particular type of head injury in 37 patients. Brain 100: 287–298
2. Lauritzen M (1987) Cortical spreading depression as a putative migrain mechanism. Trends Neurosci 10: 8–13
3. Barkley GL, Tepley N, Nagel-Leiby S, Moran JE, Simkins RT, Welch KM (1990) Magnetoencephalographic studies of migraine. Headache 30: 428–434
4. Nicoli F, Milandre L, Lemarquis P, Bazan M, Jau P (1990) Chronic subdural hematoma and transient neurologic deficits. Rev Neurol 146: 256–263
5. Mayevsky A, Doron A, Manor T, Meilin S, Zarchin N, Ouaknine GE (1996) Cortical spreading depression recorded from the human brain using a multiparametric monitoring system. Brain Res 740: 268–274
6. Nedergaard M, Hansen AJ (1988) Spreading depression is not associated with neuronal injury in the normal brain. Brain Res 449: 395–398

7. Kocher M (1990) Metabolic and hemodynamic activation of postischemic rat brain by cortical spreading depression. J Cereb Blood Flow Metab 10: 564–571
8. Back T, Kohno K, Hossmann K-A (1994) Cortical negative DC deflections following middle cerebral artery occlusion and KCl-induced spreading depression: effect on blood flow, tissue oxygenation, and electroencephalogram. J Cereb Blood Flow Metab 14: 12–19
9. Kawahara N, Croll SD, Wiegand SJ, Klatzo I (1997) Cortical spreading depression induces long-term alterations of BDNF levels in cortex and hippocampus distinct from lesion effects: implications for ischemic tolerance. Neurosci Res 29: 37–47
10. Hossmann K-A (1996) Periinfarct depolarizations. Cereb Brain Metab Rev 8: 195–208
11. Dietrich WD, Alonso O, Busto R, Prado R, Dewanjee MK, Ginsberg MD (1996) Widespread hemodynamic depression and focal platelet accumulation after fluid percussion brain injury: a double-label autoradiographic study in rats. J Cereb Blood Flow Metab 16: 481–489
12. Ginsberg MD, Zhao W, Alonso OF, Loor-Estades JY, Dietrich WD, Busto R (1997) Uncoupling of local cerebral glucose metabolism and blood flow after acute fluid-percussion injury in rats. Am J Physiol 272:H2859–H2868
13. Siesjö BK, Katsura K-I, Kristián T (1996) Acidosis-related damage. Adv Neurol 71: 209–236
14. Yang K, Mu XS, Xue JJ, Whitson J, Salminen A, Dixon CE, Liu PK, Hayes RL (1994) Increased expression of c-*fos* mRNA and AP-1 transcription factors after cortical impact injury in rats. Brain Res 664: 141–147
15. Raghupathi R, Welsh F, Lowenstein DH, Gennarelli TA, McIntosh TK (1995) Regional induction of c-*fos* and heat shock protein-72 mRNA following fluid-percussion brain injury in the rat. J Cereb Blood Flow Metab 15: 467–473
16. Mikawa S, Sharp FR, Kamii H, Kinouichi H, Epstein CJ, Chan PH (1995) Expression of c-fos and hsp70 mRNA after traumatic brain injury in transgenic mice overexpressing CuZn-superoside dismutase. Brain Res Mol Brain Res 33: 288–294
17. Mies G, Djuricic B, Paschen W, Hossmann KA (1997) Quantitative measurement of cerebral protein synthesis in vivo: theory and methodological considerations. J Neurosci Methods 76: 35–44
18. Lowry OH, Passonneau JV (1972) A flexible system of enzymatic analysis. Academic Press, New York
19. Csiba L, Paschen W, Hossmann K-A (1983) A topographic quantitative method for measuring brain tissue pH under physiological and pathophysiological conditions. Brain Res 289: 334–337
20. Kogure K, Alonso OF (1978) A pictorial representation of endogenous brain ATP by a bioluminescent method. Brain Res 154: 273–284
21. Paschen W, Mies G, Kloiber O, Hossmann K-A (1985) Regional quantitative determination of brain glucose in tissue sections: a bioluminescent approach. J Cereb Blood Flow Metab 5: 465–468
22. Paschen W (1985) Regional quantitative determination of lactate in brain sections: a bioluminescent approach. J Cereb Blood Flow Metab 5: 609–612
23. Mies G, Kohno K, Hossmann K-A (1993) MK-801, a glutamate antagonist, lowers threshold for inhibition of protein synthesis after middle cerebral artery occlusion of rat. Neurosci Lett 155: 65–68
24. Neumann-Haefelin T, Wiessner C, Vogel P, Back T, Hossmann K-A (1994) Differential expression of the immediate early genes c-*fos*, c-*jun*, *jun*B, and NGFI-B in the rat brain following transient forebrain ischemia. J Cereb Blood Flow Metab 14: 206–216
25. Wiessner C, Neumann-Haefelin T, Vogel P, Back T, Hossmann K-A (1995) Transient forebrain ischemia induces an immediate-early gene encoding the mitogen-activated protein kinase phosphatase 3CH134 in the adult rat brain. Neuroscience 64: 959–966
26. Hermann DM, Mies G, Hossmann K-A (1998) Effects of a traumatic neocortical lesion on cerebral metabolism and gene expression of rats. Neuroreport 9: 1917–1921
27. Dhillon HS, Dose JM, Scheff SW, Renuka Prasad M (1997) Time course of changes in lactate and free fatty acids after experimental brain injury and relationship to morphologic damage. Exp Neurol 146: 240–249
28. Hovda DA, Becker DP, Katayama Y (1992) Secondary injury and acidosis. J Neurotrauma 9[Suppl 1]:47–60
29. Inao S, Marmarou A, Clarke GD, Andersen BJ, Fatouros PP, Young HF (1988) Production and clearance of lactate from brain tissue, cerebrospinal fluid, and serum following experimental brain injury. J Neurosurg 69: 736–744
30. Kawamata T, Katayama Y, Hovda DA, Yoshino A, Becker DP (1995) Lactate accumulation following concussive brain injury: the role of ionic fluxes induced by excitatory amino acids. Brain Res 674: 196–204
31. McIntosh TK, Faden AI, Bendall MR, Vink R (1987) Traumatic brain injury in the rat: alterations in brain lactate and pH as characterized by ^{1}H and ^{31}P nuclear magnetic resonance. J Neurochem 49: 1530–1540

32. Renuka-Prasad M, Ramaiah C, McIntosh TK, Dempsey RJ, Hipkens S, Yurek D (1994) Regional levels of lactate and norepinephrine after experimental brain injury. J Neurochem 63: 1086–1094
33. Mies G, Ishimaru S, Xie Y, Seo K, Hossmann K-A (1991) Ischemic thresholds of cerebral protein synthesis and energy state following middle cerebral artery occlusion in rat. J Cereb Blood Flow Metab 11: 753–761
34. Iijima T, Mies G, Hossmann K-A (1992) Repeated negative DC deflections in rat cortex following middle cerebral artery occlusion are abolished by MK-801: effect on volume of ischemic injury. J Cereb Blood Flow Metab 12: 727–733
35. Mies G, Iijima T, Hossmann K-A (1993) Correlation between peri-infarct DC shifts and ischaemic neuronal damage in rat. Neuroreport 4: 709–711
36. Wolf AL, Levi L, Marmarou A, Ward JD, Muizelaar P, Choi S, Young H, Rigamonti D, Robinson WL (1993) Effect of THAM upon outcome in severe head injury: a randomized prospective clinical trial. J Neurosurg 78: 54–59
37. Marmarou A, Holdaway R, Ward JD, Yoshida K, Choi SC, Muizelaar JP (1993) Traumatic brain tissue acidosis: experimental and clinical studies. Acta Neurochir Suppl (Wien) 57: 160–164
38. Dragunow M, Preston K (1995) The role of inducible transcription factors in apoptotic nerve cell death. Brain Res Brain Res Rev 21: 1–28
39. Lau LF, Nathans D (1987) Expression of a set of growth-related immediate early genes in BALB/c 3T3 cells: coordinate regulation with c-*fos* or c-*myc*. Proc Natl Acad Sci U S A 84: 1182–1186
40. Edwards DR, Mahadevan LC (1992) Protein synthesis inhibitors differentially superinduce c-*fos* and c-*jun* by three distinct mechanisms: lack of evidence for labile respressors. EMBO J 11: 2415–2424
41. Baskin DS, Zhang YJ, Widmayer MA (1998) C-*fos* antisense oligonucleotide administration prior to cerebrovascular occlusion exacerbates tissue damage. Stroke [Suppl] (in press)
42. Eriskat J, Schurer L, Kempski O, Baethmann A (1994) Growth kinetics of a primary brain tissue necrosis from a focal lesion. Acta Neurochir Suppl (Wien) 60: 425–427

Protein Expression and Brain Plasticity After Transient Middle Cerebral Artery Occlusion in the Rat

M. Chopp, Y. Li, and Z. G. Zhang

Summary. After a stroke, both animals and humans can regain lost function. The molecular basis of this functional plasticity is unknown. In this manuscript, we describe developmental protein expression in the ischemic brain after stroke. We present data on the expression and localization of select cell-cycle proteins, a cytoskeletal protein [microtubule-associated protein-2 (MAP-2)], a growth-associated protein (GAP-43) and a neurofilament protein (nestin) in ischemic rat brain. These proteins are upregulated and selectively localized to periinfarct regions of brain for at least 4 weeks after middle cerebral artery occlusion in the rat. The expression of these developmentally regulated proteins suggests that the ischemic brain reverts to a fetal stage after stroke, possibly in an attempt to restructure and regain function.

Introduction

The overwhelming focus of research directed toward improving outcome after stroke has been the reduction of the volume of cerebral infarction. Acute intervention after stroke by a number of pharmaceutical agents can spare tissue. However, in order to be effective, interventions must be instituted immediately, often within the first hour after stroke. Treatment of stroke with recombinant tissue plasminogen activator (rtPA), the only Food and Drug Administration (FDA)-approved therapeutic agent for stroke, has a window of therapeutic opportunity of 3 h [22]. Acute therapies will not benefit most stroke patients and other approaches must be considered to reduce neurological deficits after stroke.

Neurological function is restored within days after stroke [20] to many patients and to animals subjected to middle cerebral artery (MCA) occlusion. What is the basis for this restoration? What are some of the molecular markers of neurologic recovery? We hypothesize that the brain responds to stroke by cellular expression of proteins, reflecting a return to an embryonic stage of development. Proteins associated with the developing brain are upregulated. These proteins provide machinery driving phenotypic change and dendritic and axonal extension.

In this manuscript, we outline our studies on experimental focal cerebral ischemia and present data on the expression of developmental proteins after stroke. We direct attention to four proteins: cyclin D1, a growth-associated protein (GAP-43), microtubule-associated protein-2 (MAP-2) and nestin.

Maturation Phenomenon in Cerebral Ischemia III
U. Ito et al. (Eds.)
© Springer-Verlag Berlin Heidelberg 1999

Methods

All measurements were performed on 3-month-old male Wistar rats weighing 270–300 g ($n=20$). Rats were subjected to 2 h of MCA occlusion by means of intracarotid insertion of a flared tipped nylon thread (4–0 suture) [3, 34]. Animals were sacrificed at various time points between 6 h and 28 days after MCA occlusion. Brains were subjected to immunohistochemical analysis for cellular protein localization and double-labeled-immunohistochemical analysis for protein and cellular identification and to identify apoptotic cells. Coronal tissue sections were also labeled with hematoxylin and eosin (H&E) for evaluation of cellular morphological changes.

Results

Cell-Cycle Proteins, p53 and Apoptosis

Cerebral ischemia induces genomic instability in the brain. DNA damage and repair ensue, and these processes tend to be localized to neurons after a stroke. Evidence of genomic instability following human stroke is found in the significantly elevated risk of brain cancer in patients having experienced a stroke [19]. Associated with genomic instability is cellular mitosis. Thus, a stroke apparently activates protein machinery that both kills cells and fosters conditions that promote cellular proliferation. We have sought to reveal molecular mechanisms associated with DNA damage, DNA repair and genomic activity [4]. A focus of our work has been the expression of the p53 protein [6]. Wild-type p53 is a tumor-suppressor protein and a potent transcription factor that engenders families of proteins that decrease the threshold for genomic activity, both repair and damage [8, 10, 13, 24]. p53 is expressed in ischemic brain, as are many of the proteins that vie to repair and damage parenchymal cells [16–18]. Among p53 response proteins expressed, are DNA-repair proteins, such as GADD45 and proliferating cell nuclear antigen (PCNA). These proteins are preferentially expressed within morphologically intact cells and in reversibly damaged cells within ischemic tissue areas. Proteins associated with DNA damage, such as the Bax family of proteins, are also expressed and are primarily localized to apoptotic cells.

p21 (WAF-1) is a p53 response protein [10]. This protein is an inhibitor of the cell-cycle process and also interacts with PCNA [32]. Using immunohistochemical methods, we detected p21 localized in the boundary of the ischemic lesion [16]. In control non-ischemic animals, p21 was slightly expressed within the cytoplasm of neurons. After stroke, there is an increased expression and translocation of p21 to the nucleus of cells in the boundary of the ischemic lesion. Thus, expression of p21 evokes the possibility that cell-cycle proteins are expressed within the ischemic brain. Cell-cycle regulation is associated with DNA damage and repair. We, therefore, investigated whether cell-cycle proteins are expressed in ischemic brain. We focused on two cell-cycle proteins and their respective cyclin-dependent kinases: cyclin A, cyclin D1 and, respectively, cdk2 and cdk4. Measurements were performed to identify which cells express these proteins [16, 17]. In addition, we sought to identify the morphological characteristics of cells expressing these proteins, whether these cells were intact, damaged, necrotic or apoptotic. Our data revealed a robust expression of these cell-

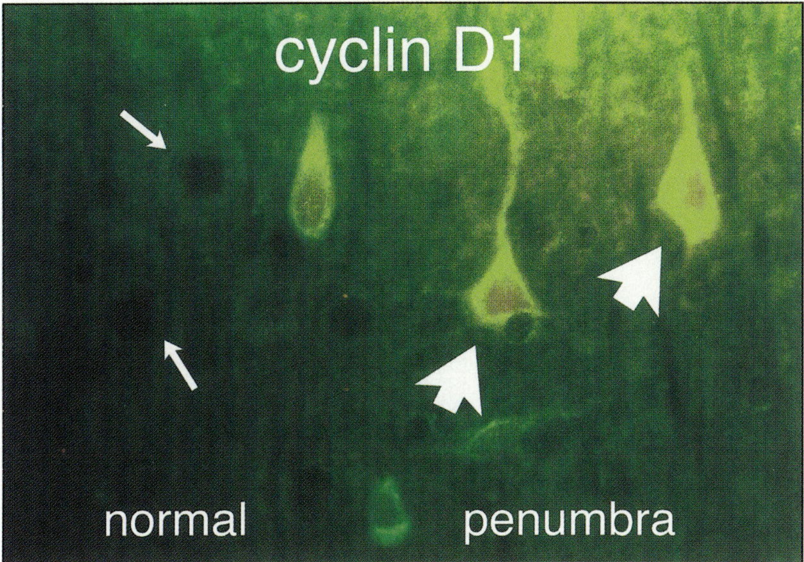

Fig. 1. Immunohistochemical reactivity of cyclin D1 localized to the penumbra of the ischemic cortex. The rat was subjected to 2 h of middle cerebral artery occlusion and sacrificed 48 h later

cycle proteins, as well as their dependent kinases, localized primarily to morphologically intact or reversibly damaged neurons within the boundary zone of the ischemic lesion (Fig. 1). However, a striking finding was that these proteins were not expressed in apoptotic cells.

Figure 2 shows ischemic cortical tissue 48 h after 2 h of MCA occlusion, double labeled for apoptosis (terminal deoxynucleotidyl transferase-mediated dUTP nick-end labeling [TUNEL]) and cyclin D1. Cyclin D1 is not colocalized with apoptotic cells. An inverse relationship is apparent between the expression of these proteins and apoptotic cells, as if cell-cycle proteins protect cells from apoptosis. It is possible that these proteins contribute to DNA repair, prevent apoptosis, or inhibit families of proapoptotic caspase proteins that promote apoptotic death. The issue of apoptotic cell death and the expression of proteins associated with the cell cycle raises intriguing possibilities. Although proteins may play multiple roles in different cells, the observation that under an ischemic insult the brain chooses to express cell-cycle proteins, proteins that are responsible for mitosis, is enigmatic; even more enigmatic is the fact that these proteins are expressed in post-mitotic cells, i.e., neurons. We speculate that the expression of these proteins is associated with an attempt by the brain to return to an earlier stage of development, a stage in which neuronal numbers are increased.

Apoptosis is associated with the developing brain and may be a signal for brain-tissue plasticity. Apoptosis is primarily found in the developing brain. More than half the neurons generated in the embryonic stage undergo apoptosis [5]. Apoptosis may be essential for enhancing neuronal circuitry. It is, therefore, possible that the presence of apoptosis itself in the injured ischemic brain is a reversion to an earlier stage of development, and apoptosis may signal repair processes that may promote neurite outgrowth.

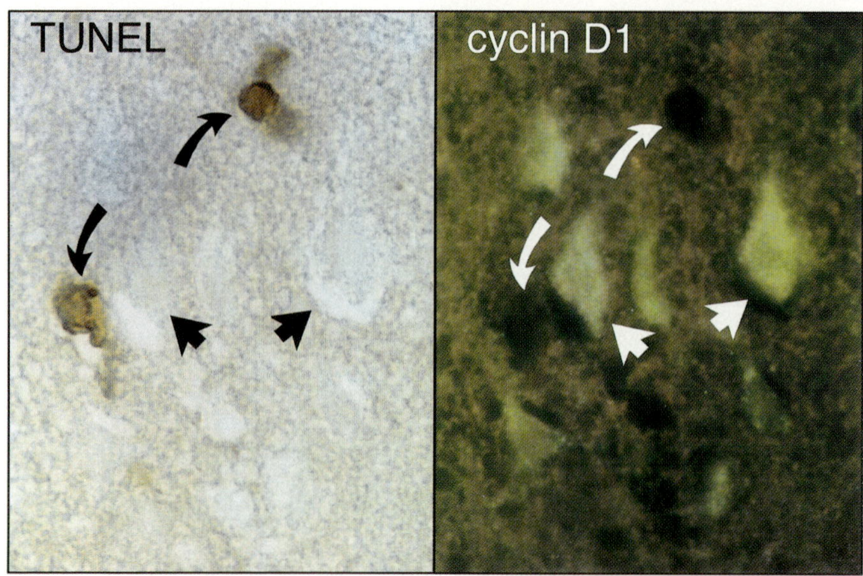

Fig. 2. Double-labeled immunohistochemistry from a cortical coronal section of brain from a rat subjected to 2 h of middle cerebral artery occlusion and sacrificed 48 h later. Terminal deoxynucleotidyl transferase-mediated dUTP nick-end labeling (TUNEL) staining labels apoptotic cells. *Arrow heads* indicate an absence of TUNEL reactivity with a concomitant cyclin D1 reactivity. Curved arrows indicate TUNEL reactivity and an absence of cyclin D1 reactivity

GAP-43/MAP-2

The 43-kDa growth associated protein (GAP-43) is central nervous system (CNS) specific. GAP-43 is synthesized at high levels during neuronal development and regeneration [11, 27]. It is primarily expressed and associated with axonal outgrowth. GAP-43 has been employed as an index of axonal sprouting and reflects enhancement of neuronal plasticity [2, 26]. GAP-43 has been detected after cortical and striatal ischemic insult in the adult rat [12, 28, 29]. Thus, GAP-43 may be a marker of axonal growth and neuronal plasticity. GAP-43 is expressed primarily in the developing brain and appears to be reactivated after stroke and injury. Figure 3 shows expression of GAP-43 in the penumbral cortical tissue of rat brain 48 h after MCA occlusion.

Although not necessarily a developmental protein, MAP-2 is a structural protein whose primary function is to maintain neuronal architecture along with other cytoskeletal proteins, such as actin, and neurofilaments [31]. MAP-2 is an early and sensitive indicator of neuronal damage [14, 33]. MAP-2 is primarily localized to dendrites within neurons, and scattered glia may also express this protein. Although the focus of much of the research associated with MAP-2 in ischemia has been in the degradation of this protein and its interaction with calpain, little attention has been paid to the ramifications of increased expression of this protein after stroke. We measured the expression of the MAP-2 dendritic protein and the GAP-43 axonal developmental neuron-specific protein before and after stroke. Modification and rearrangement of

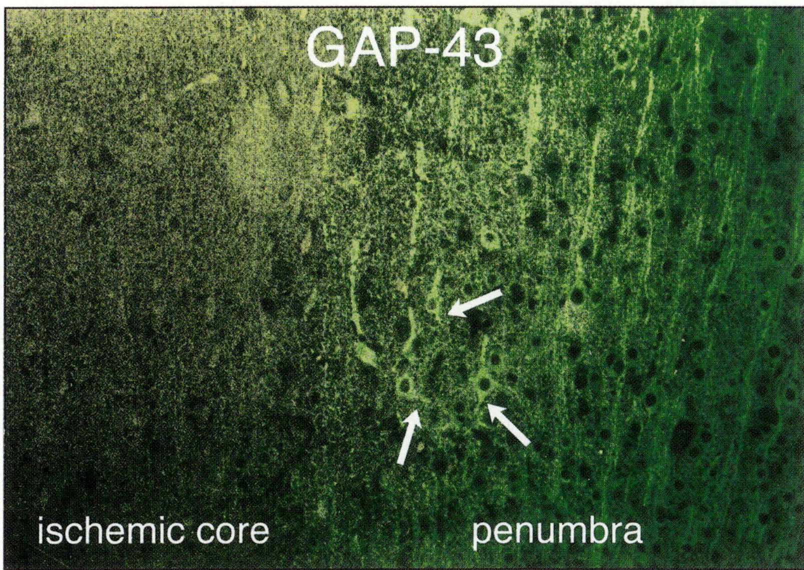

Fig. 3. Growth-associated protein-43 (GAP-43) labeling of a coronal section from ischemic brain from a rat subjected to 2 h of middle cerebral artery occlusion and sacrificed at 48 h. GAP-43 is expressed in the axon and cytoplasm within the penumbral regions

these proteins in neurons may be indicative of processes that modify neuronal connections and, hence, function. The hypothesis tested was that the penumbral regions express both GAP-43 and MAP-2 proteins after stroke, and the expression of these proteins are indicative of tissue plasticity and an attempt by the CNS to reformat the brain to increase synaptogenesis and to extend and repair axons [18].

In non-ischemic brain, MAP-2 and GAP-43 were colocalized in the soma of morphologically intact neurons. A reciprocal staining pattern for both proteins was evident in neurites. In non-ischemic brain, expression of GAP-43 was low and expressed primarily in the cytoplasm and axon. MAP-2 immunoreactivity showed smooth uniform labeling of soma and dendrites. Acutely (6 h) after MCA occlusion, a rapid degradation of MAP-2 reactivity was present in dendrites within the core of the lesion and MAP-2 staining was lost. Likewise, degradation and loss of GAP-43 was also detected within 6 h of MCA occlusion, with progressive loss of protein within the core of the lesion [18].

However, an increase in protein expression occurs within the boundary zones of the lesion. The boundary zone of an ischemic lesion is a complex structure and likely constitutes an array of regions, a continuity of tissue at various stages of repair and plasticity that is dynamic with time. For ease of presentation, we divide the boundary of the lesion into two primary zones, an inner and an outer zone. These regions are defined based on proximity to the core of the lesion and have selected differential protein expression. Very acutely after stroke, the entire lesion is penumbra; however, we employ the term penumbra when a well-defined core of a lesion is present, usually at 24 h after stroke. In contrast to the loss of MAP-2 within the core of the lesion,

MAP-2 reactivity is greatly increased throughout the boundary of the lesion, both inner and outer boundary zones. Intense labeling is present and is in marked contrast to the light MAP-2 immunoreactivity localized with non-ischemic neurons.

Morphologically, the immunoreactive neurons show a pattern of lengthened fibers at extended time points after ischemia, such as 28 days, compared with expression at 2 days after stroke [18]. However, neurite lengths were not quantified. A somewhat-similar pattern was observed for GAP-43 after stroke. Immunoreactivity for GAP-43 was rapidly lost after stroke within the core of the lesion. In contrast to the loss of reactivity in the core of the lesion, a large and intense increase of GAP-43 is present and localized primarily to the outer boundary of the lesion. Intense labeling is present in the soma and axons within this outer region. We emphasize that the selective increase of GAP-43 is localized to the outer boundary zone of the lesion. As for MAP-2, radial fibers appeared obviously extended at 28 days compared with earlier (7 days) expression.

Our data indicate that cytoskeletal proteins, such as MAP-2, and the developmental protein GAP-43 are possibly associated with restructuring of the brain within the penumbral regions after stroke. The decreased expression of these proteins is a sensitive and early marker for damage, but what is most interesting is the large increase in immunoreactivity specifically localized to morphologically intact neurons. These neurons with extended axons and dendrites are immunoreactive in the penumbral tissue, suggesting that tissue plasticity may be ongoing within this tissue. The parallel architecture of the axons and dendrites suggest that a purposeful restructuring of cerebral connection occurs within the boundaries of the ischemic lesion. It is also interesting to note that MAP-2 reactivity is upregulated within the inner boundary zone of the ischemic lesion; however, GAP-43 is only upregulated in the outer boundary zone. This may suggest that axons are more vulnerable to the ischemic insult and a greater distance between the lesion and viable neurons are needed for axonal function.

The observation of enhanced protein expression, particularly cytoskeletal-and growth-associated-protein expression in the penumbra is evidence of reversible tissue damage in this region. The overriding hypothesis that is supported by these data is that proteins primarily expressed in the developing brain are increased in viable periischemic tissue, which suggests, as does the expression of the cell-cycle proteins, an effort to recapture the early stage of development.

Astrocyte Vascular Endothelial Growth Factor

Glia function in multifaceted roles to promote as well as to block brain-tissue plasticity. Astrocytes circumscribe and likely limit the region of tissue damage. The glial scar formed around the core lesion protects the non-ischemic tissue from progressive and expanding damage from the original injury. The scar may also block new circuitry from developing in the ischemic brain [1, 23]. It, thus, may be reasonable to rapidly activate the astrocyte to encircle and contain the lesion. When the progress of damage is slowed, the intensity of this response is reduced to allow for neuronal circuit building and synaptogenesis. The astrocyte may also play a prominent role in enhancing brain-tissue plasticity. Acutely after stroke, astrocytes express vascular

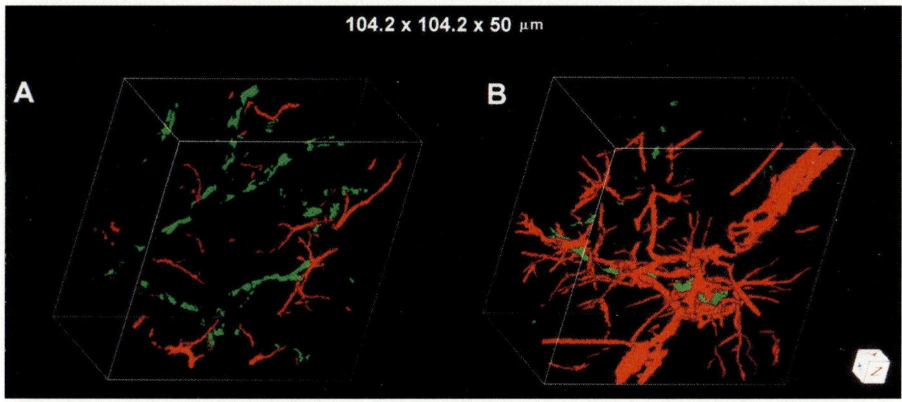

Fig. 4A, B. A three-dimensional figure obtained with a laser scanning confocal microscope of vascular perfusion and vascular endothelial growth factor (VEGF). High-molecular-weight dextran-labeled fluorescein isothiocyanate was employed to measure vascular perfusion. The voxel of tissue was obtained from rat brain 2 h after induction of embolic stroke. **A** Contralateral (non-ischemic) hemisphere, showing perfused vessels and low VEGF expression. **B** Homologous tissue from the ipsilateral hemisphere, showing intense VEGF expression concomitant with low tissue perfusion

endothelial growth factor (VEGF; unpublished results). Figure 4 shows vascular perfusion and VEGF expression at 2 h after onset of embolic stroke in the rat.

VEGF has pluripotent roles in the brain. It can promote blood–brain barrier (BBB) breakdown and the associated neovascularization. The relationship between the generation of new vessels and synaptogenesis is unknown. However, we speculate that new blood vessels are required to activate the process of brain-tissue plasticity.

Nestin

Nestin is an intermediate filament protein which is highly expressed in multipotential stem cells of the CNS during embryogenesis [15]. It is either absent or expressed primarily in endothelial and subventricular cells in the mature brain. In the maturing brain, nestin is replaced by cell-specific-type intermediate filaments, such as glial fibrillary acidic protein (GFAP) [21, 30]. Nestin is also present in CNS tumors [30]. Kainic acid hippocampal lesions [7] as well as focal and global cerebral ischemia induce nestin expression [9, 25]. Reactive astrocytes and scattered cortical neurons have also been shown to express nestin after induction of global cerebral ischemia. Since nestin is primarily expressed in the developing brain, and is re-expressed in the brain after injury, and because it is specifically localized to astrocytes, we performed a series of experiments to measure the temporal profile and cellular expression of nestin after MCA occlusion in rats (M. Chopp et al., unpublished results).

In non-ischemic brain, only endothelial cells and ependymal cells are nestin reactive. Acutely (within the first 12 h) after ischemia, nestin reactivity is present within astrocytes and endothelial cells within the lesion. At later times after onset of ischemia, nestin expression rings the boundary of the ischemic lesion and clearly demarcates the cerebral infarct. At 2 days after ischemia, nestin expression extends throughout the ischemic hemisphere. Over time, however, nestin localization becomes restricted to the boundary of the lesion. Intense nestin immunoreactivity is observed in astrocytes and in scattered oligodendrocytes. Neurons express nestin only within the outer boundary zone to the penumbra. Nestin is present within vascular endothelial cells within the core as well as in the boundary of the ischemic lesion.

Nestin is a developmentally regulated protein and its expression in neurons and astrocytes suggests a return to an immature state in these activated neurons and astrocytes. These data also indicate that mature cells within injured tissue can alter their phenotype and revert to a phenotype typical of a developing cell. The expression of nestin within astrocytes and endothelial cells may be related to cellular proliferation. Nestin in neurons was only found within the outer boundary zone of the lesion within areas of little or no glial activation, while, in the inner boundary zone to the ischemic lesion (an area with intense glial activation), no neuronal expression of nestin was detected. This suggests that activation of neuronal plasticity occurs in regions without activated glia, and is consistent with the hypothesis that neuronal plasticity can be suppressed or overwhelmed by reactive astrocytes.

Conclusions

We have demonstrated that brain responds to a stroke by expressing developmental proteins. Some of these proteins are important for structural integrity of the cell and are cytoskeletal and intermediate-filament proteins. Likewise, proteins needed for cell mitosis are localized in morphologically intact neurons. These data suggest that brain ischemia promotes a return to early development. After a stroke, neurological function returns in many patients and in animals. Although tissue has been infarcted, compensatory mechanisms are active, with varying degrees of success. Some patients fully recover and others do not. We speculate that the brain responds to a stroke by recapitulating development. Tissue plasticity is engendered by a return to an early developmental stage. Protein markers of development may be associated with the compensatory response to stroke. Our goal is to enhance this compensatory response. A possible pathway would be to promote the expression of developmental proteins in the ischemic brain.

Acknowledgements. The authors wish to thank Denice Janus for manuscript preparation. This work was supported by National Institute of Neurological Disorders and Stroke grants PO1 NS23393 and RO1 NS35504.

References

1. Berry M, Maxwell WL, Logan A, Mathewson A, McConnell P, Ashhurst DE, Thomas GH (1983) Deposition of scar tissue in the central nervous system. Acta Neurochir Suppl (Wien) 32: 31–53
2. Buffo A, Holtmaat AJDG, Savio T, Verbeek JS, Oberdick J, Oestreicher AB, Gispen WH, Verhaagen J, Rossi F, Strata P (1997) Targeted overexpression of the neurite growth-associated protein B-50/ GAP-43 in cerebellar purkinje cells induces sprouting after axotomy but not axon regeneration into growth-permissive transplants. J Neurosci 17: 8778–8791
3. Chen H, Chopp M, Zhang ZG, Garcia JH (1992) The effect of hypothermia on the transient middle cerebral artery occlusion in the rat. J Cereb Blood Flow Metab 12: 621–628

4. Chopp M, Chan PH, Hsu HY, Cheung ME, Jacobs TP (1990) DNA damage and repair in central nervous system injury. National Institute of Neurological Disorders and Stroke Workshop summary. Stroke 27: 363–369
5. Chopp M, Li Y (1996) Apoptosis in focal cerebral ischemia. In: Baethmann A, Kempski O, Plesnila N, Staub F (eds) Mechanisms of secondary brain damage in cerebral ischemia and trauma. Springer, Berlin Heidelberg New York, pp 21–26
6. Chopp M, Li Y, Zhang ZG, Freytag SO (1992) p53 expression in brain after middle cerebral artery occlusion in the rat. Biochem Biophys Res Commun 182: 1201–1207
7. Clarke SR, Shetty AK, Bradley JL, Turner DA (1994) Reactive astrocytes express the embryonic intermediate neurofilament nestin. Neuroreport 5: 1885–1888
8. Cox LS, Lane DP (1995) Tumor suppressors, kinases and clamps: how p53 regulates the cell cycle in response to DNA damage. Bioessays 17: 501–506
9. Duggal N, Schmidt-Kastner R, Hakim AM (1997) Nestin expression in reactive astrocytes following focal cerebral ischemia in rats. Brain Res 768: 1–9
10. El-Deiry WS, Harper JW, O'Connor PM, Velculescu VE, Canman CE, Jackman J, Pietenpol JA, Burrell M, Hill DE, Wang Y, Wiman KG, Mercer WE, Kastan MB, Kohn KW, Elledge SJ, Kinzler KW, Vogelstein B (1994) WAF1/CIP1 is induced in p53-mediated G1 arrest and apoptosis. Cancer Res 54: 1169–1174
11. Goslin K, Schreyer DJ, Skene JHP, Banker G (1988) Development of neuronal polarity: GAP43 distinguishes axonal from dendritic growth cones. Nature 336: 672–674
12. Goto S, Yamada K, Inoue N, Nagahiro S, Ushio Y (1994) Increased expression of growth-associated protein GAP-43/B-50 following cerebral hemitransection or striatal ischemic injury in the substantia nigra of adult rats. Brain Res 647: 333–339
13. Kastan MB, Onyekwere O, Sidransky D, Vogelstein B, Craig RW (1991) Participation of p53 protein in the cellular response to DNA damage. Cancer Res 51: 6304–6311
14. Kitagawa K, Matsumoto M, Niinobe M, Mikoshiba K, Hata R, Ueda H, Handa N, Fukunaqa R, Isaka Y, Kimura K, Kamada T (1989) Microtubule-associated protein 2 as a sensitive marker for cerebral ischemic damage–immunohistochemical investigation of dendritic damage. Neuroscience 31: 401–411
15. Lendahl U, Zimmerman LB, McKay RDG (1990) CNS stem cells express a new class of intermediate filament protein. Cell 60: 585–595
16. Li Y, Chopp M, Powers C, Jiang N (1997) Apoptosis and protein expression after focal cerebral ischemia in rat. Brain Res 765: 301–312
17. Li Y, Chopp M, Powers C, Jiang N (1997) Immunoreactivity of cyclin D1/cdk4 in neurons and oligodendrocytes after focal cerebral ischemia in rat. J Cereb Blood Flow Metab 17: 846–856
18. Li Y, Jiang N, Powers C, Chopp M (1998) Neuronal damage and plasticity identified by MAP-2, GAP-43 and cyclin D1 immunoreactivity after focal cerebral ischemia in rat. Stroke 29: 1972–1981
19. Lindvig K, Moller H, Mosbeck J, Jensen OM (1990) The pattern of cancer in a large cohort of stroke patients. Int J Epidemiol 19: 498–504
20. McDowell FH (1991) Activation of rehabilitation. Arzneimittelforschung 41: 355–359
21. Morshead CM, Reynolds BA, Craig CG, McBurney MW, Staines WA, Morassutti D, Weiss S, van der Kooy D (1994) Neural stem cells in the adult mammalian forebrain: a relatively quiescent subpopulation of subependymal cells. Neuron 13: 1071–1082
22. The National Institute of Neurological Disorders and Stroke rt-PA Stroke Study Group (1995) Tissue plasminogen activator for acute ischemic stroke. N Engl J Med 333: 1581–1587
23. Reier PJ, Stensaas LJ, Guth L (1983) Spinal cord reconstruction. In: Kao CC, Bunge RP, Reier PJ (eds) Raven, New York, pp 163–195
24. Sanchez Y, Elledge SJ (1995) Stopped for repairs. Bioessays 17: 545–548
25. Schmidt-Kastner R, Garcia I, Busto R, Ginsberg MD (1997) Nestin antibodies label reactive glial cells and some cortical neurons after global brain ischemia in adult rat (abstract). J Cereb Blood Flow Metab 17[Suppl 1]:S727
26. Skene H (1989) Axonal growth-associated proteins. Annu Rev Neurosci 12: 127–156
27. Skilbeck CE, Wade DT, Langton Hewer RL, Wood VA (1983) Recovery after stroke. J Neurol Neurosurg Psychiatry 46: 5–8
28. Stroemer RP, Kent TA, Hulsebosch CE (1993) Acute increase in expression of growth associated protein GAP43 following cortical ischemia in rat. Neurosci Lett 162: 51–54
29. Stroemer RP, Kent TA, Hulsebosch CE (1995) Neocortical neural sprouting, synaptogenesis and behavioral recovery after neocortical infarction in rats. Stroke 26: 2135–2144
30. Tohyama T, Lee VM-Y, Rorke LB, Marvin M, McKay RDG, Trojanowski JQ (1992) Nestin expression in embryonic human neuroepithelium and in human neuroepithelial tumor cells. Lab Invest 66: 303–313

31. Wiche G (1989) High-M_r microtubule-associated proteins: properties and functions. Biochem J 259: 1–12
32. Xiong Y, Zhang H, Beack D (1992) D type cyclins associate with multiple protein kinases and the DNA replication and repair factor PCNA. Cell 71: 505–514
33. Yamashita T, Tada K, Sobue D, Niigawa H, Suzuki H, Hariguchi S, Nishimura T (1986) Effect of transient ischemia on brain proteins in mongolian gerbil. Neurochem Res 11: 1728–1729
34. Zea Longa E, Weinstein PR, Carlson S, Cummins R (1989) Reversible middle cerebral artery occlusion without craniectomy in rats. Stroke 20: 84–91

Alteration of Cyclic Adenosine Monophosphate Binding in Ischemic Brain: Sensitive Metabolic Marker for Early Ischemic Tissue Damage

K. Tanaka, Y. Fukuuchi, T. Shirai, H. Nozaki, E. Nagata, S. Suzuki, and T. Dembo

Summary. Binding of cyclic adenosine monophosphate (cAMP) to the regulatory subunit of cAMP-dependent protein kinase (PKA) is an essential step for cAMP-mediated signal transduction in neuronal cells. Various neuroprotective effects of activated PKA have recently been demonstrated. In the acute phase of cerebral ischemia, the cAMP content of the brain tissue has been found to increase markedly. In spite of these facts, the alterations in the binding capacity of PKA with cAMP have not yet been examined in cerebral ischemia. We, therefore, undertook an autoradiographic study of the binding capacity of PKA and the local cerebral blood flow (lCBF) during cerebral ischemia using [^{3}H]cAMP and [^{14}C] iodoantipyrine, respectively. After occlusion of the common carotid artery in the gerbil, a significant reduction in cAMP binding began to manifest itself in the dendritic subfields in the hippocampus CA1 at 15 min, then proceeded centrally to the pyramidal cell bodies. In contrast, other brain regions did not reveal any significant changes in cAMP binding until 30 min of ischemia. Between 30 min and 6 h of ischemia, the cAMP binding decreased progressively in various regions in response to a reduction in CBF. The ischemic CBF threshold for a reduction in cAMP binding in the hippocampus CA1 was significantly higher than that in other regions at each time point. The level of the above threshold increased progressively during the time course of ischemia. Western-blot analysis of PKA revealed that each subunit protein of PKA was preserved even at 6 h of ischemia. In focal ischemia, induced by occlusion of the middle cerebral artery in the rat, the reduction in cAMP binding in the cerebral cortex and striatum in the ischemic hemisphere at 5 h after occlusion was extensive and severe, but restricted to localized parts of the striatum and the temporal cerebral cortex at 3 h. However, each subunit protein of PKA was preserved in the ischemic tissue even after 5 h of ischemia. These data suggest that reductions in binding capacity of PKA with cAMP in the acute phase of cerebral ischemia may be caused by conformational changes of the PKA protein, and may precisely reflect the ischemic vulnerability of each brain region. The duration and degree of ischemia exert a definite influence on the cAMP binding, suggesting that the binding capacity of PKA with cAMP represents a good indicator of the viability of ischemic neuronal cells. The implementation of measures to maintain the binding ability of PKA with cAMP is expected to help cAMP to exert its neuroprotective effects in acute cerebral ischemia.

Maturation Phenomenon in Cerebral Ischemia III
U. Ito et al. (Eds.)
© Springer-Verlag Berlin Heidelberg 1999

Introduction

Cyclic adenosine monophosphate (cAMP) plays a vital role as one of the cardinal intracellular signaling systems of the central nervous system [9]. A large number of neurotransmitters and neuropeptides stimulate neuronal cells through cAMP. cAMP binds to the regulatory subunit of cAMP-dependent protein kinase (PKA), followed by dissociation of the catalytic subunit of PKA, which then promotes the phosphorylation of various substrates. Binding of cAMP to the regulatory subunit of PKA is, therefore, an essential step for cAMP-mediated signal transduction in neuronal cells.

Activation of PKA induced by an intracellular increase in cAMP content has been reported to be neuroprotective by (1) reducing Ca^{2+} release from the endoplasmic reticulum via inositol 1, 4, 5-trisphosphate receptor [15], (2) enhancing presynaptic release of the inhibitory amino acid, γ-aminobutyric acid (GABA) [14], (3) activating the high-affinity uptake of glutamate [13], (4) inhibiting the cytokine-induced expression of adhesion molecules [1], (5) suppressing the activity of neuronal nitric-oxide synthase [4], and (6) opposing the reaction induced by the stimulated N-methyl-D-aspartate (NMDA) receptor via activation of dopamine- and cAMP-regulated phosphoprotein with a molecular weight of 32 kDa (DARPP-32) [6]. As has recently been shown, cAMP also regulates a number of genes through a conserved cAMP response element (CRE). Upon phosphorylation of nuclear CRE-binding protein (CREB) by PKA, the CREB binds to CRE and stimulates the transcription of cAMP-responsive genes such as c-fos, tyrosine hydroxylase, etc. [11]. It has been suggested that phosphorylation of CREB may be involved in the process of neuroprotection against hypoxic/ischemic insult [17].

Lust et al. [8] found that the cAMP level in the brain tissue increases markedly for several hours after induction of severe cerebral ischemia. As mentioned above, various intracellular functions of cAMP manifest themselves only via binding of this substance to the regulatory subunit of PKA. Nevertheless, the alterations in binding capacity of PKA with cAMP have not yet been examined in cerebral ischemia. Recently, several PKA-anchoring proteins, which may play a pivotal role in the localization of the intracellular-cAMP action, have been identified in neurons [5]. The binding capacity of PKA with cAMP in each region, therefore, represents one of the important aspects of the fundamental metabolic integrity of the brain tissue, and analysis of the binding capacity of PKA in cerebral ischemia is expected to provide insight into the pathophysiological mechanisms of ischemic brain damage.

In this context, we examined the cAMP binding and local cerebral blood flow (lCBF) in the same brains, which were obtained from hemispheric-ischemia and focal-ischemia models. The binding protocol with [^{3}H] cAMP employed in the present study can be assumed to reflect, specifically, the binding capacity of intracellular membrane-bound PKA with cAMP [16].

Materials and Methods

Hemispheric Ischemia Model of Gerbils

A total of 67 Mongolian gerbils weighing $60\sim100$ g were employed and divided into eight groups: (1) a 15-min ischemia group ($n=10$), (2) a 30-min ischemia group ($n=14$), (3) a 2-h ischemia group ($n=15$), (4) a 6-h ischemia group ($n=9$), (5) a 15-min sham group ($n=3$), (6) a 30-min sham group ($n=3$), (7) a 2-h sham group ($n=5$), and (8) a 6-h sham group ($n=8$). The right common carotid artery was occluded in each ischemia group, whereas the artery was only exposed in each sham group. At the end of each experiment, the lCBF was measured by means of the $[^{14}C]$ iodoantipyrine (IAP) method. The body temperature was maintained at $37\pm0.5\,°C$ throughout the experiments. Serial brain sections were cut on a cryostat, and one set of sections was exposed to X-ray films to obtain lCBF autoradiograms. The sections of another set were incubated in buffer to wash out $[^{14}C]$ IAP from the tissue, then incubated with 5 nM $[^{3}H]$ cAMP [16]. Autoradiograms were generated by apposing the sections on to tritium-sensitive films. The sets of autoradiograms obtained were analyzed using a digital image-processing system to correlate the changes in lCBF and cAMP binding.

Western-blot analysis of PKA was also performed in a 6-h ischemia group ($n=3$) and a sham group ($n=3$). At the end of each experiment, the brain was quickly removed and divided into three blocks: the cerebral hemispheres on the operated side and non-operated side, and the cerebellum. Each block was homogenized in a glass Teflon-Potter homogenizer. The homogenate was centrifuged at $1000{\cdot}g$ for 5 min at $4\,°C$. The supernatant obtained was centrifuged at $10,500{\cdot}g$ for 60 min at $2\,°C$, and the pellets were collected. Protein concentration was determined with a Protein Assay Kit (Bio-Rad) employing bovine serum albumin as a standard. The pellets were subjected to 10 % sodium dodecyl sulfate/polyacrylamide gel electrophoresis (SDS-PAGE) in the buffer system of Laemmli. Proteins were then transferred onto nitrocellulose membranes and, subsequently, incubated with anti-PKA type-IIα regulatory subunit antibody (Santa Cruz Biotechnology) or anti-PKA-α catalytic subunit antibody (Santa Cruz Biotechnology). The blots were then incubated with horseradish peroxidase-labeled anti-rabbit immunoglobulin G (IgG) and developed by means of an enhanced chemiluminescence procedure (Amersham).

Focal Ischemia Model of Rats

A total of 17 Sprague-Dawley rats weighing 290–350 g were employed and divided into three groups: (1) a 3-h ischemia group ($n=5$), (2) a 5-h ischemia group ($n=7$), and (3) a sham group ($n=5$). In the ischemia groups, the origin of the middle cerebral artery was occluded by the intraluminal-suture method for 3 h or 5 h [2]. At the end of each experiment, lCBF was measured by means of the $[^{14}C]$-IAP method. The procedures for $[^{3}H]$-cAMP binding were the same as those described for the gerbil study.

Western-blot analysis of PKA was also performed in a 5-h ischemia group ($n=3$) and a sham group ($n=3$). The procedures of analysis were similar to those described above. In addition, the presence of phosphorylated CREB was examined by Western-blot analysis in the nuclear fraction of the brain homogenate, using the rabbit poly-clonal anti-phosphorylated CREB antibody (Upstate Biotechnology).

The protocols described above had been approved as meeting the Animal Experimentation Guidelines of Keio University School of Medicine.

Results

Hemispheric Ischemia Model of Gerbils

Physiological Parameters

The blood gases and arterial blood pressure were within the normal ranges in each group and none of them differed significantly among the groups.

Alteration of cAMP Binding after 15-min and 30-min Ischemia in the Hippocampus CA1

We utilized gerbils with CBF levels of less than 50 ml/100 g/min in the lateral nuclei of the thalamus in order to assess the effects of severe ischemia. Since the data for the cAMP binding and CBF obtained in the 15-min and 30-min sham groups did not differ from each other, the data for these two groups were combined together and are presented here as those of the sham groups.

Representative autoradiograms of the CBF and cAMP binding magnified for the hippocampus region are shown in Fig. 1A and 1B, respectively. A severe and diffuse reduction in CBF was noted in the right hemisphere of both the 15-min (middle image) and 30-min (bottom image) ischemia groups. In the sham group (top image), the CBF was symmetrical on both sides. The autoradiograms of the cAMP binding revealed a moderate reduction in the dendritic subfields of the hippocampus CA1 (middle and bottom images), while the 30-min ischemic group showed a definite reduction in cAMP binding, not only in each dendritic subfield of the hippocampus CA1, but also in the layer of pyramidal cell bodies.

The CBF in each ischemia group demonstrated a significant and homogeneous decrease in each subfield of the hippocampus CA1 and other regions on the ischemic side. However, the cAMP binding was significantly reduced only in the dendritic subfields of the hippocampus CA1, such as the strata oriens, radiatum and lacunosum-moleculare in the 15-min ischemia group. In the 30-min ischemia group, the cAMP binding was significantly reduced, not only in each dendritic subfield of the hippocampus CA1, but also in the layer of the pyramidal cell bodies (stratum pyramidale). Other brain regions did not exhibit any definite changes in cAMP binding. Figure 2 summarizes the results for the CBF and cAMP binding in the stratum radiatum (representative dendritic subfield of the hippocampus CA1) and the stratum pyramidale in each ischemia group and the sham group.

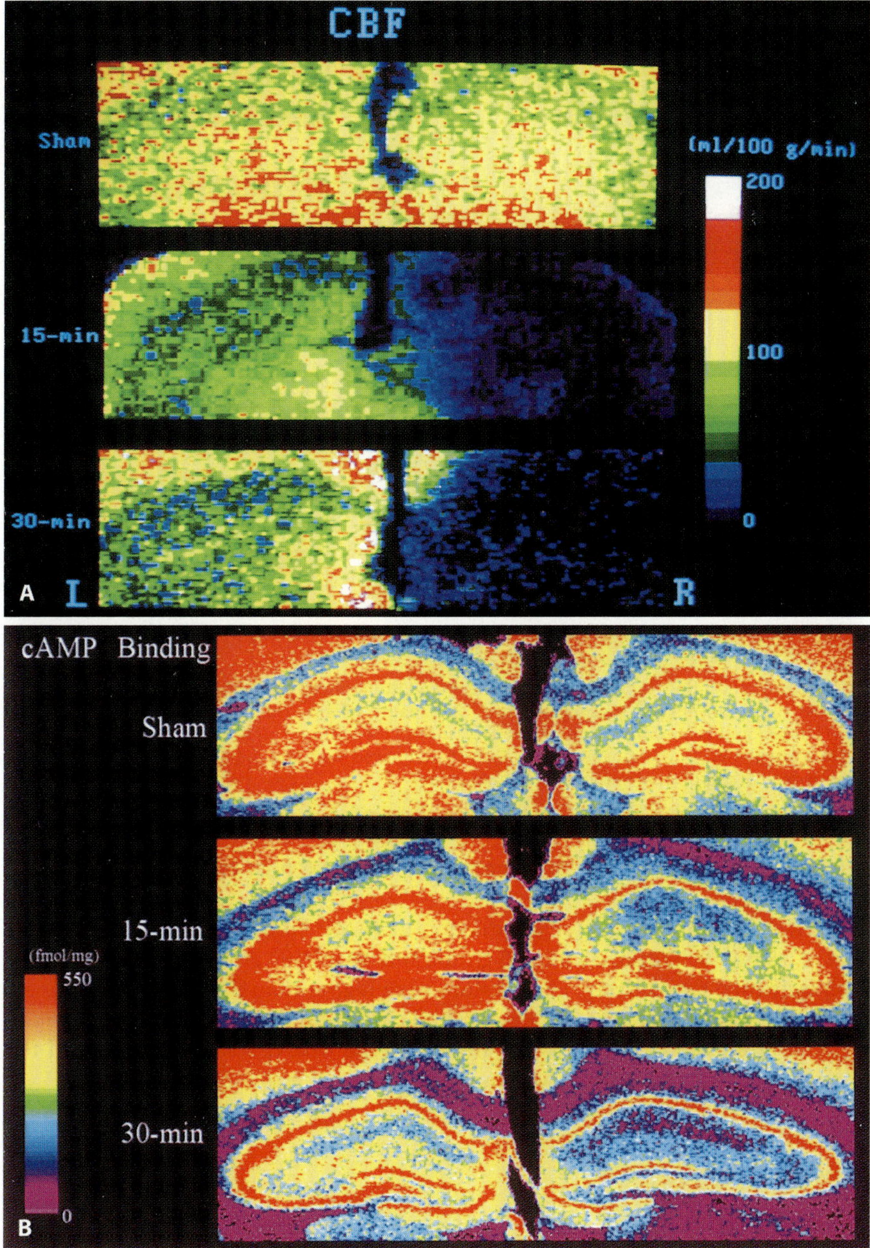

Fig. 1A, B. Representative autoradiograms of cerebral blood flow (CBF) images (**A**) and [³H] cyclic AMP (cAMP) binding (**B**) magnified for the hippocampal region of the gerbil. Ischemia was induced by ligating the right common carotid artery. The *middle* and *bottom* images were obtained from the 15-min and 30-min ischemia groups, respectively. The *top* image was obtained from the sham group. Each image in **B** derives from the same animal as that shown in **A**. The viewer's right side is the operated side on the autoradiograms

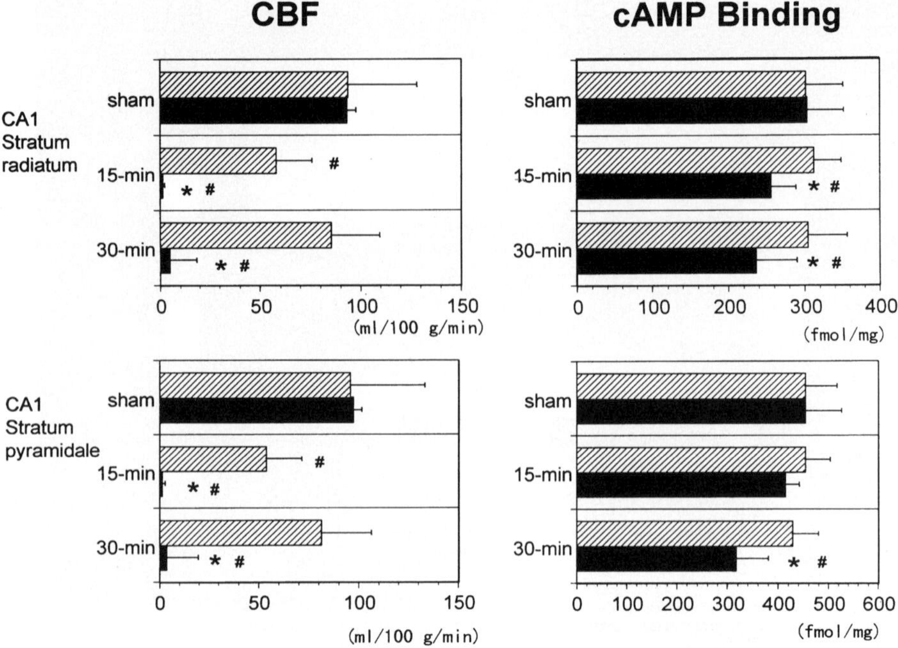

Fig. 2. Cerebral blood flow (CBF) and cyclic adenosine monophosphate (cAMP) binding in the sub-field of the hippocampus CA1 obtained from the sham, 15-min ischemia and 30-min ischemia groups. *Hatched* and *solid bars* represent the left (non-occluded) and right (occluded) sides, respectively. Data are shown as the means ± SD. $^*P<0.05$ compared with the opposite side. $^\#P<0.05$ compared with the corresponding value in the sham group

Alteration of cAMP Binding Between 30 min and 6 h of Ischemia

The ischemic CBF thresholds for a reduction in cAMP binding in the hippocampus CA1 were 18 ml/100 g/min, 34 ml/100 g/min and 49 ml/100 g/min after 30-min, 2-h and 6-h ischemia, respectively. These values were higher than those in other regions, such as the hippocampus CA3 and the cerebral cortex, for each duration of ischemia.

Western-blot analysis revealed that the PKA type-IIα regulatory subunit and the PKA α-catalytic subunit protein were preserved even after 6 h of ischemia.

Focal Ischemia Model of Rats

Physiological Parameters

The blood gases and arterial blood pressure were within the normal ranges in each group. None of the parameters differed significantly among the groups, although $PaCO_2$ in the 3-h ischemia group was slightly higher than that in the other groups.

Alteration of cAMP Binding

Representative autoradiograms of the CBF and cAMP binding in the 3-h and 5-h ischemia groups are shown in Fig. 3A and 3B, respectively. Although the reduction in CBF was similar in both groups, the topographical range, as well as the degree of reduction in cAMP binding, was much more extensive in the 5-h ischemia group than the 3-h group.

In the 3-h ischemia group, a significant reduction in cAMP was noted only in the temporal cortical region, with CBF amounting to less than 8 ml/100 g/min, and in the lateral striatum, with CBF amounting to less than 5 ml/100 g/min. The values for the cAMP binding in other brain regions, which surrounded the above ischemic core, were within the normal range.

In the 5-h ischemia group, a significant reduction in cAMP binding was noted, not only in the ischemic cortical region with CBF lower than 8 ml/100 g/min, but also in the surrounding cortical regions with CBF lower than 30 ml/100 g/min, where the tissue was stained normal by 2 % 2, 3 and 5 triphenyltetrazolium chloride (TTC) at 37 °C for 10 min. Similarly, an extensive striatal region with CBF lower than 15 ml/100 g/min revealed a significant reduction in cAMP binding.

The proportion of brain area with CBF amounting to less than 20 ml/100 g/min (top image) and the proportion of brain area with cAMP binding amounting to less than 180 fmol/mg (bottom image), respectively, is shown in Fig. 4. The area data are presented as the percent of the number of pixels on the autoradiograms showing values of less than 20 ml/100 g/min for the CBF or 180 fmol/mg for the cAMP binding, relative to the number of whole pixels on the autoradiograms of each structure at the level of the striatum (10.2 mm anterior to the interaural line) [12]. The brain area with CBF lower than 20 ml/100 g/min was similar in both ischemia groups, whereas the brain area with cAMP binding lower than 180 fmol/mg was significantly larger in the 5-h than in the 3-h ischemia groups.

Western-Blot Analysis of PKA and Phosphorylated CREB

Western-blot analysis revealed that the regulatory and catalytic subunits of PKA existed normally in both the ischemic and non-ischemic regions. However, the level of phosphorylated CREB was clearly decreased in the ischemic region, compared with that in the non-ischemic region.

Discussion

The present findings obtained with a hemispheric-ischemia model of the gerbil suggest that derangement of PKA may begin in the dendritic subfields of the hippocampus CA1 after as little as 15 min of severe ischemia, and proceed centrally to the neuronal cell bodies of the hippocampus CA1. At the same time, no definite alteration in cAMP binding was evident in other regions. Early inhibition of PKA-dependent signal transduction may be closely linked with the ischemic vulnerability of the hippocampus CA1, especially the dendritic subfields of this region. High amounts of aden-

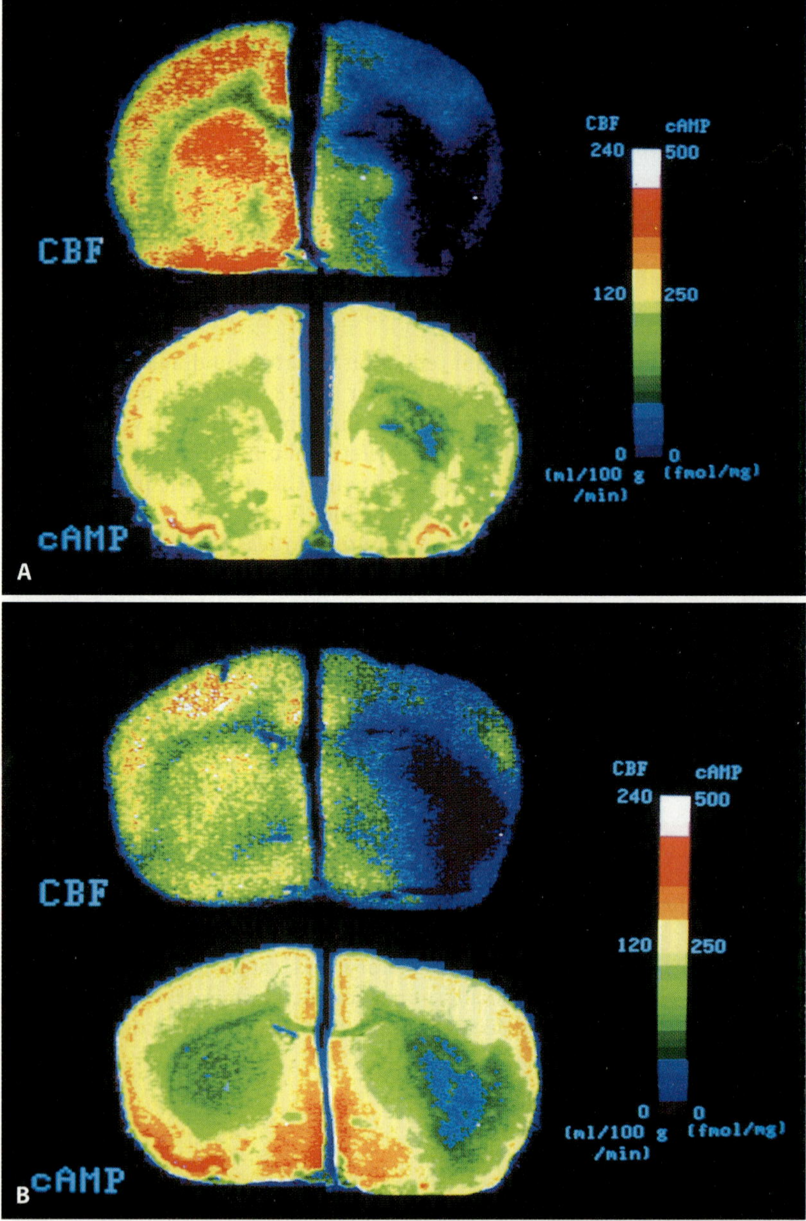

Fig. 3A, B. Representative autoradiograms of cerebral blood flow (CBF) and [^{3}H] cyclic AMP (cAMP) binding in the 3-h ischemia (**A**) and 5-h ischemia (**B**) groups of rats. Ischemia was induced by occluding the right middle cerebral artery by the suture method. A mild reduction in cAMP binding was observed in localized parts of the striatum and temporal cerebral cortex in the 3-h ischemia group, whereas a severe and extensive decrease in cAMP binding was noted in these structures in the 5-h ischemia group. The reduction in CBF was comparable between both groups, or even milder in the 5-h ischemia group, compared with the 3-h ischemia group

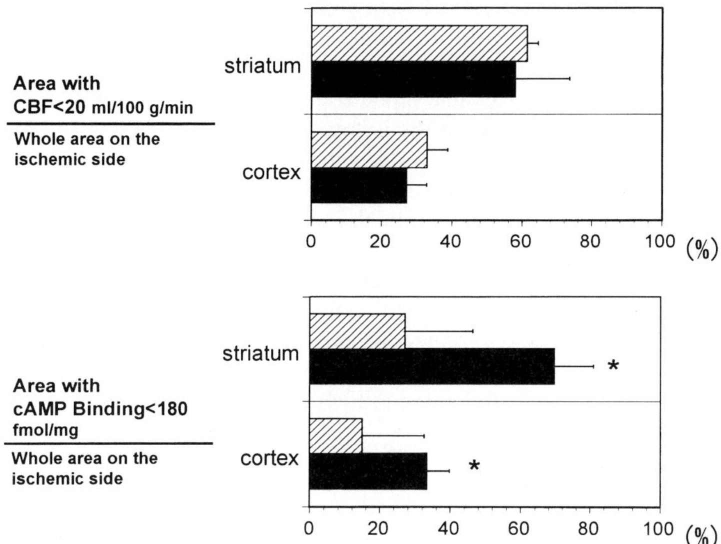

Fig. 4. Bar graphs showing the proportion of brain area with cerebral blood flow (CBF) amounting to less than 20 ml/100 g/min (*top image*) and the proportion of brain area with cyclic adenosine monophosphate (cAMP) binding amounting to less than 180 fmol/mg (*bottom image*). The area data are presented as the percentage versus the whole area of each structure on the ischemic side. *Hatched* and *solid bars* represent the 3-h and 5-h ischemia groups, respectively. Data are shown as the means ±SD. *$P<0.05$, compared with the 3-h ischemia group

ylate cyclase and PKA in the hippocampus CA1 coincide with the dense localization of NMDA receptors occurring in this region [10]. In fact, a significant influx of Ca^{2+} into the hippocampus CA1 region through NMDA receptors has been observed in response to ischemic insult [7]. Light- and electron-microscopic immunocytochemical studies have revealed that PKA may be strongly associated with microtubular networks in dendrites, and bound to microtubule-associated protein 2 (MAP2) [3]. Taken together, these and the present findings suggest a rapid functional disintegration of microtubules in the dendrites of the hippocampus CA1 during the acute phase of ischemia.

In addition, the present data indicate that the ischemic CBF threshold for perturbation of the cAMP–PKA system may be higher in the hippocampus CA1 than in other regions, implying that the hippocampus CA1 may be especially vulnerable to acute ischemic stress. Our results also revealed that the level of the above-mentioned threshold increased progressively during the time course of ischemia, suggesting that the duration of ischemia exerts a definite influence on the viability of ischemic neuronal cells. Based on Western-blot analysis, the alterations of cAMP binding observed in the present experiments may be attributable to conformational changes of the PKA protein, and not to a loss of PKA protein itself from the ischemic tissue. Various neuroprotective roles have been reported for activated PKA [1, 4, 6, 13–15, 17]. Certain interventions to restore the binding capacity of PKA with cAMP could, therefore, help to rescue the dying brain tissue in the early phase of ischemia.

The present data obtained from the focal-ischemia study on the rat indicate that perturbation of PKA is restricted to the ischemic core after 3 h of ischemia, but clearly extends to the penumbral regions by 5 h of ischemia, where TTC staining does not yet reveal any abnormality. Intracellular signal transduction via PKA may, therefore, be significantly inhibited, not only in the ischemic core at 3 h of ischemia, but also in the penumbral region at 5 h of ischemia, despite an increased content of cAMP in the ischemic brain tissue [8]. In fact, phosphorylation of CREB was inhibited in the ischemic region. Accordingly, 3 h may represent the time limit for restricting ischemic neuronal damage to the ischemic core.

In conclusion, our findings suggest that PKA-dependent intracellular signal transduction is prone to early ischemic damage, and analysis of PKA function by cAMP binding may provide a useful method for detecting early ischemic intracellular injury. A recirculation study is currently in progress to examine the time window within which PKA function can be restored following ischemic insult.

References

1. Ballestas ME, Benveniste EN (1997) Elevation of cyclic AMP levels in astrocytes antagonizes cytokine-induced adhesion molecule expression. J Neurochem 69: 1438–1448
2. Belayev L, Alonso OF, Busto R, Zhao W, Ginsberg MD (1996) Middle cerebral artery occlusion in the rat by intraluminal suture. Stroke 27: 1616–1623
3. De Camilli P, Moretti N, Donini SD, Walter U, Lohmann SM (1986) Heterogeneous distribution of the cAMP receptor protein RII in the nervous system: evidence for its intracellular accumulation on microtubules, microtubule-organizing centers, and in the area of the Golgi complex. J Cell Biol 103: 189–203
4. Dinerman JL, Steiner JP, Dawson TM, Dawson V, Snyder SH (1994) Cyclic nucleotide dependent phosphorylation of neuronal nitric oxide synthase inhibits catalytic activity. Neuropharmacology 33: 1245–1251
5. Faux MC, Scott JD (1996) More on target with protein phosphorylation: conferring specificity by location. Trends Biochem Sci 21: 312–315
6. Halpain S, Girault J-A, Greengard P (1990) Activation of NMDA receptors induces dephosphorylation of DARPP-32 in rat striatal slices. Nature 343: 369–372
7. Lobner D, Lipton P (1993) Intracellular calcium levels and calcium fluxes in the CA1 region of the rat hippocampal slice during in vitro ischemia: relationship to electrophysiological cell damage. J Neurosci 13: 4861–4871
8. Lust WD, Mrsulja BB, Mrsulja BJ, Passonneau JV, Klatzo I (1975) Putative neurotransmitters and cyclic nucleotides in prolonged ischemia of the cerebral cortex. Brain Res 98: 394–399
9. Mons N, Cooper DMF (1995) Adenylate cyclases: critical foci in neuronal signaling. Trends Neurosci 18: 536–542
10. Mons N, Harry A, Dubourg P, Premont RT, Iyengar R, Cooper DM (1995) Immunohistochemical localization of adenylyl cyclase in rat brain indicates a highly selective concentration at synapses. Proc Natl Acad Sci U S A 92: 8473–8477
11. Montminy MR, Gonzalez GA, Yamamoto KK (1990) Regulation of cAMP-inducible genes by CREB. Trends Neurosci 13: 184–188
12. Paxinos G, Watson C (1986) The rat brain in stereotaxic coordinates, 2nd edn. Academic Press, San Diego
13. Pisano P, Samuel D, Nieoullon A, Goff LK-L (1996) Activation of the adenylate cyclase-dependent protein kinase pathway increases high affinity glutamate uptake into rat striatal synaptosomes. Neuropharmacology 35: 541–547
14. Sciancalepore M, Cherubini E (1995) Protein kinase A-dependent increase in frequency of miniature GABAergic currents in rat CA3 hippocampal neurons. Neurosci Lett 187: 91–94
15. Supattapone S, Danoff SK, Theibert A, Joseph SK, Steiner J, Snyder SH (1988) Cyclic AMP-dependent phosphorylation of a brain inositol trisphosphate receptor decreases its release of calcium. Proc Natl Acad Sci U S A 85: 8747–8750

16. Tanaka K, Gomi S, Mihara B, Shirai T, Nogawa S, Nozaki H, Nagata E, Kondo T, Fukuuchi Y (1996) Flow threshold for reduction of cyclic AMP binding in the hippocampus CA1 and other brain regions during stroke development in gerbils. J Cereb Blood Flow Metab 16: 468–473
17. Walton M, Sirimanne E, Williams C, Gluckman P, Dragunow M (1996) The role of the cyclic AMP-responsive element binding protein (CREB) in hypoxic-ischemic brain damage and repair. Mol Brain Res 43: 21–29

IV Ischemic Infarction: Threshold, Experimental and Clinical Dynamics and Therapeutic Design for Prevention or Reduction of Intensity

Role of Mitochondria in Immediate and Delayed Reperfusion Damage

B. K. Siesjö, Y. Ouyang, T. Kristián, E. Elmér, P.-A. Li, and H. Uchino

Summary. Ischemia leads to mitochondrial dysfunction. This is reversible if ischemia is of brief duration, but secondary mitochondrial damage is observed after longer periods of ischemia, particularly in selectively vulnerable neuronal populations. This damage is triggered during the period of ischemia, but secondary factors lead to its "maturation". Probably, the most important of these factors is gradual accumulation of calcium in the mitochondria. The mechanisms involved encompass phospholipase A_2-mediated breakdown of the lipid skeleton of membranes, and free-radical-mediated oxidation of its lipid and protein components. However, the immediate trigger may be the opening ("assembly") of a mitochondrial permeability transition (MPT) pore, which is followed by calcium release, collapse of the electrochemical gradient for H^+ and a burst of production of reactive oxygen species (ROS). The ensuing bioenergetic compromise and the mitochondrial production of ROS probably constitute important causes of cell death. Recent results suggest that mitochondrial dysfunction is a leading event in the cascade of events that cause apoptotic and necrotic cell death. Very likely, the trigger is the release of cytochrome c from depolarized or otherwise compromised mitochondria. By activating caspase-3, cytochrome c can initiate terminal events encompassing activation of proteases, endonucleases and poly (ADP-ribose) polymerase. Therefore, the type of enzyme activated may determine whether cell death is of the apoptotic or necrotic type.

Introduction

Ischemia leads, almost by definition, to mitochondrial dysfunction (for brief reviews and further literature, see [23, 25, 36]). This is because unsaturation of cytochrome-c oxidase at the terminus of the electron-transport chain disrupts mitochondrial respiratory functions, including the synthesis of adenosine triphosphate (ATP). The important question is whether recirculation can reverse the changes induced by ischemia, i.e., whether the mitochondrial structure is intact. Even if this were the case, experience predicts that mitochondria, like other component parts of the cell, may suffer secondary damage during reperfusion.

Recent results of postischemic mitochondrial metabolism have brought forward an additional aspect of the role played by mitochondrial dysfunction. This concerns the secondary consequences of such dysfunction. Extensive results suggest that functionally perturbed mitochondria release substances, e.g., cytochrome c, which trigger reactions leading to cell death [21, 22, 43]. We will discuss the general subject, i.e., the role of mitochondria in immediate and delayed reperfusion damage, under three

Maturation Phenomenon in Cerebral Ischemia III
U. Ito et al. (Eds.)
© Springer-Verlag Berlin Heidelberg 1999

headings. The first relates to the new role that mitochondrial dysfunction has been given in the pathogenesis of cell death, the second to maturation of neuronal necrosis after brief periods of global (or forebrain) ischemia, and the third to characteristics of mitochondrial dysfunction following long periods of ischemia, as in stroke.

Mitochondria and Cell Death: an Expanded Concept

The traditional concept is that primary and secondary mitochondrial damage is due to breakdown of the lipid skeleton of mitochondrial membranes by activation of phospholipase A_2 (PLA_2), and by oxidation of their lipid and protein components by free-radical-mediated reactions (for overviews on ischemia, and literature references see [23, 25, 36]). Another related concept is that the consequences of mitochondrial damage encompass failure of mitochondrial respiratory functions and, thereby, of ATP synthesis. Since PLA_2 activation and generation of reactive oxygen species (ROS) are calcium dependent, one can envisage a coupling among loss of calcium homeostasis, mitochondrial dysfunction, bioenergetic failure and cell death. Such a coupling has been envisaged to exist, not only in anoxia/ischemia, but also in chronic neurodegenerative disease [2, 3].

The last 10 years of research have brought new insight into the role played by mitochondria in ischemic cell death. In fact, the mitochondria are now considered the primary affected organelle in a signal-transduction chain, which orchestrates cell death in a variety of systems, in which cells die by apoptosis or necrosis, following such diverse insults, such as exposure to dexamethasone, e.g., thymocytes or glutamate, e.g., neurons, growth-factor deprivation, or anoxia/ischemia [18, 34, 46].

The first aspect of this concept was unraveled when it was found that, under certain circumstances, mitochondrial membranes can open ("assemble") a large conductance channel, which allows Ca^{2+} to leave the mitochondria; in fact, this mitochondrial-permeability-transition (MPT) pore has such a large conductance that it causes the potential across the inner mitochondrial membrane ($\Delta\psi_m$) to collapse and the ion gradients to be dissipated [5, 14, 15, 31, 48]. Since this will uncouple oxidative phosphorylation, the result is a burst of production of ROS by the mitochondria. From a physiological point of view, the MPT pore can be regarded as a voltage-sensitive and Ca^{2+}-activated channel, which is more or less specifically blocked by cyclosporin A (CsA). Its function may be to allow the mitochondria to dispose of a large calcium load with little energy expenditure. However, the MPT is potentially harmful since it is accompanied by Ca^{2+} release, uncoupling of oxidative phosphorylation, production of ROS and cessation of ATP synthesis. The MPT is triggered by multiple inducers, which include mitochondrial calcium accumulation and oxidative stress [8, 35]. It seems natural, therefore, that the MPT is considered of pathogenetic importance in ischemia reperfusion [4, 10, 13].

According to this general concept [16], different inducers trigger an MPT, which, by reducing the mitochondrial membrane potential, causes calcium release, uncoupling of oxidative phosphorylation and enhanced production of ROS. This view is not shared by all, though, since Richter and his collaborators maintain that the initial event is oxidation of reduced nicotinamide adenine dinucleotide (NADH) and reduced nicotinamide adenine dinucleotide phosphate (NADPH), which then triggers release and membrane cycling of Ca^{2+} and, secondary to that, enhanced production of ROS [35].

Results obtained on thymocytes and other rapidly proliferating cells, which were committed to apoptosis by exposure to dexamethasone, demonstrated that a fall in ΔY_m preceded the enhanced production of ROS, which, in turn, preceded cell death [44]. In these experiments, CsA blocked the fall in mitochondrial-membrane potential, ruthenium red, a blocker of mitochondrial Ca^{2+} uptake, reduced the production of ROS, while cell death was ameliorated by the spin trap α-phenyl-*N*-tert butyl nitrone (PBN) and by Trolox, a vitamin-E analogue.

Subsequent results obtained by the same group [18, 46] demonstrated that the membrane depolarization, associated with an MPT, caused the release of an apoptosis-inducing factor (AIF), probably a protease, which induced morphological and biochemical signs of apoptosis in isolated nuclei or cell-free systems. The results, thus, suggested the existence of a signal-transduction pathway that is initiated by mitochondrial-membrane depolarization, which then leads to cell death by inducing nuclear pathology. However, another mediator than AIF has been incriminated; mitochondrial-membrane depolarization was found to cause release of cytochrome c [22, 43]. It could also be shown that the protoncogene bcl-2, which is known to suppress apoptosis in several cell systems [19, 20], acts by preventing the release of cytochrome c into the cytosol [21, 43].

It was subsequently shown that cytochrome c, released from the mitochondria, induces apoptosis by activating caspase-3, a cysteine protease of the interleukin-1β-converting enzyme (ICE) family [28, 34]. Activation of caspase-3 represents a commitment to cell death, since the enzyme activates other proteases as well as endonucleases and poly (ADP-ribose) polymerase (PARP).

Although the scheme of events discussed illustrates the general case, it is not necessarily valid for all conditions in which apoptosis is induced. First, if the AIF is a protease, one must envisage that mitochondrial dysfunction leads to the release or activation of different proteases. Since these include calpains, with an activation that causes breakdown of α-spectrin and, thereby, of cytoskeletal components, the targets are both nuclear and extranuclear [33]. Second, conditions exist in which cytochrome-c release occurs in the absence of a decrease in ΔY_m, in fact, since cytochrome c activates caspase-3 and this enzyme is known to trigger an MPT, the decrease in ΔY_m may be secondary to cytochrome-c release [34].

It has recently become evident that apoptosis and necrosis may share the same inducers, and both are commonly preceded by an MPT [18, 46]. A speculative deduction is that the choice between the two modalities is determined by the availability of apoptogenic and other proteases [18, 34]. Regardless of the explanation, in vitro experiments on glutamate-stimulated cells demonstrate that, depending on the severity of the insult, the same stimulus can trigger either apoptosis or necrosis [1, 6].

Maturation of Cell and Mitochondrial Damage After Brief Periods of Global (or Forebrain) Ischemia

The maturation of neuronal cell damage after brief periods of ischemia shows the typical sequence of events with an insult, a free interval and delayed cell death. A similar sequence characterizes mitochondrial damage. Thus, while a decrease of ADP- and uncoupler-stimulated respiration during ischemia is usually followed by normalization of mitochondrial function, a secondary decline in ADP-stimulated and uncoupled respiration rates is observed [38, 39]. However, the results obtained did not show whether deterioration of mitochondrial function preceded bioenergetic failure and cell death, or whether mitochondrial dysfunction was the result of cell damage by other causes.

A clue to the problem emerged when it could be shown that CsA, given systematically in a setting that allowed its translocation across the blood–brain barrier, dramatically ameliorated CA1 damage after 7–10 min of forebrain ischemia in rats [42]. The results obtained after 7 min of ischemia are illustrated in Fig. 1. Subsequent results showed that CsA also ameliorated the aggravated damage, which is observed in hyperglycemic subjects and suppressed the postischemic seizures, which are observed in these rats [27].

It is tempting to speculate that CsA ameliorated neuronal damage by preventing the assembly of an MPT pore. It is equally tempting to suggest that the delayed assembly of such a pore is related to the gradual increase in tissue and mitochondrial calcium content, which is observed during recirculation (for discussion and further literature references see [23, 37]). However, contradictory results exist, which inspire caution in interpretation. Most importantly, the immunosuppressant drug FK506 also partially ameliorates CA1 damage [9]. Since FK506 does not block the MPT pore, and both CsA and FK506 inhibit calcineurin, a protein phosphatase involved in nitric oxide metabolism, it seems logical to conclude that the effects of CsA and FK506 are related to their immunosuppressant activities. In view of results obtained in other systems, though, this conclusion is of uncertain validity. For example, in thymocytes, the non-immunosuppressant CsA analogue N-methyl-Val-4-CsA prevents apoptotic ΔY_m disruption [31, 45]. Furthermore, the results of Steiner et al. [40] demonstrate that non-immunosuppressive analogues of CsA and FK506 promote neurite outgrowth in P12 cells and sensory neuronal cultures of dorsal root ganglia, with a potency equal to their immunosuppressive homologues. A non-immunosuppressive analogue of FK506 also enhanced both functional and morphological recovery of crushed sciatic nerves. The immunosuppressive drugs (and their analogues) bind to receptor proteins called immunophilins, i.e., cyclophilins for CsA and FK506-binding proteins (FKBPs) for FK506. Since the non-immunosuppressive immunophilin

Fig. 1A, B. Histopathological outcome in the CA1 sector of hippocampus at 7 days of recovery following 7 min of ischemia in animals pretreated (**A**) or posttreated (**B**) with CsA or vehicle. Intraperitoneal administration of CsA exerts significant neuroprotection only in combination with disruption of the blood–brain barrier. Damage is given as percentage of the total neuronal population in CA1 (at bregma –3.8). *Filled circles* denote the mean values of the left and right CA1 regions, which are shown as *outlined symbols* to the left and right, respectively. Group mean values are represented by *horizontal bars*. *** $P<0.001$; one-way ANOVA with post-hoc Scheffé. Data from Uchino et al. (1995) [42]

A
7 min ischemia, pre-treatment
CA1 neuronal necrosis (%)
***
Vehicle
Vehicle and barrier disruption
CsA
CsA and barrier disruption
B
7 min ischemia, post-treatment
CA1 neuronal necrosis (%)
***
Vehicle and barrier disruption
CsA
CsA and barrier disruption

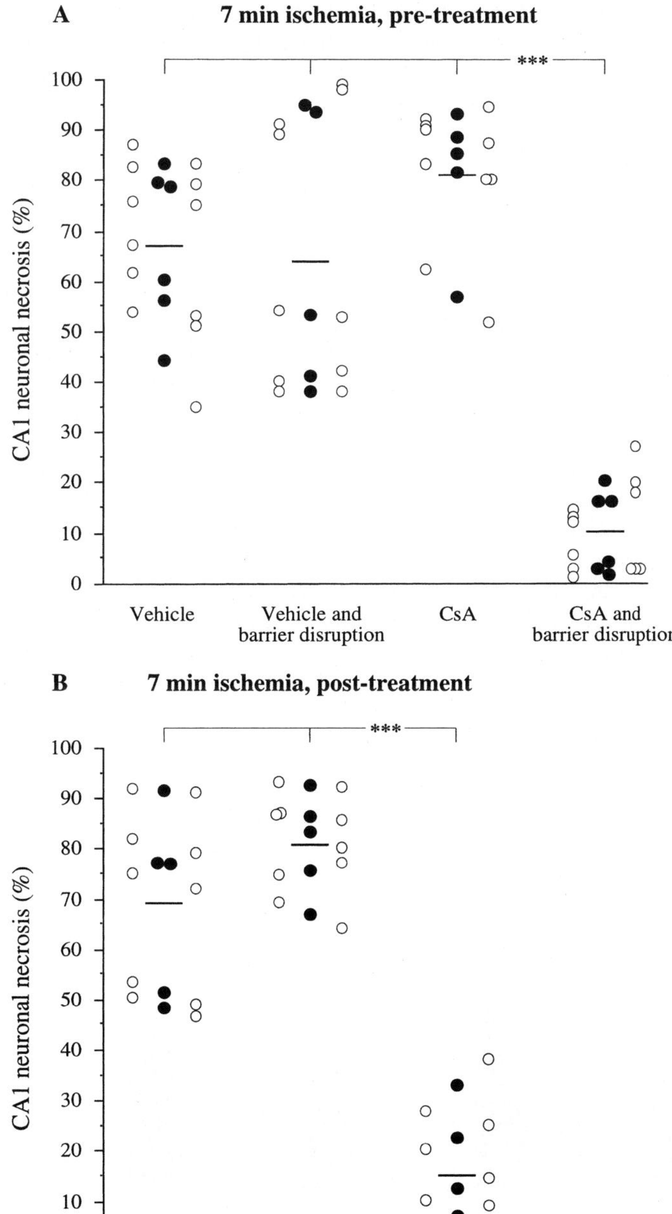

Fig. 1. A, B

ligands have no calcineurin inhibitory activity, the neurotrophic effects could not have been mediated by modulation of calcineurin activity. The mechanisms remain to be clarified. It also remains to be seen to what extent the effect of CsA reflects its ability to prevent the assembly of an MPT pore.

Mitochondrial Dysfunction During and Following Focal Ischemia of Long Duration

When ischemia is of long duration, recirculation predictably leads to mitochondrial dysfunction. This is illustrated in Fig. 2, which gives respiratory characteristics of mitochondria isolated after 2 h of focal ischemia, as well as after 1, 2, and 4 h of recirculation [26]. The respiratory control ratio (RCR), which is the ADP-stimulated divided by the unstimulated respiratory rates, decreased markedly after 2 h of ischemia. Recirculation data showed two important features. First, the RCR never returned to control values, suggesting sustained mitochondrial dysfunction. Second, following the partial recovery after 1 h of recirculation, RCR showed a secondary decline. The RCR values shown are in excellent agreement with data on changes in the bioenergetic state of focal and penumbral tissues [12]. Thus, recirculation led to only partial recovery of ATP values and the sum of adenine nucleotides, with secondary deterioration being observed after 4 h. Furthermore, lactate concentrations never normalized and a secondary increase occurred after 4 h.

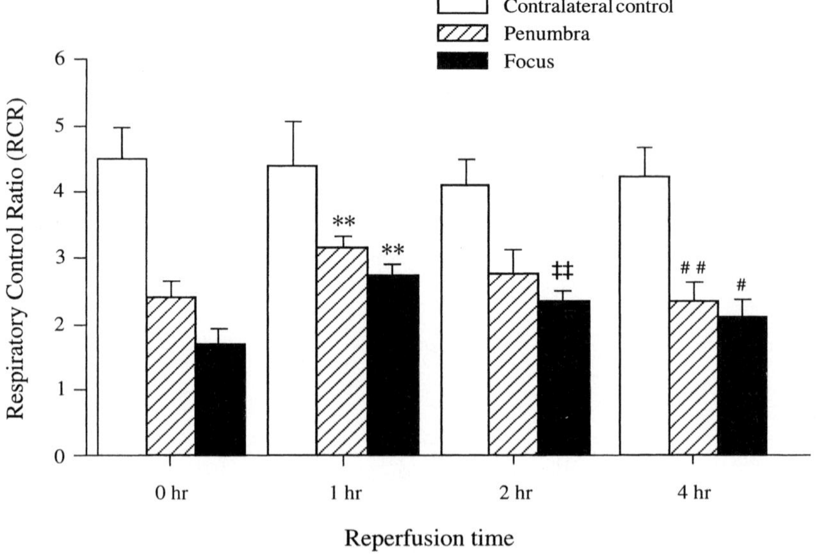

Fig. 2. Respiratory control ratio (RCR) of mitochondria during different reperfusion times after 2 h of middle cerebral artery (MCA) occlusion in rat. Values are mean ±SD. ** $P<0.01$ against ischemic group (0 h), #, ## against 1-h reperfusion group, and #, ## against 1-h reperfusion group ($P<0.05$ and $P<0.01$ respectively); one factor ANOVA with post-hoc Scheffé. Data from Kuroda et al. (1995) [26]

The combined results, thus, demonstrate that, following a long period of ischemia, mitochondrial function never returns to normal and secondary deterioration is observed after 2–4 h. The molecular mechanisms behind this failure of mitochondrial function in vivo and in vitro are not known. The reduction in ADP-stimulated (and uncoupled) respiratory rates suggests inactivation of one or more of the respiratory complexes. However, the activities of complexes I–V remain unchanged during ischemia and recirculation, compared with control [7]. A change in the permeability of mitochondrial membranes seems to be at hand, though, since the mitochondrial isoform of aspartate aminotransferase leaks out into the cytosol during the first hour of reperfusion [32]. It is tempting to conclude that MPT is induced during ischemia and that recirculation triggers adverse reactions, encompassing enhanced production of ROS and release of cytochrome c, but definitive results are lacking.

The pharmacology of this type of ischemia is fascinating and gives hints to the mechanisms of damage involved. A decrease in infarct size has been observed in animals injected intracerebroventricularly with ICE-like protease inhibitors [17], with those treated with a central-nervous-system-penetrating calpain inhibitor [29] and in those either given a PARP inhibitor i.p. [41] or subjected to genetic deletion of PARP [11]. We recognize that each of these therapeutic interventions is directed toward steps in the cascade, which is triggered by mitochondrial release of cytochrome c, or of proteases (see above).

Two drugs have been found to markedly ameliorate the ischemic damage and prevent the secondary deterioration of mitochondrial function, even when given 1 h after the start of recirculation, following 2 h of ischemia: the spin trap PBN and the immunosuppressant FK506 [26, 30]. Their targets of attack are unknown, and we do not know how any extra-mitochondrial effect could secondarily improve mitochondrial function. Both drugs work within a therapeutic window of about 3 h following the start of recirculation [24, 47]. This suggests that they block steps in a signal-transduction chain, which is gradually recruited during recirculation. One can envisage that the role of the mitochondria in this series of events is primarily that of an initiator. However, secondary events (such as caspase-3 activation) may maintain mitochondrial-membrane depolarization, thereby leading to rapidly developing bioenergetic failure. If this is the case, the mitochondria may be both inducers of damage and executors of cell death.

Acknowledgements. Work from our own laboratory was supported by grants from the NIH (NINDS), The Swedish Medical Research Council, and Centaur Pharmaceuticals Inc., Sunnyvale, CA. E. E. has a postdoctoral grant from the Swedish Brain Foundation (Hjärnfonden).

References

1. Ankarcrona M, Dypbukt JM, Bonfoco E, Zhivotovsky B, Orrenius S, Lipton SA, Nicotera (1995) Glutamate-induced neuronal death: a succession of necrosis or apoptosis depending on mitochondrial function. Neuron 15: 961–973
2. Beal MF (1992) Does impairment of energy metabolism result in excitotoxic neuronal death in neurodegenerative illnesses? Ann Neurol 31: 119–130
3. Beal MF, Hyman BT, Koroshetz W (1993) Do defects in mitochondrial energy metabolism underlie the pathology of neurodegenerative diseases? Trends Neurosci 16: 125–131

4. Bernardi P (1996) The permeability transition pore. Control points of a cyclosporin A-sensitive mitochondrial channel involved in cell death. Biochim Biophys Acta 1275: 5–9
5. Bernardi P, Broekemeier KM, Pfeiffer DR (1994) Recent progress on regulation of the mitochondrial permeability transition pore; a cyclosporin-sensitive pore in the inner mitochondrial membrane. J Bioenerg Biomembr 26: 509–517
6. Bonfoco E, Krainc D, Ankarcrona M, Nicotera P, Lipton SA (1995) Apoptosis and necrosis: two distinct events induced, respectively, by mild and intense insults with N-methyl-D-aspartate or nitric oxide/superoxide in cortical cell cultures. Proc Natl Acad Sci U S A 92: 7162–7166
7. Canevari L, Kuroda S, Bates TE, Clark JB, Siesjö BK (1997) Activity of mitochondrial respiratory chain enzymes after transient focal ischemia in the rat. J Cereb Blood Flow Metab 17: 1166–1169
8. Crompton M, Costi A (1988) Kinetic evidence for a heart mitochondrial pore activated by Ca^{2+}, inorganic phosphate and oxidative stress. A potential mechanism for mitochondrial dysfunction during cellular Ca^{2+} overload. Eur J Biochem 178: 489–501
9. Drake M, Friberg H, Boris Möller F, Sakata K, Wieloch T (1996) The immunosuppressant FK506 ameliorates ischaemic damage in the rat brain. Acta Physiol Scand 158: 155–159
10. Duchen MR, McGuinness O, Brown LA, Crompton M (1993) On the involvement of a cyclosporin A sensitive mitochondrial pore in myocardial reperfusion injury. Cardiovasc Res 27: 1790–1794
11. Endres M, Wang ZQ, Namura S, Waeber C, Moskowitz MA (1997) Ischemic brain injury is mediated by the activation of poly(ADP-ribose)polymerase. J Cereb Blood Flow Metab 17: 1143–1151
12. Folbergrová J, Zhao Q, Katsura K, Siesjö BK (1995) N-tert-butyl-α-phenylnitrone improves recovery of brain energy state in the rats following transient focal ischemia. Proc Nat Acad Sci, USA 92: 5057–5061
13. Griffiths EJ, Halestrap AP (1995) Mitochondrial non-specific pores remain closed during cardiac ischaemia, but open upon reperfusion. Biochem J 307: 93–98
14. Gunter TE, Pfeiffer DR (1990) Mechanisms by which mitochondria transport calcium. Am J Physiol 258:C755–C786
15. Gunter TE, Gunter KK, Sheu SS, Gavin CE (1994) Mitochondrial calcium transport: physiological and pathological relevance. Am J Physiol 267:C313–C339
16. Haletrap AP, Connern CP, Griffiths EJ, Kerr PM (1997) Cyclosporine A binding to mitochondrial cyclophilin inhibits the permeability transition pore and protects hearts from ischemia/reperfusion injury. Mol Cell Biochem 174: 167–172
17. Hara H, Friedlander RM, Gagliardini V, Ayata C, Fink K, Huang Z, Shimizu-Sasamata M, Yuan J, Moskowitz MA (1997) Inhibition of interleukin 1β converting enzyme family proteases reduces ischemic and excitotoxic neuronal damage. Proc Natl Acad Sci U S A 94: 2007–2012
18. Hirsch T, Marchetti P, Susin SA, Dallaporta B, Zamzami N, Marzo I, Geuskens M, Kroemer G (1997) The apoptosis-necrosis paradox. Apoptogenic proteases activated after mitochondrial permeability transition determine the mode of cell death. Oncogene 15: 1573–1581
19. Hockenbery DM, Oltvai ZN, Yin XM, Milliman CL, Korsmeyer SJ (1993) Bcl-2 functions in an antioxidant pathway to prevent apoptosis. Cell 75: 241–251
20. Kane DJ, Sarafian TA, Anton R, Hahn H, Gralla EB, Valentine JS, Ord T, Bredesen DE (1993) Bcl-2 inhibition of neural death: decreased generation of reactive oxygen species. Science 262: 1274–1277
21. Kluck RM, Bossy Wetzel E, Green DR, Newmeyer DD (1997) The release of cytochrome c from mitochondria: a primary site for Bcl-2 regulation of apoptosis. Science 275: 1132–1136
22. Kluck RM, Martin SJ, Hoffman BM, Zhou JS, Green DR, Newmeyer DD (1997) Cytochrome c activation of CPP32-like proteolysis plays a critical role in a Xenopus cell-free apoptosis system. EMBO J 16: 4639–4649
23. Kristián T, Siesjö BK (1998) Calcium in ischemic cell death. Stroke 29: 705–718
24. Kuroda S, Siesjö BK (1996) Postischemic administration of FK506 reduced infarct volume following transient brain ischemia. Neurosci Res Com 19: 83–90
25. Kuroda S, Siesjö BK (1997) Reperfusion damage following focal ischemia: pathophysiology and therapeutic windows. Clin Neurosci 4: 199–212
26. Kuroda S, Katsura K, Hillered L, Bates TE, Siesjö BK (1996) Delayed treatment with α-phenyl-N-tert-butyl nitrone (PBN) attenuates secondary mitochondrial dysfunction after transient focal cerebral ischemia in the rat. Neurobiol Dis 3: 149–157
27. Li PA, Uchino H, Elmér E, Siesjö BK (1997) Amelioration by cyclosporin A of brain damage following 5 or 10 min of ischemia in rats subjected to preischemic hyperglycemia. Brain Res 753: 133–140
28. Liu X, Kim CN, Yang J, Jemmerson R, Wang X (1996) Induction of apoptotic program in cell-free extracts: requirement for dATP and cytochrome c. Cell 86: 147–157
29. Markgraf CG, Velayo NL, Johnson MP, McCarty DR, Medhi S, Koehl JR, Chmielewski PA, Linnik MD (1998) Six-hour window of opportunity for calpain inhibition in focal cerebral ischemia in rats. Stroke 29: 152–158

30. Nakai A, Kuroda S, Kristián T, Siesjö BK (1997) The immunosuppressant drug FK506 ameliorates secondary mitochondrial dysfunction following transient focal cerebral ischemia in the rat. Neurobiol Dis 4: 288–300
31. Nicolli A, Basso E, Petronilli V, Wenger RM, Bernardi P (1996) Interactions of cyclophilin with the mitochondrial inner membrane and regulation of the permeability transition pore, a cyclosporin A-sensitive channel. J Biol Chem 271: 2185–2192
32. Ouyang YB, Kuroda S, Kristián T, Siesjö BK (1997) Release of mitochondrial aspartate aminotransferase (mAST) following transient focal cerebral ischemia suggests the opening of a mitochondrial permeability transition pore. Neurosci Res Commun 20: 167–173
33. Pike RB, Zhao X, Newcomb JK, Wang KK, Postmantur RM, Hayes RL (1998) Temporal relationships between de novo protein synthesis, calpain and caspase 3-like protease activation, and DNA fragmentation during apoptosis in septo-hippocampal cultures. J Neurosci Res (in press)
34. Reed JC (1997) Cytochrome c: can't live with it-can't live without it. Cell 91: 559–562
35. Richter C, Gogvadze V, Laffranchi R, Schlapbach R, Schweizer M, Suter M, Walter P, Yaffee M (1995) Oxidants in mitochondria: from physiology to diseases. Biochim Biophys Acta 1271: 67–74
36. Siesjö BK (1992) Pathophysiology and treatment of focal cerebral ischemia. Part I: Pathophysiology. J Neurosurg 77: 169–184
37. Siesjö BK, Kristián T, Katsura K (1995) The role of calcium in delayed postischemic brain damage. In: Moskowitz M, Caplan LR (eds) Cerebrovascular diseases. Butterworth-Heinemann, Boston, pp 353–370
38. Sims NR (1991) Selective impairment of respiration in mitochondria isolated from brain subregions following transient forebrain ischemia in the rat. J Neurochem 56: 1836–1844
39. Sims NR, Pulsinelli WA (1987) Altered mitochondrial respiration in selectively vulnerable brain subregions following transient forebrain ischemia in the rat. J Neurochem 49: 1367–1374
40. Steiner JP, Connolly MA, Valentine HL, Hamilton GS, Dawson TM, Hester L, Snyder SH (1997) Neurotrophic actions of nonimmunosuppressive analogues of immunosuppressive drugs FK506, rapamycin and cyclosporin A. Nat Med 3: 421–428
41. Takahashi A, Goldschmidt Clermont PJ, Alnemri ES, Fernandes Alnemri T, Yoshizawa Kumagaya K, Nakajima K, Sasada M, Poirier GG, Earnshaw WC (1997) Inhibition of ICE-related proteases (caspases) and nuclear apoptosis by phenylarsine oxide. Exp Cell Res 231: 123–131
42. Uchino H, Elmér E, Uchino K, Lindvall O, Siesjö BK (1995) Cyclosporin A dramatically ameliorates CA1 hippocampal damage following transient forebrain ischaemia in the rat. Acta Physiol Scand 155: 469–471
43. Yang J, Liu X, Bhalla K, Kim CN, Ibrado AM, Cai J, Peng TI, Jones DP, Wang X (1997) Prevention of apoptosis by Bcl-2: release of cytochrome c from mitochondria blocked. Science 275: 1129–1132
44. Zamzami N, Marchetti P, Castedo M, Decaudin D, Macho A, Hirsch T, Susin SA, Petit PX, Mignotte B, Kroemer G (1995) Sequential reduction of mitochondrial transmembrane potential and generation of reactive oxygen species in early programmed cell death. J Exp Med 182: 367–377
45. Zamzami N, Marchetti P, Castedo M, Hirsch T, Susin SA, Masse B, Kroemer G (1996) Inhibitors of permeability transition interfere with the disruption of the mitochondrial transmembrane potential during apoptosis. FEBS Lett 384: 53–57
46. Zamzami N, Hirsch T, Dallaporta B, Petit PX, Kroemer G (1997) Mitochondrial implication in accidental and programmed cell death: apoptosis and necrosis. J Bioenerg Biomembr 29: 185–193
47. Zhao Q, Pahlmark K, Smith ML, Siesjö BK (1994) Delayed treatment with the spin trap α-phenyl-N-tert-butyl nitrone (PBN) reduces infarct size following transient middle cerebral artery occlusion in rats. Acta Physiol Scand 152: 349–350
48. Zoratti M, Szabò I (1995) The mitochondrial permeability transition. Biochim Biophys Acta 1241: 139–176

Temporal Profile of Cortical Injury Following Ischemic Insult Just Below and at the Threshold Level for Induction of Infarction: Light and Electron Microscopic Study

U. Ito, S. Hanyu, Y. Hakamata, K. Arima, K. Oyanagi, T. Kuroiwa, and I. Nakano

Summary. By unilaterally occluding the carotid artery of Mongolian gerbils twice for 10 min, with an interval of 5 h, we affected ischemic insults of just below or at the threshold level needed to induce infarction in cerebral cortex that had been sectioned coronally at the level of the infundibulum or at the chiasma. The temporal profile of cortical tissue injuries was compared by light- and electron microscopy at 15 min, 5 h, 12 h, 24 h, 4 days and 7 days following both intensities of the above insults. We have found that:

1. Following ischemic insults just below the threshold level to induce infarction, only disseminated selective neuronal necrosis (DSNN) progresses. Following ischemic insults of threshold level to induce infarction, DSNN develops first, followed by an evolution to a gradually enlarging infarcted focus.
2. Swelling, glycogen accumulation and an increase in the size and number of mitochondria are observed in astrocytes associated with DSNN, and no astrocytic necrosis is found.
3. When astrocytic cell processes degenerate and perivascular end-feet disappear, the cortical tissue demonstrates infarction
4. Astrocytes appear to protect against post-ischemic neuronal and cortical tissue injuries. A therapeutic window exists to rescue the cortical tissue evolving from DSNN to infarction.
5. Surviving astrocytes proliferate, extending and widening their cell processes, which are rich in astrocytic fibrils. The processes are intercalated among the neuropil and surround blood vessels as astrocytic end-feet.

Introduction

In the previous study [4], using a repetitive unilateral carotid-occlusion model in gerbils, we found that with an increase in the number of small repetitive insults and a decrease in the repetitive intervals, ischemic injury progresses from less extensive to more extensive disseminated selective neuronal necrosis (DSNN), and then to cerebral infraction. Therefore, the maturation phenomenon of ischemic insults is expressed by a continuum from selective neuronal necrosis to infarction upon reaching a critical threshold of intensity of ischemic insults [4, 10].

In the present study, we have compared the temporal profile of cortical tissue injuries after ischemic insults, just under the level and at the level required to induce focal infarction. We have found that only DSNN develops in the former; in the latter, DSNN

Maturation Phenomenon in Cerebral Ischemia III
U. Ito et al. (Eds.)
© Springer-Verlag Berlin Heidelberg 1999

develops first and focal infarction appears later and further increases in size in the cortical tissue where DSNN is progressing.

Materials and Methods

We occluded the left carotid artery of the Mongolian gerbil twice, each for a 10-min period, at an interval of 5 h. Ischemia-positive animals were selected during the first 10-min period of ischemia [15]. In this model, following reperfusion, focal infarction develops in the coronal section sectioned at the chiasmatic level, and only DSNN progresses in the coronal section sectioned at the infundibular level [5]. All animals were sacrificed at 15 min, 5 h, 12 h, 24 h, 48 h, 4 days and 7 days after the second ischemic insult by intracardiac perfusion with 10 % phosphate-buffered formalde-hyde for light microscopy (five animals in each group) or with glutaraldehyde fixative (three animals in each group) for electron microscopic (EMS) study. Paraffin sections were obtained from coronal sections cut at the chiasmatic (face A) and infundibular (face B) levels and were stained with hematoxylin and eosin (H&E) and periodic acid–Schiff stain (PAS), and for glial fibrillary acidic (GFA) protein. Ultrathin sections, including the third through the fifth cortical layers, were prepared from the left ischemic cerebral hemisphere at the midpoint between the interhemispheric (IH) and rhinal fissures (RF) of coronal sections cut at the chiasmatic and infundibular levels. Alternative sections were double stained with uranyl acetate and lead solutions, and observed using a JEM-2000 EX electron microscope.

Results

A temporal profile of the cortical tissue showed progression of DSNN at the infundib-ular level (face B). Progression of DSNN followed the evolving infarction in the corti-cal tissue at the chiasmatic level (face A), while DSNN continued to progress in the cortical tissue around the infarction. No astrocytic necrosis was found associated with DSNN.

Fifteen minutes after the last ischemic insult, in both faces A and B, no morpho-logical changes were observed except for moderate swelling of astrocytic cell bodies, cell processes and perivascular end-feet (EF), without an increase in number of glyco-gen granules; mitochondria were moderately increased in number and size.

No infarction evolved 5 h after the last ischemic insult in the cerebral cortex. In the infundibular level (face B), some neurons became swollen, losing ribosomes from their rough-surfaced endoplasmic reticulum. Dark neurons (DN) with condensed cytoplasm and nuclear chromatin condensations were occasionally observed in the third and fifth cortical layers where glycogen granules were increased in number (Fig. 1a, b). All astrocytic cell bodies, cell processes and perivascular EF were moder-ately swollen, with an increase in the number of glycogen granules and elongated mitochondria containing an electron-dense matrix (Fig. 2a, b). The number of GFA protein-positive astrocytes was slightly increased in the post-ischemic cortex. At the chiasmatic level (face A), the above changes were more prominent than those observed at the infundibular level. Astrocytic cell processes with cystic degeneration

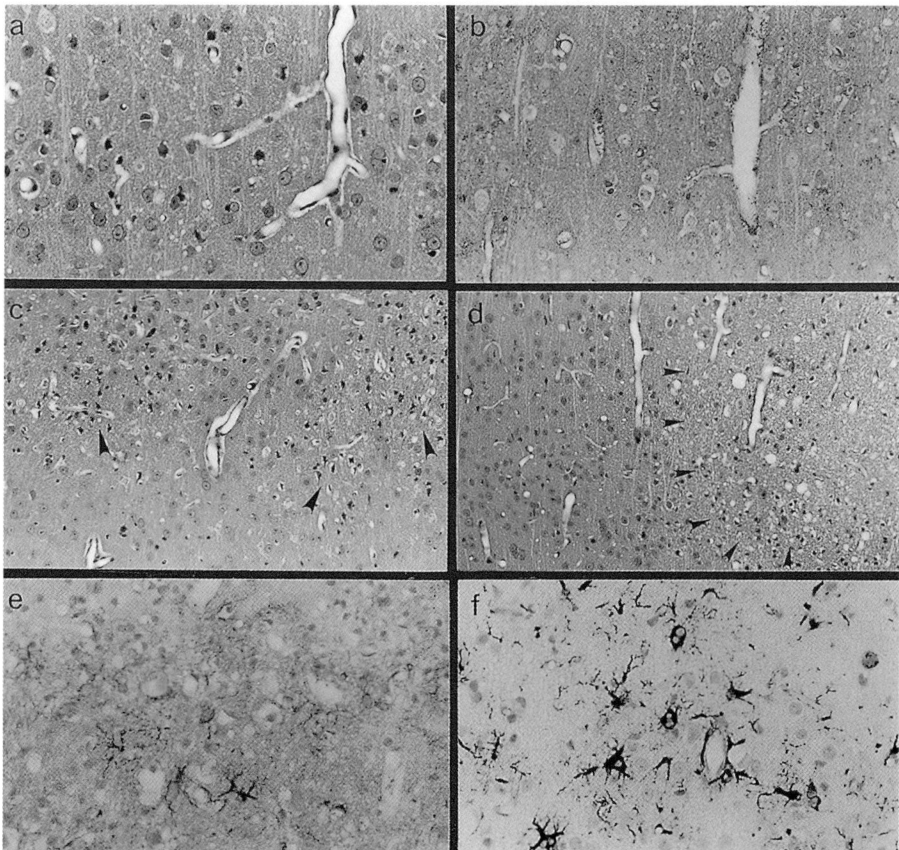

Fig. 1a–f. Light microscopic pictures. **a** In the cerebral cortex of the infundibular level (face B), 5 h after the last ischemic insult, dark neurons (DN) are disseminated among the normal looking neurons. Small vesicles are seen scattered in the neuropil. H&E × 200. **b** In the same cortex as A, glycogen granules are increased in number in the neuropils, especially around the small vessels. PAS × 200. **c** Patchy infarctions (*arrows*) evolve at 12 h, in the chiasmatic level (face A), involving the third and fifth cortical layers. H&E × 100. **d** The patchy small infarctions fused to become a larger infarcted focus (IF) at 24 h. In the margin of the infarcted focus (*arrows*), same tissue necrosis as C, is still progressing. Surrounding the infarcted focus, disseminated selective neuronal necrosis (DSNN) continues to progress. H&E × 100. **e** Glial fibrillary acidic (GFA) protein-positive astrocytes in the patchy small infarctions (12 h) and at the periphery of the growing focal infarction (24 h) show interrupted astrocytic cell processes compatible with Cajal's clasmatodendrosis. GFAP × 400. **f** Surrounding the infarcted focus at the chiasmatic level (face A), GFA protein-positive astrocytes having two or three nuclei are observed. GFAP × 400

containing degenerated mitochondria were occasionally observed (Fig. 2c). Otherwise, no ultrastructural destruction of astrocytes was seen in face A or B.

At 12–24 h, only DSNN progressed in the infundibular level (face B), while patchy infarctions evolved in the chiasmatic level (face A) in the third and fifth cortical layers. In the infundibular level (face B), scattered swollen neurons (SN) and condensed DN with nuclear chromatin condensation were increased in number, especially in the

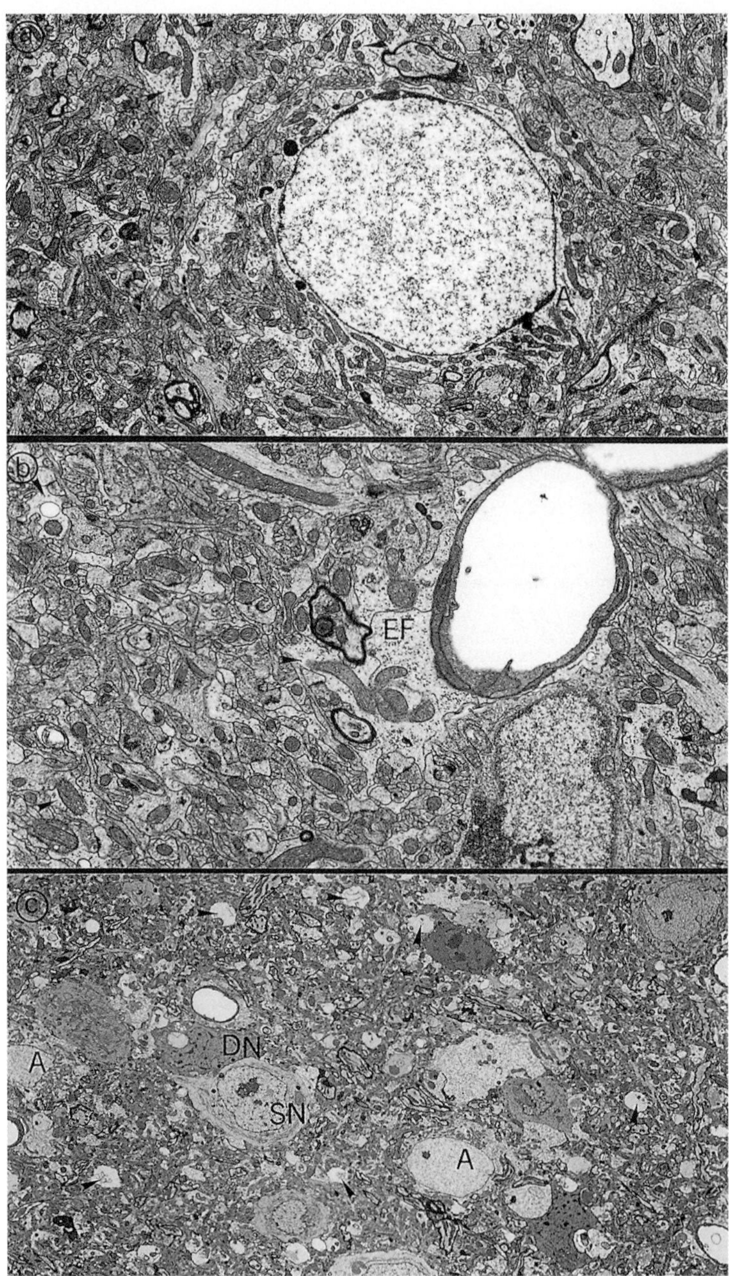

Fig. 2a–c

third and fifth cortical layers (Fig. 2c). Astrocytic swelling was more prominent than that observed at 5 h. However, no ultrastructural disintegration occurred in astrocytes, except for occasional cystic degeneration of the astrocytic cell processes associated with degenerated mitochondria. At the chiasmatic level (face A), patchy small infarctions appeared at 12 h involving the third and fifth cortical layers (Fig. 1c) and fused to become a larger infarcted focus at 24 h (Fig. 1d). In the former and the periphery of the latter, all neurons were necrotic, with nuclear chromatin condensation; all astrocytic cell processes degenerated into cystic fragments containing degenerated mitochondria (Fig. 3a), and most of the perivascular EF disappeared, occasionally leaving cystic EF containing degenerated mitochondria (Fig. 3b). Glycogen granules were not found in the degenerated astrocytic cell processes or EF. Some of the astrocytic cell bodies with cystic degeneration of their processes remained, attached to the vascular wall (Fig. 3c). GFA protein-positive astrocytes in the patchy small infarctions (12 h) and in the periphery of the growing focal infarction (24 h) showed interrupted astrocytic cell processes compatible with Cajal's clasmatodendrosis (a morphologic term for astrocytic cell degeneration) (Fig. 1e). Almost all astrocytes and neurons in the larger infarcted foci became swollen and underwent degenerative changes, with multiple sites of infiltration by macrophages and monocytes. Surrounding the infarcted focus, DSNN continued to progress, with an increased number of glycogen granules in astrocytes (Fig. 1d).

At 48 h and 4 days, in both faces A and B, all astrocytic cell bodies, cell processes and EF were thickened and were rich in bundles of glial fibrils. The GFA protein-positive astrocytes increased in number and were especially prominent in the zone surrounding the infarcted focus in face A, where mitotic figures and GFA protein-positive astrocytes having two or three nuclei were observed (Fig. 1f). In the infarcted focus, numerous foamy phagocytic cells were seen close to ultrastructurally well-preserved small vessels. Although DSNN continued to progress at both levels, including the cortical tissue surrounding the infarcted focus in face A, most of the surviving neurons appeared normal.

Discussion

The two different morphological types of ischemic injuries have been considered to have different fates following ischemic insults; DSNN as induced by a mild ischemia, and cerebral infarction, pan-necrosis or coagulation necrosis involving all compo-

---

Fig. 2a–c. Electron microscopic pictures. **a** All astrocytic cell bodies (*a*) and cell processes (*arrows*) are moderately swollen in face B at 5 h, with an increase in number of glycogen granules and of elongated mitochondria containing an electron-dense matrix × 6800. **b** Perivascular end-feet (*EF*) and all astrocytic cell processes (*arrows*) are moderately swollen in face B at 5 h, with an increase in number of glycogen granules and of elongated mitochondria containing an electron-dense matrices × 10,200. **c** In face B, at 12 h, scattered swollen neurons (*SN*) and condensed dark neurons(*DN*) with nuclear chromatin condensation are increased in number, especially in the third and fifth cortical layers. Astrocytic (*A*) swelling is more prominent than that observed at 5 h. No ultrastructural disintegration occurred in astrocytes except for occasional cystic degeneration of the astrocytic cell processes associated with degenerated mitochondria (*arrows*) × 1800

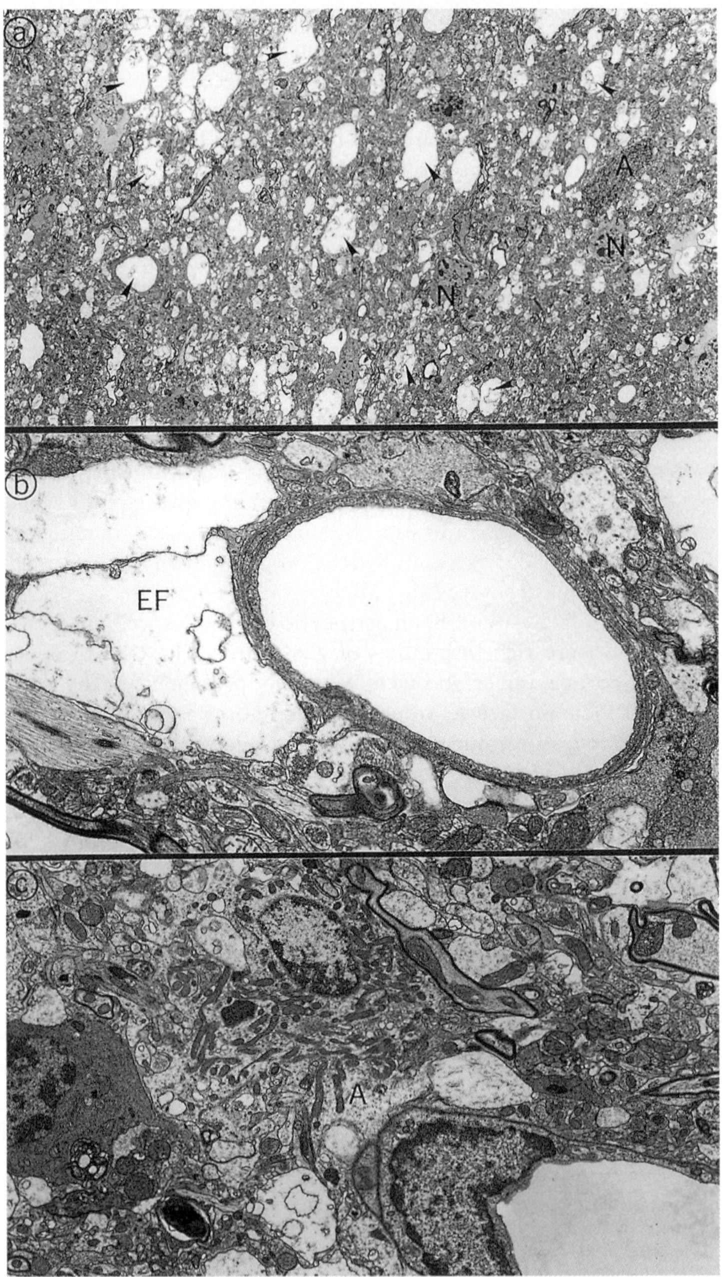

Fig. 3 a–c

nents of the cerebral tissue (infarction) as induced by intensive ischemia [1, 3, 7, 8, 10, 14, 17]. The pathogenesis of the two types of ischemic injuries are considered to be different [16]. In the present study, using the model of ischemic insult around the threshold level for the induction of infarction, we found that only DSNN developed after the ischemic insults just under the threshold level. At the level to induce focal infarction, DSNN developed first and focal infarction appeared later and enlarged in size in the cortical tissue where DSNN was continuing to progress [10]. No astrocytic necrosis was observed associated with DSNN.

As DSNN progressed, astrocytes became swollen and accumulated glycogen granules and increasing numbers of elongated mitochondria, without showing ultrastructural disintegration of the cytoplasm. In the early stage of evolution of the infarction (12 h in the chiasmatic level), as well as in the margin of the enlarging infarcted focus (24–48 h in the chiasmatic level), astrocytic cell processes degenerated, displaying multiple cystic swellings containing degenerated mitochondria [9]. These changes of the astrocytic processes are compatible with Cajal's clasmatodendrosis. Simultaneously, most of the perivascular EF disappeared except for the occasionally remaining degenerated cystic EF [9]. These findings suggest that the maturation phenomenon of ischemic cortical injury [7, 8, 10] progresses continuously from less extensive to more extensive DSNN, and then evolves into cerebral infarction with the destruction of astrocytic cell processes [9]. Therefore, astrocytic swelling associated with progressive DSNN is considered to protect the viability of neurons [11–13, 18, 19].

In contrast to the mitochondrial swelling observed in the degenerating cortical neurons in areas where DSNN is progressing, the increase of number and size of astrocytic mitochondria with electron-dense matrices [9] suggests an activated astrocytic compartmentation of the cortical-energy metabolism used for housekeeping the extracellular neuronal environment and for processing plants for the generation of fuel molecules that can be used by their neighboring neurons [6]. In our other study using the same experimental model, adenosine triphosphate content and succinic dehydrogenase (SDH) activity did not decrease following the last ischemic episode, even though DSNN was progressing until the evolution of infarction (see chap, by Kuroiwa et al.). This suggested that the activated astrocytic energy metabolism counterbalanced the declining neuronal one, and retained a constant energy metabolism in the cortical tissue as a whole.

Increasing astrocytic-glycogen granules [9] might be considered a reaction to deranged glucose metabolism after reperfusion [20] and/or to represent astrocytic gluconeogenesis [2], a process consuming lactic acid formed in the cortical tissue during anaerobic glycolysis. Perturbed glucose metabolism may be an expression of the disturbed glucose utilization induced by an altered metabolism of the mitochon-

---

Fig. 3a–c. Electron microscopic pictures. **a** In face A, in the patchy small infarctions (12 h; Fig. 1c), and in the periphery of the enlarged infarcted focus (24 h; Fig. 1d), all neurons are necrotic, with nuclear chromatin condensation (*N*) and all astrocytic cell processes are degenerated into cystic fragments containing degenerated mitochondria (*arrows*). A astrocytic cell body containing increased number of mitochondria × 1360. **b** In the same cortex as A, most of the perivascular end-feet (*EF*) disappeared, occasionally leaving cystically enlarged EF containing degenerated mitochondria × 13,600. **c.** In the same cortex as A, some of the astrocytic cell bodies (*A*) with cystic degeneration of their processes remained, attached to the vascular wall × 7600

drial electron-conducting energy system. Further study is necessary to clarify the interaction of these mitochondrial changes with the increased glycogen granules in post-ischemic astrocytes [6, 19].

In the early evolution of infarction and in the periphery of the enlarging infarcted focus in the cortical tissue, some astrocytic cell bodies survived, although their processes had degenerated [9]. These cells remained attached to the vascular wall and some of them appeared to proliferate by mitosis, becoming reactive astrocytes rich in astrocytic glial fibers and occasionally showing multinucleation.

Conclusions

1. Following ischemic insults just under the threshold level required to induce infarction, only DSNN progresses. Following ischemic insults at the threshold levels needed to induce infarction, initially only DSNN develops, followed by the evolution of a gradually enlarging infarcted focus. Therefore, a therapeutic window exists to rescue cortical tissue evolving from DSNN to infarction by slowing down the evolution and/or upraising the threshold.
2. Astrocytic swelling, glycogen accumulation and an increase in mitochondrial size and number are observed to be associated with progressive DSNN. No astrocytic necrosis is found with DSNN.
3. When astrocytic cell processes degenerate and perivascular EF disappear, the cortical tissue has undergone infarction.
4. The surviving astrocytes proliferate, extending and widening their cell processes, which are rich in astrocytic fibrils into the neuropil, and again surrounding blood vessels as astrocytic EF.

References

1. DeGirolami U, Crowell RM, Marcoux FW (1984) Selective necrosis and total necrosis in focal cerebral ischemia. Neuropathologic observations on experimental middle cerebral artery occlusion in the macaque monkey. J Neuropathol Exp Neurol 43: 57–71
2. Dringen R, Schmoll D, Cesar M, Hamprecht B (1993) Incorporation of radioactivity from [14 C] lactate into the glycogen of cultured mouse astroglial cells. Evidence for gluconeogenesis in brain cells. Biol Chem Hoppe-Seyler 374: 343–347
3. Garcia JH, Yoshida Y, Chen H, Li Y, Zhang ZG, Lian J, Chen S, Chopp M (1993) Progression from ischemic injury to infarct following middle cerebral artery occlusion in the rat. Am J Pathol 142: 623–635
4. Hanyu S, Ito U, Hakamata Y, Yoshida M (1995) Transition from ischemic neuronal necrosis to infarction in repeated ischemia. Brain Res 686: 44–48
5. Hanyu S, Ito U, Hakamata Y, Nakano I (1997) Topographical analysis of cortical neuronal loss associated with disseminated selective neuronal necrosis and infarction after repeated ischemia. Brain Res 767: 154–157
6. Hamprecht B, Dringen R (1995) Energy metabolism. In: Kettenmann H, Ransom, B (eds) Neuroglia. Oxford University Press, New York, pp 473–487
7. Ito U, Spatz M, Walker J, Jr., Klatzo I (1975) Experimental cerebral ischemia in mongolian gerbils. Light microscopic observations. Acta Neuropathol (Berl) 32: 209–223
8. Ito U, Yamaguchi T, Tomita H, Tone O, Shishido T, Hayashi H, Yoshida M (1992) Maturation phenomenon of ischemic injuries observed in Mongolian gerbils: introductory remarks. In: Ito U, Kirino T, Kuroiwa T, Klatzo I (eds) Maturation phenomenon in cerebral ischemia I. Springer, Berlin Heidelberg New York, pp 1–13

9. Ito U, Hanyu S, Hakamata Y, Nakamura M, Arima K (1996) Ultrastructure of astrocytes associated with progressing selective neuronal death or impending infarction after repeated ischemia. In: Krieglstein J (ed) Pharmacology of cerebral ischemia. Medpharm Scientific, Stuttgart, pp 385–392
10. Ito U, Hanyu S, Hakamata Y, Kuroiwa T, Yoshida M (1997) Features and threshold of infarct development in ischemic maturation phenomenon. In: Ito U, Kirino T, Kuroiwa T, Klatzo I (eds) Maturation phenomenon in cerebral ischemia II. Springer, Berlin Heidelberg New York, pp 115–121
11. Kempski O, Staub F, von-Rosen F, Zimmer M, Neu A, Baethmann A (1988) Molecular mechanisms of glial swelling in vitro. Neurochem Pathol 9: 109–125
12. Kempski O, Volk C (1997) Glial protection against neuronal damage. In: Ito U, Kirino T, Kuroiwa T, Klatzo I (eds) Maturation phenomenon in cerebral ischemia II. Springer, Berlin Heidelberg New York, pp 143–150
13. Kimelberg HK, Rutledge E, Goderie S, Charniga C (1995) Astrocytic swelling due to hypotonic or high K+ medium causes inhibition of glutamate and aspartate uptake and increases their release. J Cereb Blood Flow Metab 15: 409–416
14. Marcoux FW, Morawetz RB, Crowell RM, DeGirolami U, Halsey J, Jr (1982) Differential regional vulnerability in transient focal cerebral ischemia. Stroke 13: 339–346
15. Ohno K, Ito U, Inaba Y (1984) Regional cerebral blood flow and stroke index after left carotid artery ligation in the conscious gerbil. Brain Res 297: 151–157
16. Siesjo BK (1992) Pathophysiology and treatment of focal cerebral ischemia. Part II: mechanisms of damage and treatment. J Neurosurg 77: 337–354
17. Smith ML, Auer RN, Siesjo BK (1984) The density and distribution of ischemic brain injury in the rat following 2–10 min of forebrain ischemia. Acta Neuropathol (Berl) 64: 319–332
18. Sokoloff L (1992) Energy metabolism and effects of energy depletion or exposure to glutamate. Can J Physiol Pharmacol 70:S107–S112
19. Sokoloff L, Gotoh J, Law MJ, Takahashi S (1996) Functional activation of energy metabolism in nervous tissue: roles of neurons and astroglia. In: Krieglstein J (ed) Pharmacology of cerebral ischemia. Medpharm Scientific, Stuttgart, pp 259–270
20. Swanson RA, Choi DW (1993) Glial glycogen stores affect neuronal survival during glucose deprivation in vitro. J Cereb Blood Flow Metab 13: 162–169

Mitochondrial Dysfunction and Maturation Phenomenon in Ischemic Gerbil Cortex

T. Kuroiwa, G. Mies, Y. Hakamata, S. Hanyu, R. Okeda, and U. Ito

Summary. We examined the time course of energy impairment in the cerebral cortex, which develops cerebral infarction after repeated ischemia. Cerebral ischemia was induced in the gerbil by repeated unilateral carotid-artery occlusion (two 10-min periods of ischemia separated by a 5-h interval). Histological examination of the cortex at the stereotaxic levels of chiasma and infundibulum revealed infarction and disseminated selective neuronal necrosis (DSNN), respectively, 7 days after transient ischemia. Cortical glucose content increased at both levels 5 h after the second transient ischemia. At the infundibular level, cortical succinic dehydrogenase (SDH) activity remained within the normal range after ischemia. The cortical activity at the chiasmal level remained within normal range during the initial 12 h. However, the activity gradually reduced thereafter to 28±7.6 % of the control level at 2 days of recirculation. The time course of cortical adenosine triphosphate content paralleled the change in SDH. Lactate and tissue pH changes indicated lactoacidosis at the chiasmal level, but not at the infundibular level. Thus, energy metabolism slowly deteriorated over the 2 days of recirculation in the area of the cortex that developed infarction. Mitochondrial dysfunction appears to play a crucial role in the recruitment into the infarction process of postischemic tissue, which is developing DSNN.

Introduction

Cortical infarction, as well as selective neuronal necrosis, develops very slowly in gerbils after repeated cerebral ischemia (maturation phenomenon) [4–7]. The process of slow infarction may take as long as 2 weeks following a mild ischemic insult [3]. Thus, in comparison with postischemic neuronal necrosis, cerebral infarction is not a process characterized by rapid development. Various different mechanisms, such as abnormal gene expression and impairment of protein synthesis and energy metabolism, play causative roles in the neuronal necrosis. In the infarction process, it is known that energy impairment is important. However, the precise temporal profile of the evolution of energy failure has not been fully elucidated. Assuming that energy impairment is as important in the slowly progressing as in the rapidly developing infarction, we have attempted to elucidate the temporal and spatial profile of energy impairment in cortical infarction, using a gerbil model of slowly developing cortical infarction.

Maturation Phenomenon in Cerebral Ischemia III
U. Ito et al. (Eds.)
© Springer-Verlag Berlin Heidelberg 1999

Materials and Methods

Adult Mongolian gerbils weighing 60–80 g were used. The animals were subjected to two occlusions of the left common carotid artery for 10 min each, separated by a 5 h recovery interval. Animals showing positive stroke symptoms [10] were sacrificed at 15 min, 5 h, 12 h, 1 day, 2 days, 4 days or 7 days after the second episode of ischemia. For quantitative imaging of tissue adenosine triphosphate (ATP) and glucose levels by means of the substrate-induced bioluminescence method, 20-μm-thick cryostat sections at the stereotaxic levels of the chiasma and infundibulum were covered with a 60-μm section of frozen reaction mix containing all enzymes, coenzymes and substrates necessary for evoking the bioluminescence reaction. The sandwich was placed in the dark on photographic film, and the optical-density sandwich was scanned with an image-processing system [11].

Regional tissue pH was measured quantitatively on cryostat sections at the same levels by the umbelliferone method of Csiba et al.[2], in which the sections were brought into contact with umbelliferone-soaked paper strips and the fluorescence (450 nm) following excitation at 370 nm and 340 nm was recorded photographically. The 340-nm excitation image was subtracted from the 370-nm picture. For the quantitative imaging of succinic dehydrogenase (SDH) activity [9], gerbil brain was cut into coronal slices at the same stereotaxic levels in a cool moist chamber and submerged for 3 min in 1 % triphenyl tetrazolium solution maintained at 35 °C. Red coloration of the cut surface, resulting from the accumulation of formazan, was recorded using a charge-coupled device (CCD) camera, and regional activity of SDH was calculated from the speed of formazan production using an image-processing system.

For histological examination, the animal was perfused transcardially with 10 % buffered formalin. Coronal sections at the same levels were stained with hematoxylin and eosin and Kluever Barrera.

Quantitative evaluations were carried out in the cortex at the midpoint between the interhemispheric fissure and rhinal fissure of the two stereotaxic levels.

Results

Histological examination revealed cortical infarction at the chiasmal level. The infarction was located in the left dorsolateral part of the cortex and was centered in the middle layer. At the infundibular level, many neurons showing cytoplasmic eosinophilia (ischemic neurons) were scattered among normal-appearing neurons in the left dorsolateral part of the frontal cortex. These ischemic neurons were distributed throughout cortical layers II–VI [disseminated selective neuronal necrosis (DSNN)].

The glucose level was significantly increased in the left cortex at both the chiasmal and infundibular levels at 5 h after the second period of ischemia (chiasmal level 124±5.3 %; infundibular level 130±9.8 % OD, compared with the opposite hemisphere; mean ± SEM; $P<0.05$), which was even more pronounced at 2 days (chiasmal level 251±46 %; infundibular level 181±41 %; $P<0.05$).

SDH activity declined significantly in the area developing cerebral infarction (chiasmal level, 1 day, 55±9.3 % activity of opposite cortex; 4 days, 11±2.4 %; $P<0.05$), but was only discretely affected in the area showing DSNN (infundibular level, 1 day,

Table 1. Time course of tissue glucose content, adenosine triphosphate (ATP) content, succinic dehydrogenase (SDH) activity and pH in the left frontal cortex of gerbil brain subjected to two 10-min occlusions of the left common carotid artery, separated by a 5-h interval. Note the gradual decrease in tissue ATP level and SDH activity over 2 days of recirculation. Values are expressed as a percentage of the control level. Values of glucose, ATP and SDH levels are expressed as a percentage of the levels of the right frontal cerebral cortex and are expressed as mean ± SEM

	15 min	5 h	12 h	1 day	2 days	4 days
Glucose	114±9.6	124±5.3	126±27	144±13	251±46	111±14
ATP	103±1.2	102±1.9	96±3.9	78±6.5	45±13	48±14
SDH	89±5.8	90±4.1	94±2.8	55±9.3	28±7.6	11±2.4
pH	6.94±0.08	6.76±0.12	6.81±0.14	6.85±0.12	6.26±0.19	6.06±0.19

87±1.9 %; 4 days, 68±12 %; n.s.). Reduction of SDH activity was paralleled by a significant decrease of ATP levels at the chiasmal level (1 day, 78±6.5 %; 4 days, 48±14 %; $P<0.05$). However, ATP content remained unchanged (1 day, 97±3.2 %; 4 days, 96±2.1 %; n.s.) at the infundibular level. The cortical time profile of tissue acidosis and lactate accumulation corresponded to the changes observed in the ATP and SDH measurements (Table 1).

Discussion

After a short period of ischemia, the cortex slowly develops neuronal necrosis and infarction (maturation phenomenon) [6, 7]. When ischemia is induced in the gerbil, by means of unilateral carotid-artery occlusion for 30 min, cortical neurons in the middle layer show ischemic change, with vacuolation of the neuropil at 20 h after recirculation. After repeated ischemia (three 7-min periods of occlusion of the left common carotid artery) in the gerbil, ischemic neuronal change and infarction are observed at 4 weeks after recirculation in the frontal cortex [4]. In rats subjected to a transient focal cerebral ischemia induced by 90 min of occlusion of both common carotid arteries and the right middle cerebral artery [3], infarction requires as long as 14 days of recirculation to develop. Therefore, the evolution of cerebral infarction is slow when the ischemic insult is mild.

It has been shown that acute cerebral infarction is induced by the energy failure, which rapidly develops and persists in ischemic tissue. Assuming that the mechanism of infarction is the same in both rapidly and slowly developing infarctions, we have attempted to analyze the temporal and spatial profile of the infarction process using a model of slowly developing infarction following repeated ischemia.

In the area that develops only DSNN, both tissue ATP content and SDH activity are maintained within normal ranges. Postischemic tissue shows no acidosis. In the area that develops cerebral infarction, both ATP content and SDH activity remain within the normal range during the initial 12–24 h of recirculation. However, both are gradually reduced, thereafter, over 2–4 days of recirculation. The tissue develops lactoacidosis, which parallels a decrease in ATP and SDH levels. In the area developing infarction, multiple small foci of reduced SDH activity initially appear in the middle layer

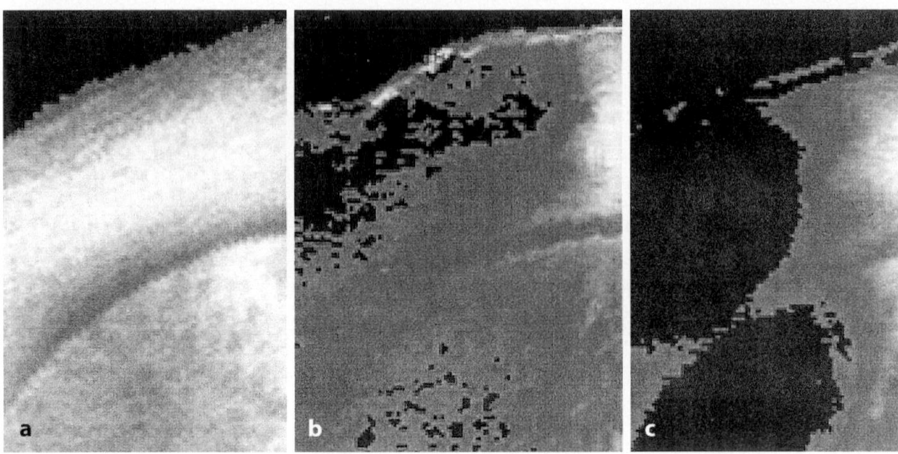

Fig. 1a–c. The area showing succinic dehydrogenase (SDH) activity less than 20 % of the control levels in the left frontal cortex of a control gerbil (**a**), and 2 days (**b**) and 4 days (**c**) after repeated ischemia in two other gerbils. Note the initial scattered foci of low SDH activity (**b**), which gradually enlarges and merges to form a large area of low SDH activity (**c**)

of the cortex, which gradually coalesce to form a large area of reduced SDH activity. Light microscopically, infarction appears in the center of the cortex showing DSNN.

It is known that tissue ATP levels promptly decrease to nearly zero levels following the onset of ischemia, and they return to the control levels shortly after recirculation, when the ischemic interval is short. SDH activity remains unchanged during a short transient ischemia. These findings, together with the present results, indicate that the ATP decrease in postischemic tissue evokes two different response mechanisms. The initial decrease, occurring shortly after the onset of ischemia, is not associated with reduced mitochondrial respiratory-enzyme activity. This decrease in ATP may have a causative role in the development of postischemic neuronal necrosis; however, it is not sufficient to induce infarction. The second decrease in ATP level takes place in the postischemic tissue, which has already started the slow process of progressive neuronal necrosis. This decrease is closely associated with the development of infarction. Light-microscopic examination in a similar transient-ischemia model demonstrates apparent ischemic change in neurons at 20 h of recirculation. These results indicate that the observed bioenergy change is not merely the result of infarction, but is also a mechanism involved in the development of infarction (Fig. 1).

Recently, Kuroda et al. have demonstrated that the cellular bioenergetic state shows partial recovery, but subsequent deterioration after a transient middle-cerebral-artery occlusion in the rat [8]. They measured the respiratory control ratio in rat brain at different time intervals following transient ischemia, and observed secondary deterioration of oxidative phosphorylation at 4 h after recirculation.

Therefore, slow progression of energy failure has been observed in different types of transient cerebral ischemia. Canevari et al. have speculated that free radicals, generated during the recirculation phase by polymorphonuclear leukocytes, may damage components of the respiratory chain [1]. However, we have not observed enhanced adhesion or extravasation of these blood cells at the time of secondary ATP decrease.

Further study is mandatory to elucidate the mechanism of slow bioenergy impairment in the postischemic cortex.

Acknowledgements. We thank Drs. M Ueki (Department of Anesthesiology, Tokyo Medical and Dental University) and S Endo (Animal research Center, Tokyo Medical and Dental University) for their cooperation in parts of this project.

References

1. Canevari L, Kuroda S, Bates TE, Clark JB, Siesjo BK (1997) Activity of mitochondrial respiratory chain enzymes after transient focal ischemia in the rat. J Cereb Blood Flow Metab 17: 1166–1169
2. Csiba L, Paschen W, Hossmann K-A(1983) A topographic quantitative method for measuring brain pH under physiological and pathophysiological conditions. Brain Res 289: 334–337
3. Du C, Hu R, Csernansky CA, Hsu CY, Choi DW (1996) Very delayed infarction after mild focal cerebral ischemia: a role for apoptosis? J Cereb Blood Flow Metab 16: 195–201
4. Hanyu S, Ito U, Hakamata Y, Yoshida M (1995) Transition from ischemic neuronal necrosis to infarction in repeated ischemia. Brain Res 686: 44–48
5. Hanyu S, Ito U, Hakamata Y, Nakano I (1997) Topographical analysis of cortical neuronal loss associated with disseminated selective neuronal necrosis and infarction after repeated ischemia. Brain Res 767: 154–157
6. Ito U, Spatz M, Walker JT, Klatzo I (1975) Experimental cerebral ischemia in Mongolian gerbils I Light microscopical observations. Acta Neuropathol 32: 209–223
7. Ito U, Hanyu S, Hakamata Y, Kuroiwa T, Yoshida M (1997) Maturation phenomenon in cerebral ischemia II. Springer, Berlin Heidelberg New York, pp 115–121
8. Kuroda S, Katsura K, Hillered L, Bates TE, Siesjo BK (1996) Delayed treatment with alpha-phenyl-N-tert-butyl nitrone (PBN) attenuates secondary mitochondrial dysfunction after transient focal cerebral ischemia in the rat. Neurobiol Dis (Japan) 3: 149–157
9. Kuroiwa T, Terakado M, Yamaguchi T, Endo S, Ueki M, Okeda R (1996) The pyramidal cell layer of sector CA 1 shows the lowest hippocampal succinic dehydrogenase activity in normal and postischemic gerbils. Neurosci Lett 206: 1–4
10. Ohno K, Ito U, Inaba Y (1984) Regional cerebral blood flow and stroke index after left carotid artery ligation in the conscious gerbil. Brain Res 297: 151–157
11. Paschen W, Mies G, Kloiber O, Hossmann K-A (1985) A bioluminescent method for the demonstration of regional glucose distribution in brain slices. J Neurochem 36: 513–517

Metabotropic Ca²⁺ Signalling and Refilling of Ca²⁺ Stores in Hippocampal Astrocytes Are Driven by Adenosine Triphosphate Supplied by Glycolysis

G. Reiser and M. Bernstein

Summary. Changes in metabotropic Ca^{2+} signalling following disturbance of the cellular energy supply were investigated in cultured hippocampal astrocytes loaded with the Ca^{2+}-sensitive fluorophore fura-2. The Ca^{2+} content of intracellular stores was estimated based on the Ca^{2+} signal elicited by cyclopiazonic acid in Ca^{2+}-free medium. Metabotropic Ca^{2+} signals were induced by stimulation of P2Y receptors with extracellular adenosine triphosphate (ATP). Inhibition of the mitochondrial ATP synthase with oligomycin did not affect the Ca^{2+} content of Ca^{2+} stores in all cells tested. Purinergic Ca^{2+} signalling also was not affected by oligomycin. Similarly, inhibition of the mitochondrial respiratory chain using cyanide had no influence on the metabotropic Ca^{2+} signalling and the store Ca^{2+} content. Therefore, energy supply by mitochondrial ATP is not essential for the Ca^{2+} release elicited by metabotropic-receptor stimulation and for refilling of the Ca^{2+} stores. The Ca^{2+} signal elicited by release from the Ca^{2+} stores in Ca^{2+}-free medium was reduced to less than 20 % after replacement of glucose with 2-deoxy-D-glucose, resulting in glycolysis inhibition, even when acetate was supplemented as mitochondrial substrate. Treatment with 2-deoxy-D-glucose in the presence of lactate as mitochondrial substrate also reduced the size of receptor-dependent Ca^{2+} signals to less than 20 %. Similarly, the glycolysis inhibitor iodoacetate caused a depletion of Ca^{2+} stores in astrocytes, even when additionally supplied with acetate or lactate. Therefore, energy supplied by glycolysis seems to be essential for loading of Ca^{2+} stores and for metabotropic-receptor-induced Ca^{2+} signalling.

Introduction

Transient interruption of the supply with nutrients to neural cells requires the cells to reduce energy [adenosine triphosphate (ATP)] consumption by downregulating metabolic pathways. Assuming that the ATP consumption of endoplasmic reticulum Ca^{2+}-ATPase reaches the same order of magnitude as the plasma membrane Na^+/K^+-ATPase (20 % of total astrocytic ATP production [19]), disturbance of the cellular energy supply is expected to inhibit signal-transduction processes, which include Ca^{2+} release from endoplasmic-reticulum cisternae [intracellular Ca^{2+} stores, (ICS)]. Astroglia express a variety of metabotropic neurotransmitter receptors, which, upon stimulation, cause an opening of Ca^{2+} channels in the membranes of ICS [8] and, consequently, intracellular-free calcium ($[Ca^{2+}]_i$) elevations (Ca^{2+} signalling).

Most of intracellular ATP is provided by oxidative phosphorylation in the mitochondria. Glycolysis contributes only about 25 % to the intracellular ATP production

Maturation Phenomenon in Cerebral Ischemia III
U. Ito et al. (Eds.)
© Springer-Verlag Berlin Heidelberg 1999

in astrocytes [19]. Nevertheless, glycolysis has a significant role for the ATP supply of some intracellular signal-transduction pathways. Thus, the plasma membrane Na^+/K^+-ATPase in neurons and glial cells is fuelled by glycolysis [11]. In a glial cell line, C6 glioma cells, capacitative Ca^{2+} influx, which follows depletion of intracellular Ca^{2+} stores, was reported to be suppressed by inhibition of glycolysis [21].

In the present work, we examined the source of intracellular ATP, which drives metabotropic Ca^{2+} signalling and filling of the Ca^{2+} stores in cultured hippocampal astrocytes. For this, we applied drugs that specifically inhibit either mitochondrial respiration or glycolysis. Metabotropic Ca^{2+} signalling was induced by stimulation of metabotropic P2Y receptors with extracellular ATP. P2Y receptors are present in about 90 % of these cells [3]. The Ca^{2+} content of intracellular stores under metabolic inhibition was assayed by recording, in Ca^{2+}-free medium, the Ca^{2+} signal of astrocytes elicited by an inhibitor of endoplasmic reticulum Ca^{2+} ATPase, cyclopiazonic acid (CPA), which has the technical advantage to inhibit reversibly.

Materials and Methods

Cell cultures were prepared from hippocampi of rats (age 1–5 days) using standard procedures [3]. Cultures were fed with a serum-containing medium every 3–4 days. Cultures were used at 7–9 days after plating, at which time about 60 % of the cells could be identified as astrocytes, according to morphological criteria. The morphological criteria were derived from cells, which were labelled by an antibody directed against the astrocyte-specific glial fibrillary acidic protein. For Ca^{2+} measurements, cells were loaded with acetoxymethyl ester of the Ca^{2+}-sensitive fluorophore fura-2 (Molecular Probes, Eugene, Ore., USA). Fluorescence changes at 510 nm following stimulation were measured with an imaging system (TILL Photonics, Planegg, Germany) attached to a Zeiss Axioscope using alternate excitation at 360 nm and 390 nm. Relative $[Ca^{2+}]$ values ($[Ca^{2+}]_R$) were calculated using the fluorescence ratios determined in Ca^{2+}-free and Ca^{2+}-containing medium at the end of experiments, after cell permeabilization for Ca^{2+} with 4 µM ionomycin. The resting $[Ca^{2+}]$ (20–50 nM) was set to 1. Absolute $[Ca^{2+}]$ was not calculated, thus avoiding the error-prone determination of the intracellular K_D value of fura-2. During the experiments, the cells were perfused with Hanks balanced salt solution (HBSS). All substances were applied by addition to the perfusate. Ca^{2+}-free HBSS was prepared by omitting $CaCl_2$ and adding 0.6 mM ethylene-glycol tetraacetic acid (EGTA). Cells were allowed to recover for 10–15 min in Ca^{2+}-containing HBSS between drug applications. Experiments were performed at 36 °C.

Results

Preliminary experiments were devised to demonstrate that repeated applications of CPA (10 µM) in Ca^{2+}-free medium elicited Ca^{2+} signals of similar size. These results, subsequently, allowed us a comparison of the Ca^{2+} content of Ca^{2+} stores, first in the absence then in the presence of a metabolic inhibitor. Similarly, repeated application of extracellular ATP (10 µM) produces comparable Ca^{2+} signals, thus enabling a reli-

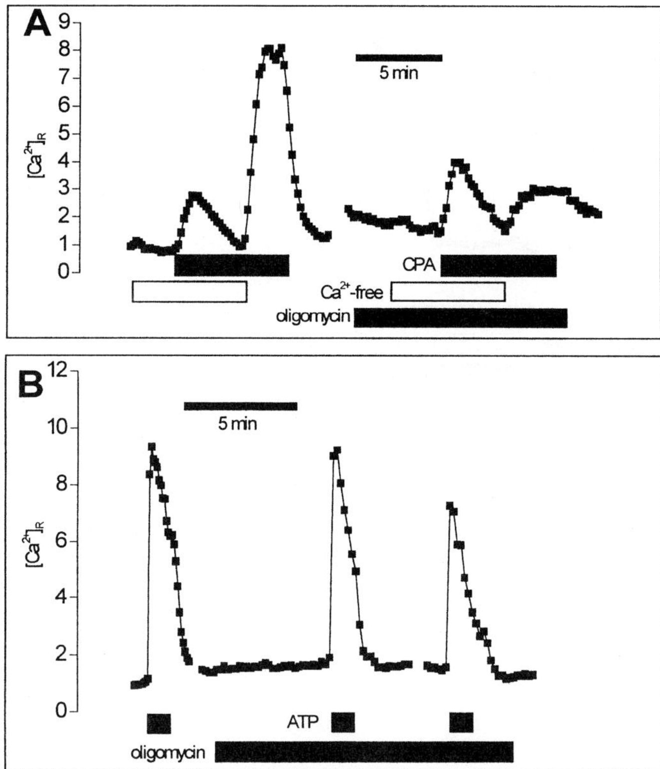

Fig. 1A, B. Astrocytic Ca²⁺ signalling under the influence of inhibition of mitochondrial adenosine triphosphate (ATP) synthesis using oligomycin (10 µM). Cyclopiazonic acid (CPA) (10 µM) was used to inhibit endoplasmic reticulum Ca²⁺ ATPase, and extracellular ATP (10 µM) was applied for purinergic receptor stimulation. **A** The size of the Ca²⁺ signal elicited by CPA in Ca²⁺-free medium was not reduced in the presence of oligomycin, indicating that the Ca²⁺ content of Ca²⁺ stores was not affected by exposure to oligomycin. The Ca²⁺ influx due to depletion of store-operated Ca²⁺ channels was reduced. **B** The amount of the metabotropic Ca²⁺ signal (P2Y-receptor activation by ATP) was not significantly changed in the presence of oligomycin, even after prolonged incubation with oligomycin. This is typical for results from all 12 [14] cells tested. For data shown here and in Fig. 2, each time point (*square*) represents the ratio of two images acquired at 510 nm, while illuminating alternately at 360 nm and 390 nm. Relative calcium concentration ([Ca²⁺]R) in the soma (excluding the nucleus) of an astrocyte was calculated from the ratio of fluorescence intensities. The time periods of substance applications are indicated by the *bars* below the trace. Between subsequent treatments, cells were allowed to recover for at least 10 min (*gaps* in the trace)

able comparison of ATP-elicited metabotropic Ca²⁺ signals in the absence and presence of an effective substance. We also found that the stores that release Ca²⁺ upon purinergic stimulation are sensitive to CPA.(Fig. 1).

Mitochondria supply most of the ATP required by brain cells. We, therefore, investigated whether the Ca²⁺ content of ICS is affected by disturbance in the mitochondrial function by use of specific inhibitors. Inhibition of the mitochondrial ATP synthase with oligomycin (10 µM) did not affect the size of the Ca²⁺ signal elicited by CPA application in Ca²⁺-free medium (Fig. 1A). Consistent with this finding, puri-

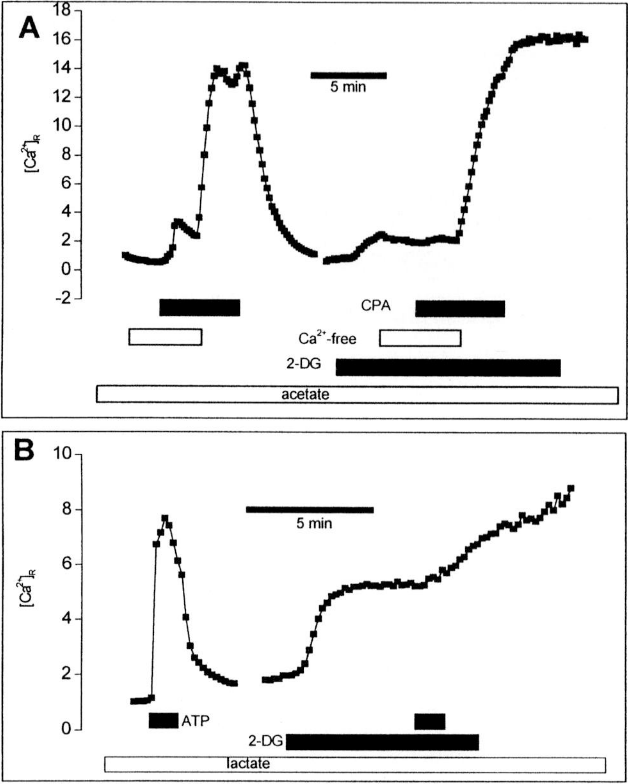

Fig. 2A, B. Effect of glycolysis inhibition using 2-deoxy-D-glucose (2-DG) (10 mM) on astrocytic Ca^{2+} signalling. Substrates (acetate, lactate), which fuel the mitochondrial respiration independently of glycolysis, were supplemented during the course of the experiment. **A** Application of 2-DG abolished the Ca^{2+} signal elicited by cyclopiazonic acid (CPA) in Ca^{2+}-free medium, which indicates emptying of CPA-sensitive stores. The Ca^{2+} elevation induced by 2-DG was irreversible within 10 min after 2-DG withdrawal. Acetate (10 mM) was applied, starting 1 h before beginning the experiment. **B** The purinergic Ca^{2+} signal was completely suppressed. 2-DG increased the resting level of cytosolic Ca^{2+}. The Ca^{2+} elevation was irreversible within 10 min after 2-DG withdrawal. Lactate (10 mM) was applied, starting 15 min before beginning the experiment. The traces in **A** and **B** are typical for 15 of 16 cells tested and all 14 cells tested, respectively

nergic Ca^{2+} signalling was also not significantly changed (Fig. 1B). The ATP supply by mitochondria does not seem to be essential for the loading of CPA-sensitive stores with Ca^{2+} and for purinergic Ca^{2+} signalling. Additional experiments were performed to substantiate this conclusion. Inhibition of the mitochondrial respiratory chain with cyanide (3 mM), or the combined application of cyanide and oligomycin, did not disturb the filling state of CPA-sensitive stores (data not shown), thus confirming our conclusion. The irreversible depletion of CPA-sensitive Ca^{2+} stores and the prevention of metabotropic Ca^{2+} signalling, which was caused by the protonophore carbonyl cyanide p-trifluoromethoxyphenylhydrazone (FCCP, 2 µM, data not shown), was attributed to nonspecific disturbance of cellular membranes (Fig. 2).

Inhibition of glycolysis is accomplished by 2-deoxy-D-glucose (2-DG). To ensure substrate delivery to the mitochondrial respiration during glycolysis inhibition, we additionally supplemented mitochondrial substrates, which are taken up by astrocytes. Cells supplied with 10 mM acetate, starting at the beginning of the experiment, displayed a 2-DG-induced rise in the resting [Ca²⁺] and a more than 80 % reduction of CPA-induced Ca²⁺ signals in Ca²⁺-free medium (in 15 of 16 cells, as shown in Fig. 2A, complete suppression in one cell). Likewise, 2-DG induced a complete suppression of the Ca²⁺ response upon stimulation with extracellular ATP, even if cells were supplied with 10 mM lactate (Fig. 2B). We conclude that failure to refill CPA-sensitive stores and, consequently, failure of purinergic Ca²⁺ signalling, may be caused by glycolysis inhibition by 2-DG. Similarly, the glycolysis inhibitor iodoacetate caused a depletion of CPA-sensitive Ca²⁺ stores in astrocytes supplied with acetate or lactate. Therefore, glycolysis is essential for the refilling of CPA-sensitive Ca²⁺ stores and for the P2-receptor-dependent Ca²⁺ signalling.

Discussion

We identified a decisive function of glycolysis in the signal transduction of glial cells, by demonstrating that glycolysis activity, rather than mitochondrial respiration, is necessary to enable filling of ICS with Ca²⁺ and to maintain the metabotropic-receptor (P2Y)-dependent Ca²⁺ signalling in hippocampus astrocytes. We obtained consistent results using two inhibitors, both of glycolysis (2-DG and iodoacetate) and of oxidative phosphorylation (oligomycin and cyanide).

We demonstrate here that Ca²⁺ filling of CPA-sensitive ICS is dependent on glycolysis; we suppose that the stores investigated by us are myo-D-inositol 1,4,5-trisphosphate (InsP₃)-sensitive stores, because only these are sensitive to CPA and thapsigargin [9, 10]. Ca²⁺ release from InsP₃-sensitive stores is involved in the Ca²⁺ signalling initiated by many neurotransmitters and hormones [8]. Therefore, our findings are of general relevance for metabotropic Ca²⁺ signalling, and we anticipate that the inhibition of metabotropic Ca²⁺ signalling by inhibition of glycolysis is also important in vivo. This conclusion holds true, even when we assume that the expression of metabotropic receptors in astrocytes in culture might be changed, compared with astrocytic cells in situ [12].

A decisive role of glycolysis activity for the active accumulation of Ca²⁺ in ICS was already elucidated in non-neural cells, namely in a macrophage cell line [5] and in quiescent fibroblasts [13]. Glucose addition to the medium was shown to stimulate the endoplasmic reticulum Ca²⁺ ATPase activity in a fibroblast cell line [15], Langerhans' islet cells [2, 18] and a kidney cell line [14], suggesting that ATP provided by glycolysis is utilised by the endoplasmic reticulum pump.

The pronounced role of glycolysis for Ca²⁺ signalling is remarkable because, under normal physiological conditions, mitochondria produce about 75 % of the cellular ATP in cultured astrocytes [19]. If a substrate for the mitochondrial respiration is provided, then the bulk cytosolic ATP concentration is not significantly decreased by glycolysis [20]. Especially in postnatal development, brain cells are able to take up and metabolise several substrates for energy production, which are not subject to glycolysis [7]. Astrocytes can use acetate [4] and lactate [1, 6] as substrates of mitochondria.

Although bulk cytosolic ATP concentrations are hardly affected by glycolysis inhibition, ATP concentrations near membranes might be strongly influenced by the activity or lack of activity of glycolysis enzymes bound to these membranes. Association of phosphoglycerate kinase and pyruvate kinase, the ATP-producing enzymes of glycolysis, with sarcoplasmic reticulum and functional coupling between glycolysis and sarcoplasmic reticulum Ca^{2+} transport were found in rabbit muscle [22]. Ca^{2+} uptake in inside-out plasma-membrane vesicles from smooth muscle [17] is fuelled by glycolysis, and ATP from plasmalemma-bound glycolysis enzymes drives the Na^+/K^+ pump in erythrocytes [16]. The emptying of CPA-sensitive ICS from Ca^{2+} induced by inhibition of glycolysis in hippocampal astrocytes, which was observed by us, could, thus, indicate that glycolytic ATP production and active Ca^{2+} uptake in the astrocytic ICS are functionally coupled.

The physiological role of this coupling still has to be elucidated. It is conceivable that emptying of ICS and the consequent suppression of metabotropic Ca^{2+} signalling protects astrocytes from injury caused by ischemia or metabolic inhibition.

Acknowledgements. This work was supported by BMBF (07NBL04 / 01ZZ9595), Land Sachsen-Anhalt (1899A) and Fonds der Chemischen Industrie.

References

1. Alves PM, McKenna MC, Sonnewald U (1995) Lactate metabolism in mouse brain astrocytes studied by [^{13}C]NMR spectroscopy. Neuroreport 6: 2201–2204
2. Asanuma N, Aizawa T, Sato Y, Schermerhorn T, Komatsu M, Sharp GW, Hashizume K (1997) Two signaling pathways, from the upper glycolytic flux and from the mitochondria, converge to potentiate insulin release. Endocrinology 138: 751–755
3. Bernstein M, Behnisch T, Balschun D, Reymann KG, Reiser G (1998) Pharmacological characterization in cultured hippocampal astrocytes of metabotropic glutamate receptors and P2 purinoceptors which are linked to Ca^{2+} signalling. Neuropharmacol 37: 169–178
4. Brand A, Richterlandsberg C, Leibfritz D (1997) Metabolism of acetate in rat brain neurons, astrocytes and cocultures: metabolic interactions between neurons and glia cells, monitored by NMR spectroscopy. Cell Mol Biol 43: 645–657
5. Darbha S, Marchase RB (1996) Regulation of intracellular calcium is closely linked to glucose metabolism in J774 macrophages. Cell Calcium 20: 361–371
6. Dringen R, Peters H, Wiesinger H, Hamprecht B (1995) Lactate transport in cultured glial cells. Dev Neurosci 17: 63–69
7. Edmond J, Robbins RA, Bergstrom JD, Cole RA, de Vellis J (1987) Capacity for substrate utilization in oxidative metabolism by neurons, astrocytes, and oligodendrocytes from developing brain in primary culture. J Neurosci Res 18: 551–561
8. Finkbeiner SM (1993) Glial calcium. Glia 9: 83–104
9. Golovina VA, Blaustein MP (1997) Spatially and functionally distinct Ca^{2+} stores in sarcoplasmic and endoplasmic reticulum. Science 275: 1643–1648
10. Inesi G, Sagara Y (1994) Specific inhibitors of intracellular Ca^{2+} transport ATPases. J Membr Biol 141: 1–6
11. Kauppinen RA, Enkvist K, Holopainen I, Akerman KE (1988) Glucose deprivation depolarizes plasma membrane of cultured astrocytes and collapses transmembrane potassium and glutamate gradients. Neurosci 26: 283–289
12. Kimelberg HK, Cai Z, Rastogi P, Charniga CJ, Goderie S, Dave V, Jalonen TO (1997) Transmitter-induced calcium responses differ in astrocytes acutely isolated from rat brain and in culture. J Neurochem 68: 1088–1098
13. Kristensen SR (1993) Removal of calcium overload caused by A23187 is more dependent on glycolysis than oxidative phosphorylation. Biochim Biophys Acta 1179: 23–26
14. Lien YH, Wang X, Gillies RJ, Martinez-Zaguilan R (1995) Modulation of intracellular Ca^{2+} by glucose in MDCK cells: role of endoplasmic reticulum Ca^{2+}-ATPase. Am J Physiol 268: F671–F679

15. Martinez GM, Martinez-Zaguilan R, Gillies RJ (1994) Effect of glucose on pH$_{in}$ and [Ca^{2+}]$_{in}$ in NIH-3T3 cells transfected with the yeast P-type H$^+$-ATPase. J Cell Physiol 161: 129–141
16. Mercer RW, Dunham PB (1981) Membrane-bound ATP fuels the Na$^+$/K$^+$ pump. Studies on membrane-bound glycolytic enzymes on inside-out vesicles from human red cell membranes. J Gen Physiol 78: 547–568
17. Paul RJ, Hardin CD, Raeymaekers L, Wuytack F, Casteels R (1989) Preferential support of Ca^{2+} uptake in smooth muscle plasma membrane vesicles by an endogenous glycolytic cascade. FASEB J 3: 2298–2301
18. Roe MW, Mertz RJ, Lancaster ME, Worley JF, Dukes ID (1994) Thapsigargin inhibits the glucose-induced decrease of intracellular Ca^{2+} in mouse islets of Langerhans. Am J Physiol 266:E852–E862
19. Silver IA, Erecinska M (1997) Energetic demands of the Na$^+$/K$^+$ ATPase in mammalian astrocytes. Glia 21: 35–45
20. Swanson RA, Benington JH (1996) Astrocyte glucose metabolism under normal and pathological conditions in vitro. Dev Neurosci 18: 515–521
21. Wu M-L, Kao E, Liu I, Wang B, Lin-Shiau S-Y (1997) Capacitative Ca^{2+} influx in glial cells is inhibited by glycolytic inhibitors. Glia 21: 315–326
22. Xu KY, Zweier JL, Becker LC (1995) Functional coupling between glycolysis and sarcoplasmic reticulum Ca^{2+} transport. Circ Res 77: 88–97

Brain-Derived Neurotrophic Factor and Ciliary Neurotrophic Factor Treatment of Focal Cerebral Ischemia in Rat

K.-A. Hossmann, K. Yamashita, C. Wiessner, and D. Lindholm

Summary. Brain-derived neurotrophic factor (BDNF) and ciliary neurotrophic factor (CNTF) are distributed widely within the central nervous system and convey neuro-protection against apoptosis and various metabolic and excitotoxic insults. We investigated whether these factors could limit infarct size in a model of permanent occlusion of the middle cerebral artery (MCA) in rat. BDNF and CNTF were infused into the territory of the occluded MCA using an osmotic minipump. The infusion was started shortly after vascular occlusion and continued for 24 h. Brains were removed at this time for determination of infarct volume and the presence and distribution of DNA-fragmented cells, using in situ end labeling with terminal deoxynucleotidyl transferase (TUNEL staining). BDNF produced a 33 % reduction of total infarct volume, compared with vehicle-treated animals ($P<0.05$), and a 37 % reduction of cortical-infarct volume ($P<0.05$). Within the striatum or anterior to the infusion side, no significant reduction was observed. CNTF reduced total infarct volume by 18 % and cortical-infarct volume by 26 %, but these changes were not statistically significant. TUNEL-stained cells were located in the center, but not in the periphery of the ischemic territory, into which infarcts expand, and there was no difference in the number and pattern of such cells in treated and untreated animals. These results demonstrate that permanent focal ischemic brain injury can be ameliorated by post-ischemic application of trophic factors, but they do not support the hypothesis that this effect is mediated by an inhibition of apoptosis.

Introduction

Brain injury induced by focal cerebral ischemia is aggravated by secondary molecular abnormalities, which result in the expansion of the ischemic lesion into the surrounding hemodynamically uncompromised tissue. Among the various mechanisms that are thought to contribute to this process, apoptosis has received particular attention. In fact, the volume of brain infarcts has been reduced using drugs that interfere with the signaling cascade leading to programmed cell death [42]. Brain infarcts produced by permanent middle cerebral artery (MCA) occlusion were also smaller in transgenic animals in which a negative mutant of interleukin-1-beta converting enzyme (ICE) was expressed [15]. This mutant acts as a dominant-negative ICE inhibitor and reduces the activity of cysteine proteases that contribute to the execution of apoptotic cell death.

Under physiological conditions, apoptosis is inhibited by trophic factors. Attempts have, therefore, been made to treat brain ischemia by the application of such mole-

Maturation Phenomenon in Cerebral Ischemia III
U. Ito et al. (Eds.)
© Springer-Verlag Berlin Heidelberg 1999

cules. Positive effects have, in fact, been obtained in transient or permanent focal ischemia using transforming growth factor (TGF)-beta 1 [17, 18, 20, 44, 49], basic fibroblast growth factor (bFGF) [14, 25, 34, 57, 58], glia-derived neurotrophic factor (GDNF) [1, 61], neurotrophin-4/5 [9], insulin-like growth factor (IGF) [19] or ciliary neurotrophic factor (CNTF) [35].

Recently, we [64] and others [52] have been interested to know whether focal ischemia can also be treated with brain-derived neurotrophic factor (BDNF), which previously has been shown to attenuate apoptosis in neuronal cultures [30, 38] and improves cell injury after various global forms of hypoxia/ischemia [4, 58]. BDNF and its receptor trkB are widely distributed within the brain [21, 59] and the cloning of the gene for this factor has opened the way for commercial production of a recombinant protein. Another trophic factor with potent neuroprotective activity is CNTF, which can also be produced by recombinant technology. In this chapter, we summarize the results of an experimental study in rats, in which these factors were applied after the onset of permanent MCA occlusion, using osmotic minipump technology for continuous topical application. A more detailed account of this investigation is presented in the original publication [65].

Material and Methods

Male CDF-344 Fischer rats were anesthetized with 0.8 % halothane and 70 % nitrous oxide. Arterial blood pressure, blood gases, blood glucose and hematocrit were monitored, and rectal temperature was kept between 37 °C and 38 °C throughout surgery and up to 1 h after recovery from anesthesia.

The left MCA was exposed and electrocoagulated proximal to the left olfactory tract, using a modification [63] of the technique described by Tamura et al. [55]. Within 15 min of MCA occlusion, a brain infusion cannula was implanted into the center of the MCA territory. Through this cannula, a bolus of 5 µl carrier solution consisting of phosphate-buffered saline (PBS) plus 0.1 % bovine serum albumin (control group, $n=7$), 5 µl carrier solution containing 10 µg BDNF (BDNF-treated group, $n=7$) or 5 µl carrier solution containing 2 µg CNTF (CNTF-treated group, $n=7$) were infused over 5 min. After bolus injection, the infusion cannula was connected to a subcutaneously implanted osmotic minipump (Alzet 2001D, Alza , Palo Alto, Calif.) loaded with 200 µl carrier solution, or neurotrophic-factor solution (0.125 µg/µl BDNF or 0.125 µg/µl CNTF in carrier-solution). The pump infusion rate was 8 µl/h, resulting in a delivery of 1 µg/h BDNF or CNTF into the brain over 24 h. The total dose (bolus plus infusion) thus amounted to 34 µg BDNF and 26 µg CNTF.

Experiments were terminated 24 h after MCA occlusion by transcardiac perfusion with 4 % paraformaldehyde in PBS under deep anesthesia. Brains were embedded in paraffin, and coronal sections (5 µm) were prepared for histological staining with cresyl-violet and hematoxylin and eosin. Infarct volume was calculated by planimetry, using edema corrections, as proposed by Swanson et al. [53]. Ischemic brain swelling was calculated by subtracting the volume of the intact from the ischemic hemisphere, and expressing it as a percentage of the non-ischemic hemisphere.

For in situ end labeling of fragmented DNA (TUNEL staining), brain sections (5 µm) were deparaffinized and incubated for 60 min at 37 °C in 14 µM biotin-16-

dUTP (Boehringer Mannheim, FRG) and 60 U/ml terminal deoxynucleotidyl transferase (Life Technologies, Eggenstein, Germany). Incorporated biotin was visualized using the ABC method (Vector Laboratories, Burlingame, Calif.), as recommended by the supplier.

All values are presented as mean ± SD. Differences of physiological variables were tested for statistical significance using two-way analysis of variance (ANOVA) followed by Scheffé's test for multiple comparisons between experimental groups. For all other statistical evaluations, one-way ANOVA followed by Fisher's protected least-squares difference test for multiple comparisons was used; $P<0.05$ was considered to indicate a statistically significant difference.

Results

Mean arterial blood pressure (MABP), arterial blood gases (PaO$_2$, PaCO$_2$, pH), blood glucose, hematocrit or rectal temperature did not change during the experiment and did not differ between control animals and BDNF- or CNTF-treated animals (Table 1). The mild degree of hypercapnic acidosis, which is typical for spontaneously breathing, halothane-anesthetized rats, was also similar in control and treated animals. Rectal temperature was monitored for 60 min into the recovery phase and remained constant during this time. In a parallel study [64], in which body temperature was recorded for 24 h after MCA occlusion, no ischemia-induced hyperthermia was found. Unspecific therapeutic effects due to temperature changes are, therefore, unlikely.

In accordance with previous studies, the coagulation model of permanent focal ischemia used in this investigation resulted in well-demarcated infarcts in the territory of the MCA at 24 h after MCA occlusion. In the untreated animals, the edema-corrected infarct volume (calculated by subtracting the volume of non-ischemic tissue on the side of vascular occlusion from that of the opposite hemisphere) amounted to 71.4±27.1 mm^3 (Table 2). About half of this volume was located in cerebral cortex and the other half in the striatum. Brain infarction resulted in swelling of the ischemic hemisphere by about 20 %. After treatment with BDNF (total dose 34 µg; $n=7$), infarct volume was reduced by 33 % (48.0±10.9 mm^3; $P< 0.05$). Cortical-infarct

Table 1. Physiological variables

Variable	Untreated ($n=7$)		BDNF ($n=7$)		CNTF ($n=7$)	
	Control	Ischemia	Control	Ischemia	Control	Ischemia
MABP (mmHg)	126±9	122±10	124±9	124±8	124±8	119±10
PaO$_2$ (mmHg)	152±17	155±16	145±12	156±14	146±15	158±14
PaCO$_2$ (mmHg)	51.5±3.0	52.4±2.5	51.7±3.2	50.2±3.2	49.8±2.4	50.7±2.7
pH	7.28±0.3	7.25±0.3	7.27±0.03	7.30±0.03	7.27±0.04	7.27±0.05
Glucose (gm/dl)	138±24	140±15	143±11	156±20	145±13	146±14
Hematocrit (percent)	45±1	45±3	45±3	46±3	45±2	46±3
Rectal temperature (°C)	37.7±0.4	37.4±0.4	37.6±0.3	37.8±0.2	37.8±0.2	37.5±0.3

Control measurements were made 5 min before and 60 min after middle cerebral artery occlusion. Values are means ± SD; no statistical differences between control and ischemia measurements or between groups

Table 2. Morphometric analysis of BDNF and CNTF treatment

Parameter	Untreated	BDNF (n=7)	CNTF (n=7)
Left hemisphere volume (mm³)	300±47	278±31	264±22
Right hemisphere volume (mm³)	246±44	231±24	220±26
Total brain volume (mm³)	546±91	509±55	484±48
Swelling (%)	22.5±8.1	20.2±5.1	20.7±9.2
Total infarct volume (mm³)	71.4±27.1	48.0±10.9* (33 % reduction)	60.2±18.6 (16 % reduction)
Cortical infarct volume (mm³)	37.2±15.1	23.4±6.8* (37 % reduction)	28.7±12.5 (23 % reduction)
Striatal infarct volume (mm³)	34.2±13.3	24.6±5.6 (28 % reduction)	31.5±10.3 (8 % reduction)

Values are means ± SD; *P<0.05 (compared to control group, Fisher's PLSD)

reduction amounted to 37 % (23.4±6.8 mm³; P < 0.05). Within the striatum, a reduction of the infarct volume by 28 % was observed, which, however, did not reach statistical significance. The slice-by-slice analysis of the cortical-infarct areas revealed that the reduction in infarct size was most obvious in the posterior parts of the brain (9.5–7.0 mm anterior to the interaural line), whereas infarct areas in the rostral parts (12–10 mm anterior to the interaural line) were of similar size (Fig. 1). This difference cannot be explained by differences in the supply of BDNF, because the cannula was implanted in the center of the infarct at 9.2 mm anterior to the interaural line.

Infusion of CNTF (total dose 26 µg; n=7) reduced mean total or cortical-infarct volume by about 20 %, but this difference was not statistically significant (Table 2). The slice-by-slice analysis of cortical infarcts revealed a similar pattern of infarct reduction as after BDNF, but this difference did not reach statistical significance either (Fig. 1).

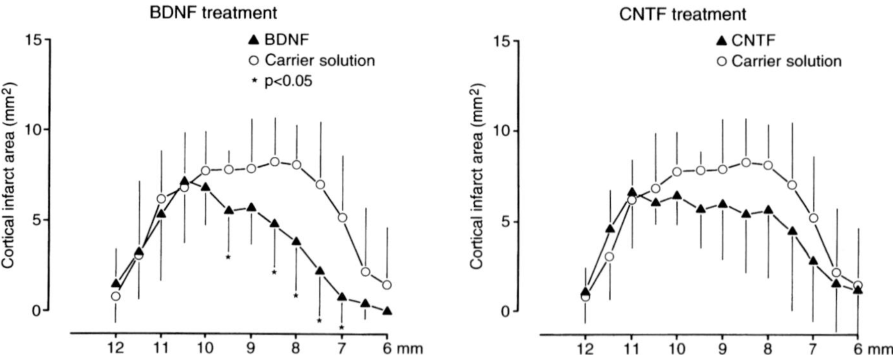

Fig. 1. Planimetric evaluation of brain infarcts after 24 h middle cerebral artery (MCA) occlusion with and without brain-derived neurotrophic factor (BDNF) and ciliary neurotrophic factor (CNTF) treatment. Values refer to cross-sectional areas of ischemic injury at the indicated stereotactic planes. Comparison of treated animals (BDNF n=7; CNTF n=7, *filled circles*) with vehicle-treated animals (n=7 *open circles*) revealed a statistically significant difference for BDNF treatment at planes 7.0–9.5 anterior to the interaural line. Values are mean ± SD; * P<0.05

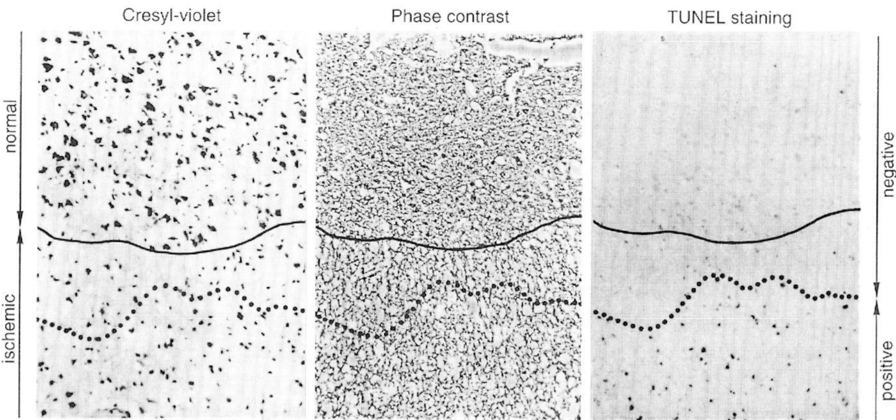

Fig. 2. Cresyl-violet and TUNEL stainings of adjacent histological sections passing through the border zone of brain infarct at 24 h after the onset of permanent middle cerebral artery (MCA) occlusion of brain-derived neurotrophic factor (BDNF)-treated rat. The TUNEL-stained section is also shown under phase contrast to highlight the demarcation between infarcted (*bottom*) and normal (*top*) brain tissue. The outer margin of the region with TUNEL-positive neurons (*dotted line*) and the outer margin of the infarcted tissue (*solid line*) is projected on all three micrographs. The data show that TUNEL-positive neurons are absent in the peripheral parts of evolving infarct, indicating that apoptosis is not a prominent feature of infarct expansion

Histological examination of cresyl-violet- and hematoxylin-and-eosin-stained sections passing through the ischemic lesion showed the typical appearance of subacute ischemic infarcts in the territory of the left MCA. Cresyl-violet staining was markedly reduced, although some shrunken neurons and other cellular elements were still present (Fig. 2). In phase-contrast microscopy, the infarcted tissue appeared spongiform. In the infarct core, numerous cells were heavily stained by in situ end-labeling with terminal deoxynucleotidyl transferase (TUNEL-staining). Between infarcted areas with TUNEL-positive cells and the intact tissue, a severely damaged transition zone with only few TUNEL-positive cells was consistently observed. In the normal brain tissue, TUNEL-positive cells were rarely found. This was also true for the intact tissue immediately adjacent to the infarct. The appearance of the infarct border zone, as exemplified in Fig. 2, was similar in all brains, irrespective of the treatment. Likewise, counting the number of TUNEL-positive cells in the center of the ischemic territory did not reveal significant differences between untreated and treated animals. No inflammatory infiltrates (macrophages, leukocytes) were observed in any of the brains.

Discussion

Our results are in line with two previous investigations, which also demonstrated neuroprotection by BDNF and CNTF during permanent focal ischemia [35, 52]. Schabitz et al. [52] delivered BNDF intraventricularly for 8 days, starting 24 h before MCA occlusion, and reported a 40 % reduction of total infarct volume. Our study revealed a slightly lesser protective effect, but we started infusion after – and not before – vascular occlusion, and we corrected infarct volume for edema formation, which, in this model, contributes substantially to the total lesion size. The results obtained in the two studies are, therefore, coherent and confirm that treatment with BDNF reliably reduces infarct size.

Successful treatment with CNTF was reported by Kumon et al. [35], who infused this molecule continuously for 4 weeks into the lateral ventricle of spontaneously hypertensive rats after the onset of permanent MCA occlusion. Similar to our study, the reduction of infarct size was less pronounced than with BDNF, but even this limited reduction in tissue injury prevented the occurrence of spatial learning disability and underlines the functional importance of this new therapeutic approach.

As far as the mechanisms of BDNF are concerned, various modes of action are conceivable. The most attractive explanation would be the prevention of an apoptotic type of ischemic cell death. It has been suggested that programmed cell death may contribute to the progression of ischemic injury after both global [5, 45] and focal ischemia [36, 42]. BDNF is a potent neuronal survival factor in vitro [2, 16, 26] and has also been shown to prevent the activation of an intrinsic death program in vitro [30, 39] and in vivo [13, 27]. During recirculation following transient global ischemia, BDNF messenger RNA (mRNA) is expressed in the resistant areas of the brain [32, 40, 41, 54] and in transient or permanent focal ischemia in the periphery of the evolving infarct [3, 23, 33, 37]. The increased expression of BDNF mRNA following ischemia could be interpreted as a protective measure against the insult, as BDNF may counteract cell death of neurons carrying the corresponding trkB receptor. This interpretation is supported by the observation that in stroke-prone spontaneously hypertensive rats, which are characterized by a high incidence of spontaneous brain infarcts, the trkB receptor is mutated [28]. Conversely, the increase in BDNF expression by preischemic conditioning with spreading depressions increases the tolerance of the brain to ischemic injury [29].

However, there are also arguments against the role of apoptosis as the major mechanism of ischemic injury, particularly after focal cerebral ischemia. Neuropathological studies have failed to document the typical morphological pattern of apoptosis, which differs distinctly from the much more common necrotic type of ischemic cell damage [7]. This is at variance with the demonstration of DNA fragmentation, which has been associated with apoptosis and can be detected by TUNEL staining [10, 12, 36, 48]. In the present study, we did not observe any differences between untreated and BDNF- or CNTF-treated animals, although the infarct size was distinctly smaller in the treated groups. Moreover, TUNEL-positive cells were located in the center and not in the periphery of the evolving infarct, where apoptosis should be expected to dominate if it contributes to infarct growth. Our data, therefore, do not support the hypothesis that BNDF or CNTF ameliorate focal ischemia by inhibiting apoptotic cell death.

An alternative explanation of the beneficial effect of BDNF could be amelioration of excitotoxicity, as previously shown in vitro [39] and in vivo [60]. Although the pathogenetic importance of excitotoxicity in ischemia has been disputed [22], glutamate must be involved in some way, because glutamate antagonists are able to reduce infarct volume [6, 43]. There are also striking similarities between the increased BDNF-mRNA expression in focal ischemia and that of various other pathologies associated with glutamate release, such as spreading depression [24, 50], hypoglycemia [31, 40] or seizures [31, 50]. However, the glutamate antagonist MK-801 decreases BDNF expression only in some parts of the brain, such as hippocampus [8], but causes prominent induction in other regions [8, 11].

BDNF may also interfere with another putative mechanism of ischemic cell injury, i.e., nitric-oxide toxicity. There is now solid evidence that inhibition of neuronal nitric-oxide synthase (nNOS) reduces infarct size [11]. This effect is the opposite of the inhibition of endothelial NOS, which tends to increase infarct volume [11] because the associated increase in vascular tone impairs autoregulation and collateral blood supply to the ischemic territory [56]. BDNF has been shown to inhibit neuronal NOS expression and to promote neuronal survival after ventral-route avulsion [46], which would be in line with the present finding of an amelioration of ischemic injury.

Finally, the possibility of a flow-promoting action has to be considered. Although the hemodynamic effects of BDNF have not been investigated so far, there is evidence that another trophic factor, bFGF, is a potent vasodilator, which decreases infarct size by improving collateral blood supply [14, 57]. This effect is probably brought about by the stimulation of endothelial NOS, because the co-administration of the NOS inhibitor N^G-nitro-L-arginine methylester (L-NAME) attenuates this response [51]. It, therefore, would be of interest to find out whether a similar mechanism could contribute to the therapeutic effect of BDNF.

The reduction of infarct volume by CNTF was less pronounced and did not reach statistical significance. This could be due to the lower initial dose, but also to a different mechanism of therapeutic intervention. CNTF is a multifunctional protein which, in addition to its trophic effect, controls neuronal and glial differentiation. However, its protective effect on excitotoxicity and selective vulnerability after global ischemia [62] is similar to that observed following BDNF and other neurotrophic factors, suggesting a common mode of action.

Although the precise mechanism of BDNF and CNTF treatment remains to be clarified, their therapeutic efficacy recommends clinical application in stroke. Obviously, direct infusion into the tissue would not be feasible under clinical conditions, but systemic application may be beneficial, as previously shown for bFGF [14]. It also remains to be seen whether the specific membrane receptors of BDNF and CNTF, trkB and CNTFR$_a$, respectively, can be activated by a barrier-permeable agonist. Finally, the possibility of trophic-factor transfection using adenovirus-mediated gene transfer [47] could be explored.

In conclusion, the present study demonstrates a marked therapeutic effect of BDNF, and to a lesser extent of CNTF, on ischemic brain infarct, which suggests that survival of ischemic tissue requires trophic support. Substitution of trophic factors is, therefore, a rational way for stroke treatment, which should be explored in more detail in the future.

Acknowledgements. BDNF and CNTF were kindly provided by Regeneron Co., Terrytown, N.Y., USA. We thank S. Krause and M. Jagodnik for competent technical assistance and Mrs. D. Schewetzky for the preparation of the manuscript.

References

1. Abe K, Hayashi T, Itoyama Y (1997) Amelioration of brain edema by topical application of glial cells line-derived neurotrophic factor in reperfused rat brain. Neurosci Lett 231: 37–40
2. Alderson RA, Alterman AL, Barde YA, Lindsay RM (1990) Brain-derived neurotrophic factor increases survival and differentiated functions of rat septal cholinergic neurons in culture. Neuron 5: 297–306
3. Arai S, Kinouchi H, Akabane A, Owada Y, Kamii H, Kawase M, Yoshimoto T (1996) Induction of brain-derived neurotrophic factor (BDNF) and the receptor trk B mRNA following middle cerebral artery occlusion in rat. Neurosci Lett 211: 57–60
4. Beck T, Lindholm D, Castren E, Wree A (1994) Brain-derived neurotrophic factor protects against ischemic cell damage in rat hippocampus. J Cereb Blood Flow Metab 14: 689–692
5. Beilharz EJ, Williams CE, Dragunow M, Sirimanne ES, Gluckman PD (1995) Mechanisms of delayed cell death following hypoxic-ischemic injury in the immature rat: evidence for apoptosis during selective neuronal loss. Mol Brain Res 29: 1–14
6. Buchan AM, Lesiuk H, Barnes KA, Li H, Huang ZG, Smith KE, Xue D (1993) Ampa antagonists – do they hold more promise for clinical stroke trials than NMDA antagonists. Stroke 24[Suppl I]:148–152
7. Campagne MV, Gill R (1996) Ultrastructural morphological changes are not characteristic of apoptotic cell death following focal cerebral ischaemia in the rat. Neurosci Lett 213: 111–114
8. Castren E, Berzaghi MD, Lindholm D, Thoenen H (1993) Differential effects of MK-801 on brain-derived neurotrophic factor messenger RNA levels in different regions of the rat brain. Exp Neurol 122: 244–252
9. Chan KM, Lam DTN, Pong K, Widmer HR, Hefti F (1996) Neurotrophin-4/5 treatment reduces infarct size in rats with middle cerebral artery occlusion. Neurochem Res 21: 763–767
10. Charriaut-Marlangue C, Margaill I, Represa A, Popovici T, Plotkine M, Benari Y (1996) Apoptosis and necrosis after reversible focal ischemia: an in situ DNA fragmentation analysis. J Cereb Blood Flow Metab 16: 186–194
11. Dalkara T, Moskowitz MA (1994) The complex role of nitric oxide in the pathophysiology of focal cerebral ischemia. Brain Pathol 4: 49–57
12. Du C, Hu R, Csernansky CA, Hsu CY, Choi DW (1996) Very delayed infarction after mild focal cerebral ischemia: a role for apoptosis? J Cereb Blood Flow Metab 16: 195–201
13. Enfors P, Vandewater T, Loring J, Jaenisch R (1995) Complementary roles of BDNF and NT-3 in vestibular and auditory development. Neuron 14: 1153–1164
14. Fisher M, Meadows ME, Do T, Weise J, Trubetskoy V, Charette M, Finklestein SP (1995) Delayed treatment with intravenous basic fibroblast growth factor reduces infarct size following permanent focal cerebral ischemia in rats. J Cereb Blood Flow Metab 15: 953–959
15. Friedlander RM, Gagliardini V, Hara H, Fink KB, Li WW, Macdonald G, Fishman MC, Greenberg AH, Moskowitz MA, Yuan JY (1997) Expression of a dominant negative mutant of interleukin-1-beta converting enzyme in transgenic mice prevents neuronal cell death induced by trophic factor withdrawal and ischemic brain injury. J Exp Med 185: 933–940
16. GhoshA, Carnahan J, Greenberg ME (1994) Requirement for BDNF in activity-dependent survival of cortical neurons. Science 263: 1618–1623
17. Gross CE, Bednar MM, Howard DB, Sporn MB (1993) Transforming growth-factor-beta-1 reduces infarct size after experimental cerebral-ischemia in a rabbit model. Stroke 24: 558–562
18. Gross CE, Howard DB, Dooley RH, Raymond SJ, Fuller S, Bednar MM (1994) TGF-beta 1 post-treatment in a rabbit model of cerebral ischaemia. Neurol Res 16: 465–470
19. Guan J, Williams C, Gunning M, Mallard C, Gluckman P (1993) The effects of IGF-1 treatment after hypoxic-ischemic brain injury in adult rats. J Cereb Blood Flow Metab 13: 609–616
20. Henrich-Noack P, Prehn JHM, Krieglstein J (1994) Neuroprotective effects of TGF-beta 1. J Neural Transm Suppl:33–45
21. Hofer M, Paglinsi SR, Hohn A, Leibrock J, Barde Y-A (1990) Regional distribution of brain derived neurotrophic factor mRNA in the adult mouse brain. EMBO J 9: 2459–2464
22. Hossmann K-A (1994) Glutamate-mediated injury in focal cerebral ischemia – the excitotoxin hypothesis revised. Brain Pathol 4: 23–36
23. Hsu CY, An G, Liu JS, Xue JJ, He YY, Lin TN (1993) Expression of immediate early gene and growth factor mRNAs in a focal cerebral ischemia model in the rat. Stroke 24: 178–181
24. Isackson PJ, Huntsman MM, Murray KD, Gall CM (1991) BDNF mRNA expression is increased in adult rat forebrain after limbic seizures: temporal pattern of induction distinct from NGF. Neuron 6: 937–948

25. Jiang N, Finklestein SP, Do TY, Caday CG, Charette M, Chopp M (1996) Delayed intravenous administration of basic fibroblast growth factor (bFGF) reduces infarct volume in a model of focal cerebral ischemia/reperfusion in the rat. J Neurol Sci 139: 173–179
26. Johnson JE, Barde YA, Schwab MA, Thoenen H (1986) Brain-derived neurotrophic factor supports the survival of cultured rat retinal ganglion cells. J Neurosci 6: 3031–3038
27. Jones KR, Farinas I, Backus C, Reichard LF (1994) Targeted disruption of the BDNF gene perturbs brain and sensory neuron development but not motor neuron development. Neuron 76: 989–999
28. Kageyama H, Nemoto K, Nemoto F, Sekimoto M, Nara Y, Nabika T, Iwayama Y, Fukamachi K, Tomita I, Senba E, Forehand CJ, Hendley ED, Ueyama T (1996) Mutation of the trkB gene encoding the high-affinity receptor for brain-derived neurotrophic factor in stroke- prone spontaneously hypertensive rats. Biochem Biophys Res Commun 229: 713–718
29. Kawahara N, Croll SD, Wiegand SJ, Klatzo I (1997) Cortical spreading depression induces long-term alterations of BDNF levels in cortex and hippocampus distinct from lesion effects – implications for ischemic tolerance. Neurosci Res 29: 37–47
30. Koh JY, Gwag BJ, Lobner D, Choi DW (1995) Potentiated necrosis of cultured cortical neurons by neurotrophins. Science 268: 573–575
31. Kokaia Z, Metsis M, Kokaia M, Bengzon J, Elmer E, Smith ML, Timmusk T, Siesjö BK, Persson H, Lindvall O (1994) Brain insults in rats induce increased expression of the BDNF gene through differential use of multiple promoters. Eur J Neurosci 6: 587–596
32. Kokaia, Z, Nawa H, Uchino H, Elmer E, Kokaia M, Carnahan J, Smith ML, Siesjö BK, Lindvall O (1996) Regional brain-derived neurotrophic factor mRNA and protein levels following transient forebrain ischemia in the rat. Mol Brain Res 38: 139–144
33. Kokaia, A Zhao Q, Kokaia M, Elmer E, Metsis M, Smith ML, Siesjö BK, Lindvall O (1995) Regulation of brain-derived neurotrophic factor gene expression after transient middle cerebral artery occlusion with and without brain damage. Exp Neurol 136: 73–88
34. Koketsu N, Berlove DJ, Moskoswitz MA, Kowall NW, Caday CG, Finklestein SP (1994) Pretreatment with intraventricular basic fibroblast growth factor decreases infarct size following focal cerebral ischemia in rats. Ann Neurol 35: 451–457
35. Kumon Y, Sakaki S, Watanabe H, Nakano K, Ohta S, Matsuda S, Yoshimura H, Sakanaka M (1996) Ciliary neurotrophic factor attenuates spatial cognition impairment, cortical infarction and thalamic degeneration in spontaneously hypertensive rats with focal cerebral ischemia. Neurosci Lett 206: 141–144
36. Li Y, Chopp M, Jiang N, Zaloga C (1995) In situ detection of DNA fragmentation after focal cerebral ischemia in mice. Mol Brain Res 28: 164–168
37. Lin TN, Chen JJ, Wang SJ, Cheng JT, Chi SI, Shyu AB, Sun GY, Hsu CY (1996) Expression of NGFI-B mRNA in a rat focal cerebral ischemia-reperfusion model. Mol Brain Res 43: 149–156
38. Lindholm D, Carroll P, Tzimagiorgis G, Thoenen H (1996) Autocrine-paracrine regulation of hippocampal neuron survival by IGF-1 and the neurotrophins BDNF, NT-3 and NT-4. Eur J Neurosci 8: 1452–1460
39. Lindholm D, Dechant G, Heisenberg C-P, Thoenen H (1993) Brain-derived neurotrophic factor (BDNF) is a survival factor for cultured granule neurons and protects them against glutamate-induced neurotoxicity. Eur J Neurosci 5: 1455–1464
40. Lindvall O, Ernfors P, Bengzon J, Kokaia Z, Smith ML, Siesjö BK, Persson H (1992) Differential regulation of mRNAs for nerve growth factor, brain-derived neurotrophic factor, and neurotrophin 3 in the adult rat brain following cerebral ischemia and hypoglycemic coma. Proc Natl Acad Sci USA 89: 648–652
41. Lindvall O, Kokaia Z, Bengzon J, Elmer E, Kokaia M (1994) Neurotrophins and brain insults. Trends Neurosci 17: 490–496
42. Linnik MD, Zobrist RH, Hatfield MD (1993) Evidence supporting a role for programmed cell death in focal cerebral ischemia in rats. Stroke 24: 2002–2008
43. McCulloch J (1994) Glutamate receptor antagonists in cerebral ischaemia. J Neural Transm Suppl:71–79
44. McNeill H, Williams C, Guan J, Dragunow M, Lawlor P, Sirimanne E, Nikolics K, Gluckman P (1994) Neuronal rescue with transforming growth factor-beta(1) after hypoxic-ischaemic brain injury. Neuroreport 5: 901–904
45. Nitatori T, Sato N, Waguri S, Karasawa Y, Araki H, Shibanai K, Kominami E, Uchiyama Y (1995) Delayed neuronal death in the CA1 pyramidal cell layer of the gerbil hippocampus following transient ischemia is apoptosis. J Neurosci 15: 1001–1011
46. Novikov L, Novikova L, Kellerth JO (1995) Brain-derived neurotrophic factor promotes survival and blocks nitric oxide synthase expression in adult rat spinal motoneurons after ventral root avulsion. Neurosci Lett 200: 45–48

47. Ooboshi H, Welsh MJ, Rios CD, Davidson BL, Heistad DD (1995) Adenovirus-mediated gene transfer in vivo to cerebral blood vessels and perivascular tissue. Circ Res 77: 7–13
48. Petito CK, Torres-Munoz J, Roberts B, Olarte JP, Nowak TS Jr, Pulsinelli WA (1997) DNA fragmentation follows delayed neuronal death in CA1 neurons exposed to transient global ischemia in the rat. J Cereb Blood Flow Metab 17: 967–76
49. Prehn JHM, Backhauss C, Krieglstein J (1993) Transforming growth-factor-beta-1 prevents glutamate neurotoxicity in rat neocortical cultures and protects mouse neocortex from ischemic injury in vivo. J Cereb Blood Flow Metab 13: 521–525
50. Rocamora N, Palacios JM, Mengod G (1992) Limbic seizures induce a differential regulation of the expression of nerve growth factor, brain-derived neurotrophic factor and neurotrophin-3, in the rat hippocampus. Mol Brain Res 13: 27–33
51. Rosenblatt S, Irikura K, Caday CG, Finklestein SP, Moskowitz MA (1994) Basic fibroblast growth factor dilates rat pial arterioles. J Cereb Blood Flow Metab 14: 70–74
52. Schabitz WR, Schwab S, Spranger M, Hacke W (1997) Intraventricular brain-derived neurotrophic factor reduces infarct size after focal cerebral ischemia in rats. J Cereb Blood Flow Metab 17: 500–506
53. Swanson RA, Morton MT, Tsao-Wu G, Savalos RA, Davidson C, Sharp FA (1990) A semiautomated method for measuring brain infarct volume. J Cereb Blood Flow Metab 10: 290–293
54. Takeda A, Onodera H, Sugimoto A, Kogure K, Obinata M, Shibahara S (1993) Coordinated expression of messenger RNAs for nerve growth factor, brain-derived neurotrophic factor and neurotrophin-3 in the rat hippocampus following transient forebrain ischemia. Neuroscience 55: 23–31
55. Tamura A, Graham DI, McCulloch J, Teasdale GM (1981) Focal cerebral ischemia in the rat: 1. description of technique and early neuropathological consequences following middle cerebral artery occlusion. J Cereb Blood Flow Metab 1: 53–60
56. Tanaka K, Fukuuchi Y, Gomi S, Mihara B, Shirai T, Nogawa S, Nozaki H, Nagata E (1993) Inhibition of nitric oxide synthesis impairs autoregulation of local cerebral blood flow in the rat. Neuroreport 4: 267–270
57. Tanaka R, Miyasaka Y, Yada K, Ohwada T, Kameya T (1995) Basic fibroblast growth factor increases regional cerebral blood flow and reduces infarct size after experimental ischemia in a rat model. Stroke 26: 2154–2158
58. Tsukahara T, Yonekawa Y, Tanaka K, Ohara O, Watanabe S, Kimura T, Nishijima T, Taniguchi T (1994) The role of brain-derived neurotrophic factor in transient forebrain ischemia in the rat brain. Neurosurgery 34: 323–331
59. Valenzuela DM, Maisonpierre PC, Glass DJ, Rojas E, Nunez L, Kong Y, Gies DR, Stitt TN, Ip NY, Yoncopoulos GD (1993) Alternative forms of rat TrkC with different functional capabilities. Neuron 10: 963–974
60. Volpe BT, Wildmann J, Altar CA (1998) Brain-derived neurotrophic factor prevents the loss of nigral neurons induced by excitotoxic striatal-pallidal lesions. Neuroscience 83: 741–748
61. Wang Y, Lin SZ, Chiou AL, Williams LR, Hoffer BJ (1997) Glial cell line-derived neurotrophic factor protects against ischemia-induced injury in the cerebral cortex. J Neurosci 17: 4341–4348
62. Wen TC, Matsuda S, Yoshimura H, Kawabe T, Sakanaka M (1995) Ciliary neurotrophic factor prevents ischemia-induced learning disability and neuronal loss in gerbils. Neurosci Lett 191: 55–58
63. Yamamoto M, Tamura A, Kirino T, Shimizu M, Sano K (1988) Behavioral changes after focal cerebral ischemia by left middle cerebral artery occlusion in rats. Brain Res 452: 323–328
64. Yamashita K, Busch E, Wiessner C, Hossmann K-A (1997) Thread occlusion but not electrocoagulation of the middle cerebral artery produces hypothalamic damage with subsequent hyperthermia. Neurologia medico-chirurgica 37: 723–729
65. Yamashita K, Wiessner C, Lindholm D, Thoenen H, Hossmann K-A (1997) Post-occlusion treatment with BDNF reduces infarct size in a model of permanent occlusion of the middle cerebral artery in rat. Metab Brain Dis 12: 271–280

Environmental Influence on Neurotrophic Gene Expression After Experimental Brain Infarction in the Rat

B. B. Johansson, L.-R. Zhao, and B. Mattsson

Summary. We have investigated whether post-ischemic housing in an activity-stimulating environment stimulates gene expression for brain-derived neurotrophic factor (BDNF), a neurotrophic factor known to stimulate brain plasticity in intact animals, in focal brain ischemia. From 30 h after a middle-cerebral-artery ligation, rats were housed in standard cages or in larger cages, allowing various activities. In situ hybridization was performed on brain from rats killed 2, 3, 7 and 12 days after the arterial ligation. Contrary to our hypothesis, rats in an enriched environment had significantly lower BDNF messenger RNA (mRNA) than rats in standard environment in the peri-infarct area, cortex contralateral to infarction and hippocampus. Determination of whether or not the lower BDNF mRNA levels in activity-stimulated rats corresponds to lower synthesis of BDNF is needed to evaluate the functional significance of the data.

Introduction

One fundamental property of the brain is its plasticity. The current concept on brain plasticity and how it can be modulated in the intact and lesioned brain is essentially based on clinical and experimental data obtained during the last decade [5, 9, 14, 15, 18, 21, 24, 26, 29–32]. Cortical representation areas, cortical maps, are modified by loss of sensory input, such as peripheral nerve block and amputation, by training and experience, as well as in response to focal brain lesions. Some changes occur rapidly, others may take weeks or months to evolve. Post-lesion plasticity is activity dependent and can be influenced by training [20, 21, 32].

Rats housed in an enriched environment with the opportunity for various activities and interaction with other rats perform significantly better than rats housed in a standard laboratory environment after an experimental brain infarction [10, 22], even when the transfer to an enriched environment is delayed for 15 days [7]. A possible explanation to the improved performance would be that an enriched environment stimulates brain plasticity. Brain-derived neurotrophic factor (BDNF) is one of the substances, which has been shown to promote neuronal plasticity in experimental studies. In the visual cortex, BDNF messenger RNA (mRNA) is rapidly regulated by sensory input during development and in adulthood [3]. Hippocampal long-term potentiation (LTP) is impaired in mice lacking BDNF [19] and can be restored by recombinant BDNF [25].

Our aim was to investigate whether gene expression for BDNF can be modified by postoperative environmental factors. Acute ischemia transiently stimulates gene

Maturation Phenomenon in Cerebral Ischemia III
U. Ito et al. (Eds.)
© Springer-Verlag Berlin Heidelberg 1999

induction in the brain for a large number of substances [1, 8, 16]. Therefore, a transient increase in gene expression for BDNF has been observed in the cortex and hippocampus during focal brain ischemia, with a peak expression 4–5 h after induction of ischemia and a return to normal values within 24 h [4, 17]. Our study was not concerned with these early changes, which are related to the acute tissue damage. We addressed the question whether environmental stimuli can modify gene expression in the days and weeks following a ligation of middle cerebral artery (MCA). With this aim, rats were individually caged for 30 h after ligation of the MCA, then either placed in standard or in enriched environment as described below. In situ hybridization for BDNF mRNA was performed on brains from rats killed 2–12 days after arterial ligation.

Methods

The experimental protocol was approved by the local ethical committee for animal research. Male 3-month old spontaneously hypertensive rats were anesthetized with 50 mg/kg IP methohexital sodium (Brietal). Body temperature was kept close to 37 °C. Using a microsurgical approach, the right MCA was occluded distal to the origin of the striatal branches. All rats were preoperatively housed in standard laboratory cages, 550·350·200 mm, each housing 4–5 rats. Postoperatively, the rats were housed in individual cages for 30 h, then either returned to standard cages or to larger cages, 820·610·450 mm, each housing 8–10 rats, with horizontal and inclined boards and equipped with various items, such as a chain, a swing board, wooden blocks or balls [7, 10, 22]. Three times a week, some objects were added and others removed. The rats were anesthetized with methohexital and decapitated 2, 3, 7 and12 days after the arterial ligation; four or five rats were used in each group and time interval. The brains were removed and frozen in isopentane chilled to –40 °C and stored at –70 °C until sectioned. Coronal brain sections, 20-μm thick, were cut in a cryostat at –18 °C.

Cryostat coronal sections through the infarcted area and dorsal hippocampus (Bregma –3.3) were processed for in situ hybridization, using a rat BDNF-mRNA antisense-oligonucleotide probe complementary to nucleotides 650–699 in the sequence of mouse BDNF [17]. Optical-density measurement of BDNF mRNA was performed in cortex surrounding the infarct, contralateral cortex and hippocampus, using a computerized image-analysis system with the software Image Grabber 2.03 (Neotech, Eastleigh, Hampshire, UK) and Image/MG 1.44b (NIH, Bethesda, MD, USA). Fifteen sections 1 mm apart were stained with hematoxylin and eosin for determination of infarct volume. The cortical-infarct volume was calculated and expressed as a percentage of contralateral cortex.

Statistical analysis for difference in gene expression was performed by two-way analysis of variance (ANOVA), with the factors group and time, and a post-hoc analysis (Scheffé's test) if a significant main difference was achieved. Paired t-test was used to compare infarct volumes.

Results

Two rats was excluded because of no infarct or a minor infarct. In the remaining rats, there was no significant difference in cortical tissue loss between the groups at the different times. In the early stage, the presence of edema within the infarct increased the apparent infarct volume. Therefore, at 2 days and 3 days, the mean infarct volume was around 30 % of the contralateral-cortex volume, and then decreased down to 22–27 %.

Rats kept in an activity-stimulating environment had significantly lower BDNF mRNA levels than rats in standard environment in the dorsomedial cortex bordering the infarct, in the contralateral hemisphere and in the hippocampus. The data obtained for rats killed 12 days after the ligation is illustrated in Fig. 1.

Discussion

Our results show that post-ischemic events can significantly alter gene expression for BDNF in the dorsomedial infarct border zone, in the contralateral cortex and bilaterally in the hippocampus, thus including areas distant from the infarct and not subjected to ischemia after ligation of the MCA.

Activation of gene expression in hippocampus is known to occur under various stressful situations including focal brain ischemia [4, 17]. It also takes place in response to environmental stimuli in intact animals [23].

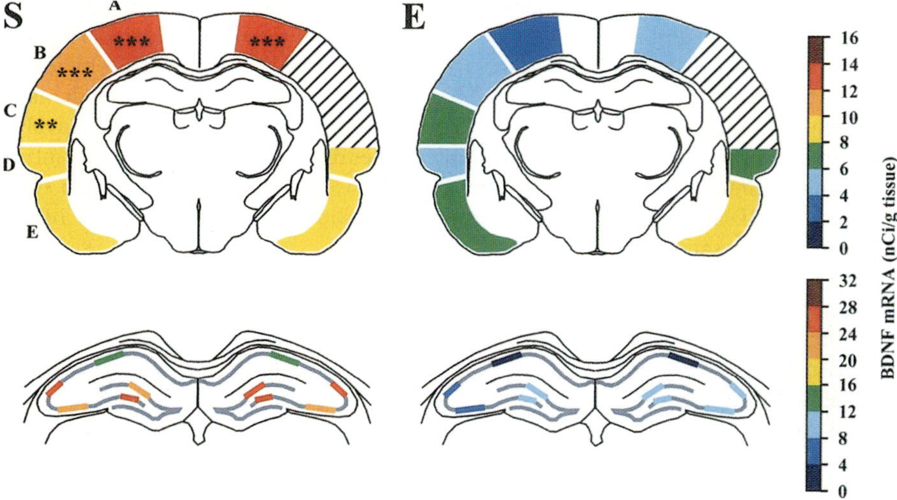

Fig. 1. Pattern of brain-derived neurotrophic factor (BDNF) messenger RNA in cortex and hippocampus 12 days after a distal ligation of the middle cerebral artery in hypertensive rats. *S* rats kept in standard laboratory cages; *E* rats transferred to activity-stimulating larger cages 30 h after the ligation. Note the different scale for cortex and hippocampus. ** $P<0.01$ and *** $P<0.001$ for significant difference from corresponding structures in the enriched group. In hippocampus, the difference was significant for CA1, CA2 and CA4 ($P<0.01$)

The potential role of the contralateral intact hemisphere for functional improvement after brain lesions is controversial. Evidence from clinical and experimental studies is not clear cut. Unilateral damage to the forelimb-representation area of the sensorimotor cortex in adult rats has been reported to increase arborization of layer V pyramidal neurons of the contralateral homotopic cortex, starting about 7 days post-lesion and with a maximum 14–18 days after the lesions [11]. Restriction of movement of the intact limb blocked the dendritic growth and aggravated functional deficits [12]. In a longitudinal ultrastructural study in the same experimental model [13], a significant increase in dendritic volume was observed 18 days after the lesions, and a significant increase in number of synapses per neuron at 30 days. Combined with other studies [5], these observations suggest that plastic changes can evolve over a long time following brain lesions. However, some studies with somewhat different designs have failed to confirm the observation of increased dendritic arborization in corticospinal motor neurons in the intact hemisphere [6, 27]. We are currently investigating dendritic morphology in the contralateral hemisphere to elucidate a possible correlation between changes in BDNF mRNA and dendritic morphology.

Electrophysiological studies in monkeys have shown that tissue surrounding a small cortical lesion in part of the hand-representation area undergoes a further territorial loss in the cortical area representing the hand, perhaps due to non-use or to disruption of local intrinsic cortical circuitry [20]. Specific hand training prevented such changes and induced functional reorganization in the peri-infarct area normally responsive to other parts of the hand [21]. Whether such reorganization can occur after large cortical infarcts remains to be seen. However, the difference in gene expression in the dorsomedial peri-infarct area suggests that this region can also be influenced by post-ischemic events.

The lower gene-expression values in hippocampus, ipsilateral and contralateral cortex in rats housed in enriched environment may seem surprising, considering the proposed role for BDNF in brain plasticity [3, 19, 25]. Pre-ischemic intraventricular administration of exogenous BDNF has been reported to reduce ischemic cell damage in global [2] and focal [28] ischemia. To promote neuronal survival may involve mechanisms other than those needed to induce neuronal plasticity. Moreover, intraventricular administration of exogenous BDNF may reach other target areas than endogenous BDNF and no studies have, thus far, shown that post-ischemic BDNF infusion has the same effect.

The functional significance of post-ischemic gene activation is not clear. The same gene can have good or bad prognostic significance under different conditions [1, 16]. A further important point is that BDNF gene expression does not necessarily correlate with BDNF synthesis. Quantification of BDNF protein is needed to establish whether the lower gene expression in rats exposed to an enriched environment corresponds to lower protein production. The main conclusion of our study is that alterations in gene expression can occur for a long time following an ischemic event and that this can be influenced by environmental stimuli. Further studies are needed to clarify whether the reduced BDNF gene expression in enriched animals is related to the well-established better outcome in such animals [7, 10, 22], or whether it is an unrelated observation.

Acknowledgements. The study was supported by grants from the Swedish Medical Research Council (Project 14x-4968), the Bank of Sweden Tercentenary Foundation, the Swedish Heart and Lung Foundation, and the Swedish Stroke Foundation.

References

1. Atkins PT, Liu PK, Hsu CY (1996) Immediate early gene expression in response to cerebral ischemia. Friend or foe? Stroke 27: 1682–1687
2. Bech R, Lindholm D, Castren E, Wree A (1994) Brain-derived neurotrophic factor protects against ischemic cell damage in rat hippocampus. J Cereb Blood Flow Metab 14: 689–692
3. Castrén E, Zafra F, Thoenen H, Lindholm D et al., (1992) Light regulated expression of brain-derived neurotrophic factor mRNA in rat visual cortex. Proc Natl Acad Sci U S A 89: 9444–9448
4. Comelli MC, Guidolin D, Seren MS, Zanoni R, Canella R, Rubini R, Manev H (1993) Time course, localization and pharmacological modulation of immediate early inducible genes, brain derived neurotrophic factor and trkB messenger RNAs in rat brain following photochemical stroke. Neuroscience 55: 473–490
5. Florence SL, Jain N, Kaas JH (1997) Plasticity of somatosensory cortex in primates. Semin Neurosci 9: 3–12
6. Forgie ML, Gibb R, Kolb B (1996) Unilateral lesions of the forelimb area of rat motor cortex: lack of evidence of use-dependent neural growth in the undamaged hemisphere. Brain Res 710: 249–259
7. Johansson BB (1996) Functional outcome in rats transferred to an enriched environment 15 days after focal brain ischemia. Stroke 27: 324–326
8. Johansson BB (1998) Neurotrophic factors and transplants. In: Goldstrein LB (ed) Restorative neurology: advances in pharmacotherapy for recovery after stroke. Futura, New York, pp 141–166
9. Johansson BB, Grabowski M (1994) Functional recovery after brain infarction: plasticity and neural transplantation. Brain Pathol 4: 85–95
10. Johansson BB, Ohlsson A-L (1996) Environment, social interaction, and physical activity as determinants of functional outcome after cerebral infarction in the rat. Exp Neurol 139: 322–327
11. Jones TA, Schallert T (1992) Overgrowth and pruning of dendrites in adult rats recovering from neocortical damage. Brain Res 581: 156–160
12. Jones TA, Schallert T (1994) Use-dependent growth of pyramidal neurons after neocortical damage. J Neurosci 14: 2140–2152
13. Jones TA, Kleim JA, Greenough WT (1996) Synaptogenesis and dendritic growth in the cortex opposite unilateral sensorimotor cortex damage in adult rats: a quantitative electron microscopic examination. Brain Res 733: 142–148
14. Kaas JH (1991) Plasticity of sensory and motor maps in adult mammals. Ann Rev Neurosci 14: 137–167
15. Kano M, Lino K, Kano M (1991) Functional reorganization of adult cat somatosensory cortex is dependent on NMDA receptors. Neuroreport 2: 77–80
16. Koistinaho J, Hökfelt T (1997) Altered gene expression in brain ischemia. Neuroreport 8: 1–8
17. Kokaia Z, Zhao Q, Kokaia M, Elmer E, Metsis M, Smith M-L, Siesjö BK, Lindvall O (1995) Regulation of brain-derived neurotrophic factor gene expression after transient middle cerebral artery occlusion with and without brain damage. Exp Neurol 136: 73–88
18. Kolb B (1995) Brain plasticity and behaviour. Lawrence Erlboum, New Jersey
19. Korte M, Carroll P, Wolf E et al., Brem G, Theonen H, Bonhoeffer T (1995) Hippocampal long-term potentiation is impaired in mice lacking brain-derived neurotrophic factor. Proc Natl Acad Sci USA 92: 8856–8860
20. Nudo RJ, Wise BM, SiFuentes F, Milliken GW (1996) Neural substrates for the effects of rehabilitative training on motor recovery after ischemic infarct. Science 272: 1791–1794
21. Nudo RJ, Plautz EJ, Milliken GW (1997) Adaptive plasticity in primate motor cortex as a consequence of behavioral experience and neuronal injury. Semin Neurosci 9: 13–23
22. Ohlsson A-L, Johansson BB (1995) Environment influences functional outcome of cerebral infarction in rats. Stroke 26: 644–649
23. Olsson T, Mohammed AH, Donaldson LF, Henriksson BG, Seckl JR (1994) Glucocorticoid receptor and NGFA-A gene expression are induced in the hippocampus after environmental enrichment in adult rats. Brain Res Mol Brain Res 23: 349–353
24. Pascual-Leone A, Torres F (1993) Plasticity of the sensorimotor cortex representation of the reading finger in Braille readers. Brain 116: 39–52

25. Patterson SL, Abel T, Deuel TA, Martin KC, Rose JC, Kandel ER (1996) Recombinant BDNF rescues deficits in basal synaptic transmission and hippocampal LTP in BDNF knockout mice. Neuron 16: 1137–1145
26. Pons TP, Garraghty PE, Mishkin M (1988) Lesion-induced plasticity in the somatosensory cortex of adult macaques. Neurobiology 85: 5279–5281
27. Prusky G, Whishaw IQ (1996) Morphology of identified corticospinal cells in the rat following motor cortex injury: absence of use-dependent change. Brain Res 714: 1–8
28. Schäbitz W-R, Schwab S, Spranger M, Hacke W (1997) Intraventricual brain derived neurotrophic factor reduces infarct size after focal cerebral ischemia in rats. J Cereb Blood Flow Metab 17: 500–506
29. Schieber MH (1995) Physiological basis for functional recovery. J Neuro Rehab 9: 65–71
30. Seitz RJ, Huang Y, Knorr U, Tellmann L, Herzog H, Freund HJ (1995) Large-scale plasticity of the human motor cortex. Neuroreport 6: 742–744
31. Steinberg BA, Augustine JR (1997) Behavioral, anatomical, and physiological aspects of recovery of motor function following stroke. Brain Res Rev 25: 125–132
32. Xerri C, Merzenich MM, Peterson BE, Jenkins W (1998) Plasticity of primary somatosensory cortex paralleling sensorimotor skill recovery from stroke in adult monkeys. J Neurophysiol 79: 2119–2148

Delayed Neuronal Death in Experimental Ischemic Stroke

J.H. Garcia, Z.-R. Ye, K.-F. Liu, and J. A. Gutierrez

Summary. The observations reported in this communication were made in an animal model of ischemic stroke. This designation applies to a syndrome characterized by an abrupt, focal neurological deficit such as monocular blindness. In most instances, these events are thought to be secondary to the thromboembolic occlusion of a large artery. In Wistar rats, the prolonged occlusion of one middle cerebral artery (MCA) produces a brain lesion, which evolves through spongiosis, pannecrosis, and cavitation. A significantly different lesion affects the brain following a transient occlusion of the same artery. Selective neuronal necrosis, astroglial and microglial activation affect the striatum within 12–24 h of the injury. A much more delayed effect is visible in the cortex 3–4 days after the brief ischemic episode. This delayed injury affects only neurons scattered through layers 3–4 of the cortex and is accompanied by microglial activation. In this review, we examine the question: could this delayed cell death be mediated by the activation of caspases, i.e., apoptosis?

Introduction

One of the earliest publications on the subject of the mechanisms responsible for the development of an infarction appeared almost 120 years ago [14]. In experiments conducted in 1880 and based on the ligation of a renal artery, Litten [14] reported two novel observations: (1) the renal artery must remain occluded approximately 2.5 h in order to produce an infarction in the kidney, and (2) the experiment must be allowed to continue for a minimum of 24 h before the first group of necrotic cells can be recognized under the microscope. Pannecrosis or signs of irreversible injury involving the entire arterial territory probably become visible only 3–4 days after the arterial occlusion.

Experiments, comparable with those conducted on the kidney, have been carried out on rats' brains. The origin of one middle cerebral artery (MCA) has been blocked by means of a nylon monofilament, introduced via the external carotid artery. Sequential observations, made at predetermined time intervals, show that for the first 4 h, only isolated foci of vacuolation (or sponginess) exist in the territory of the occluded artery. Signs of necrosis begin to affect increasing numbers of neurons after 6 h [5]. Over 90 % of the striatal neurons are necrotic 24 h after the MCA occlusion (MCAO). Intriguingly, even after this prolonged period of time, only 40 % of the cortical neurons show signs of irreversible injury [6].

Therefore, the lesion initiated by an arterial occlusion evolves over a period of days into spongiosis (first focal, then widespread), neuronal necrosis (first limited to the

Maturation Phenomenon in Cerebral Ischemia III
U. Ito et al. (Eds.)
© Springer-Verlag Berlin Heidelberg 1999

striatum, then spreading to the cortex) and, finally, becomes a wide area pannecrosis or infarction [5].

If the brain lesion consequent to the occlusion of an artery evolves through sequential stages, we asked: can the morphological features and, therefore, the pathogenesis of the lesion be modified by changing the duration of the arterial occlusion? Some observations of patients with ischemic stroke suggest that the answer to this question may be affirmative.

The syndrome of focal neurological deficit, attributed to an arterial occlusion, followed by complete functional recovery within 30–60 min of the beginning of symptoms, has been inferred to result from the restitution of the blood flow [7]. In spite of their functional recovery, a significant percentage of these patients show neuroimaging abnormalities, which are known as ischemic lesions or silent infarcts [4]. For obvious reasons, neither the histological features nor the pathogenesis of these silent ischemic lesions are known. We designed experiments in which the presumptive conditions typical of a transient ischemic attack (TIA) could be mimicked in the experimental model.

Materials and Methods

A total of 130 adult Wistar rats had the origin of one MCAO for periods of 10 min, 15 min, 20 min or 30 min. At the end of the ischemic episode, the filament occluding the artery was withdrawn. Experiments were terminated at variable intervals ranging from 1 day to 4 weeks after the ischemic episode. The features of the brain lesion, thus induced, were contrasted with those observed in two control groups. In the first, the artery was not reopened and the experiments were terminated after 7 days. A second control group had the artery occluded for a period of less than 1 min.

Serial sections of the brain from each rat were evaluated by light- and electron microscopy. Appropriate immunohistochemical methods were performed to identify astroglial and microglial components. Quantitation of many of the changes observed was completed utilizing image analysis. The results were evaluated by analysis of variance (ANOVA) and Student's t-tests.

Results

Each of the experiments involving MCAO of 7-days duration resulted in pannecrosis (infarction) (Fig. 1), involving the entire territory of the occluded artery. Brains subjected to a sham operation and 47 % of those injured by a transient occlusion (<30-min duration) had no detectable changes.

A total of 63 % of the brains exposed to the occlusion of one MCA, lasting 30 min or less, had injuries, which varied in severity as a function of topographic location, duration of the MCAO and duration of the survival after the transient occlusion. None of the 73 rats in this group developed brain infarctions or areas of pannecrosis. Spongiosis, of the type visible after permanent MCAO, was also essentially absent among the brains of rats with transient MCAO.

In the striatum, neuronal necrosis involved mostly the small neurons. Many of the large neurons in this anatomic location remained structurally intact as late as 28 days

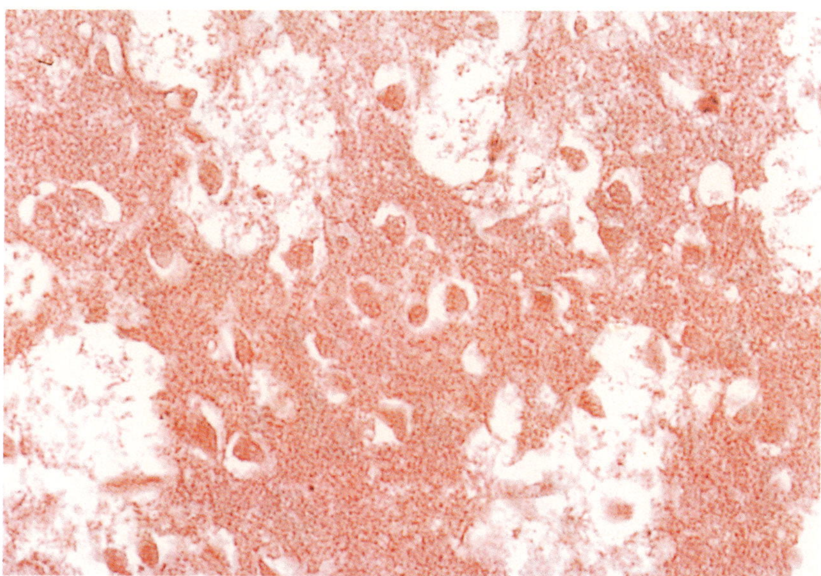

Fig. 1. Brain infarction. Coagulation necrosis as shown by the complete loss of hematoxylinophilia in this area of the striatum. The lesion is the result of the permanent middle-cerebral-artery occlusion (MCAO) of 7 days duration in a Wistar rat. (H&E; original magnification × 160)

after the ischemic episode. The dimensions of the surface area of the striatal lesion, and the number of necrotic neurons were both directly proportional to the duration of the MCAO. Accordingly, numbers of necrotic neurons were highest in the group with arterial occlusions of 30 min and lowest in the group with MCAO of 10-min duration [7]. This type of neuronal death was accompanied by astroglial and microglial activation. However, in contrast to the responses readily visible in infarcts, conversion of microglia into macrophages was not visible in the lesion produced by transient MCAO, even when these lesions were allowed to evolve for up to 28 days.

Compared with the striatum, the appearance of dead neurons in the cortex was considerably delayed. Whereas the numbers of necrotic neurons in the striatum peaked within 12–24 h of the transient ischemic episode, none were visible in the cortex at this time. Structural evidence of neuronal injury was visible in the cortex only 3–4 days after the ischemic episode. The numbers of neurons injured in this manner peaked in the cortex on day 7 after the transient MCAO. The injured neurons had a predictable distribution in layers 3–4 of the frontoparietal cerebral cortex. Frequently, one individual necrotic neuron could be seen adjacent to one or more intact ones. (Fig. 2) In contrast to the reactions observed in the striatum, this type of neuronal death was not accompanied by astrogliosis. Only a subtle, but well-defined response by microglial cells was demonstrable in the cortex. Neither conversion of microglia into macrophages, nor cavitation were observed in any of the cortical lesions induced by transient MCAO.

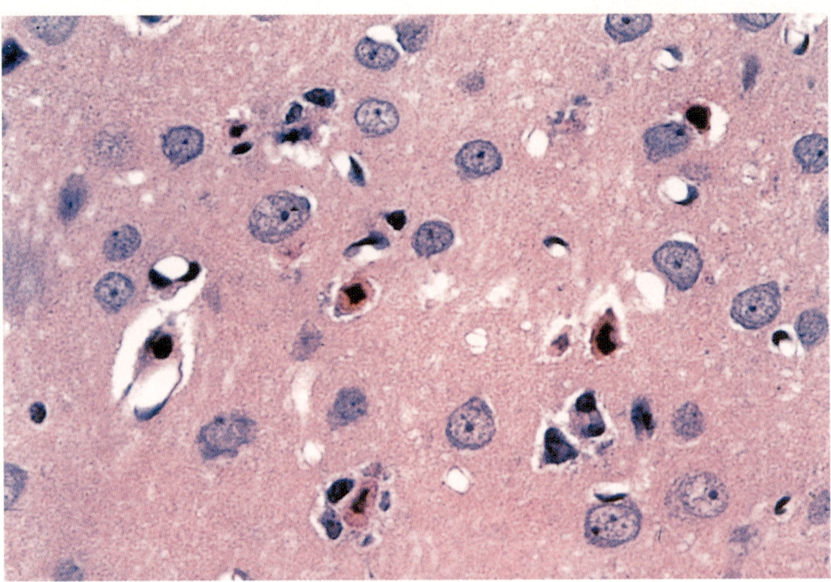

Fig. 2. Incomplete brain infarction. Selective neuronal necrosis (delayed neuronal death) in the cerebral cortex of a Wistar rat with transient middle-cerebral-artery occlusion (MCAO) of 30-min duration. The experiment was terminated 3 days later. (H&E; original magnification × 160)

Discussion

The lapse of several days between the time of the arterial occlusion and the time when dead neurons appear in the cortex, suggests that conditions different from those responsible for the death of neurons in the striatum may be responsible for the death of cortical neurons. In terms of changes in cerebral blood flow, (CBF), two different consequences have been noted at these sites (striatum, cortex) following the occlusion of one MCA. During the initial few hours after the arterial occlusion, CBF values are lower in the striatum than in the cortex. Also, after reopening the artery, the recovery of the normal blood flow is delayed in the cortex, compared with the striatum [17]. This could mean that the striatal lesion is directly related to a marked drop in CBF at this site. In contrast, the injury to the cortical neurons would be mediated by the combination of moderate ischemia, i.e., short-term arterial occlusion, and the effects of reperfusion. Siesjo and collaborators have presented evidence supporting the hypothesis that a generation of free radicals during the period of reperfusion may be one of the most important mechanisms responsible for the secondary type of brain injury, which includes delayed neuronal death [18].

An alternative explanation for the delayed neuronal death, seen in the cortex 4–7 days after transient MCA0, assumes that the short (10-min to 30-min) period of ischemia induces individual cells to express new proteins (bax) or enzymes (caspases). According to this hypothesis, the expression of these genes would be responsible for the death of cells 3–4 days later. Du and associates have asked: could this be similar to the cell death by apoptosis originally described by Kerr in liver made ischemic via the ligation of the hepatic artery? [3]. Subsequent to the publication of Kerr's paper, apoptosis has been popularized as a mechanism of cell death, which is rather easily induced in actively dividing cells, particularly lymphocytes, thymocytes and several types of neoplastic cells [11]. Cell death by apoptosis has been defined as a biologic event, which develops through mechanisms entirely different from those responsible for cell death by necrosis.

Two methods have been propounded as being capable of identifying cells undergoing death by apoptosis. The DNA of cells dying by apoptosis is cleaved into multiple 180-bp to 200-bp fragments, which result in a characteristic "ladder pattern" when separated by means of gel electrophoresis [12]. This pattern is often, but not always, coexistent with the morphological features of apoptosis [13]. Moreover, in the early stages of cell death by necrosis, the resulting DNA fragmentation is also reflected in a "ladder pattern"[19]. Therefore, gel electrophoresis is not a dependable method through which one can consistently separate necrosis from apoptosis.

The molecular endings or "nicks" of DNA fragments in cells undergoing nuclear fragmentation or karyorrhexis can be identified in histology preparations by means of an in situ end-labeling (ISEL) method [2] and by the terminal nucleotide end-labeling deoxyuridine (TUNEL) method [20]. These techniques were thought to be capable of labeling only cells dying by apoptosis. However, several publications have warned that, in appropriately conducted tests, the TUNEL assay fails to discriminate among necrosis, apoptosis and autolysis [8, 9].

Both TUNEL and ISEL detect 3'-OH terminals of DNA fragments, and DNA scission (or karyorrhexis) is common to both necrosis and apoptosis. Regardless of the mechanism by which DNA is fragmented, cell injury accompanied by nuclear fragmentation will result in an increase of 3'-OH terminals, which can be detected in tissues by either TUNEL or ISEL. Also, DNA scission is compatible with cell survival in cases in which DNA is successfully repaired [1]. Consequently, DNA fragmentation should be interpreted simply as an indication of impending cell death. The demonstration of DNA scission does not connote a specific mechanism of cell death. Nuclear fragmentation is a common consequence of lethal cell injury and, most likely, DNA scission is a relatively nonspecific expression of cell damage. A morphologic analysis of neuronal injury by glucocorticoid endangerment failed to reveal DNA cleavage [16].

Morphological alterations are considered the most accurate indicators of apoptosis [10]. The structural alterations characteristic of apoptosis have been summarized as follows [15, 21]:

1. Only individual, isolated cells are involved.
2. Chromatin granules adopt a crescent-like appearance.
3. The cytoplasm becomes condensed and protrusions appear in the form of buds; some of these may break away and become "apoptotic bodies".
4. The cellular debris is promptly phagocytosed by neighboring cells.

On average, the entire process from 1 to 4 is completed over a period of 30 min [15, 21].

Of all the morphologic features listed above, characteristic of apoptosis, we have seen only one in our preparations. Transient arterial occlusions led to the appearance of single, isolated injured neurons. However, cytoplasmic budding, formation of apoptotic bodies and prompt phagocytosis by a neighboring cell were not observed. In fact, in these experiments, dead neurons could be identified in the cortex as late as 48 days after the transient occlusion of the artery.

Based on these morphological observations, we conclude that:

1. Prolonged arterial occlusions (probably lasting longer than 3 h) produce panne-crosis (or infarction), which does not involve the entire arterial territory until 2–3 days after the injury.
2. Transient arterial occlusions produce incomplete brain infarcts [4].

The features of these lesions include: selective neuronal death (limited to a predict-able type of neuron), astrogliosis, and microglial activation. Selective neuronal death in the striatum seems to be directly linked to the initial drop in CBF. In contrast, belated neuronal death in the cortex seems to be mediated by the effects of moderate ischemia and the effects of reperfusion. Such effects may involve the generation of oxygen free radicals and wide-spread injury to the neuronal mitochondria. Astroglio-sis is limited to the striatal territory where there are abundant dead neurons. Astro-glial activation was not a part of the cellular responses at sites of cortical neuronal death. Finally, the features of neurons undergoing delayed death in the cortex are not compatible with those described by Kerr et al. [8] as being characteristic of apoptosis.

Acknowledgement. Partial financial support for this work was provided by USPHS grant NS 31631. The authors are grateful to Jun Xu, Wenji Jiang, and Kelly Ann Ran-dall for technical assistance, and to Lorraine Mayberry for secretarial support.

References

1. Charriaut-Marlangue C, Ben-Ari Y (1995) A cautionary note on the use of the TUNEL stain to determine apoptosis. Neuroreport 7: 61–64
2. Dong Z, Saikumar P, Weinberg, JM et al. (1997) Internucleosomal DNA cleavage triggered by plasma membrane damage during necrotic cell death: involvement of serine, but not cysteine proteases. Am J Pathol 151: 1205–1213
3. Du C, Hu R, Csernansky Ca, Hsu CY, Choi DW (1996) Very delayed infarction after mid focal cerebral ischemia: a role for apoptosis? J Cereb Blood Flow Metab 16: 636–643
4. Fazekas F, Fazekas G, Schmidt R, Kapeller P, Offenbacher H (1996) Magnetic resonance imaging correlates of transient cerebral ischemic attacks. Stroke 27: 607–611
5. Garcia JH, Yoshida Y, Chen H, Li Y, Zhang ZG, Lian J, Chen S, Chopp M (1993) Progression from ischemic injury to infarct following middle-cerebral-artery occlusion in the rat. Am J Pathol 142: 623–635
6. Garcia JH, Liu K-F, Ho K-L (1995) Neuronal necrosis after middle cerebral artery occlusion in Wistar rats progresses at different time intervals in the striatum and the cortex. Stroke 26: 636–643
7. Garcia JH, Liu K-F, Ye Z-R, Gutierrez JA (1997) Incomplete infarct and delayed neuronal death after transient middle cerebral artery occlusion in rats. Stroke 28: 2303–2310
8. Gavrieli Y, Sherman Y, Ben-Sasson SA (1992) Identification of programmed cell death in situ via specific labelling of nuclear DNA fragmentation. J Cell Biol 119: 493–501
9. Grasl-Kraupp B, Buttkay-Nedecky B, Koudelka H et al. (1995) In situ detection of fragmented DNA (TUNEL assay) fails to discriminate among apoptosis, necrosis and autolytic cell death: a cautionary note. Hepatology 21: 1465–1468
10. Hockenbery D (1995) Defining apoptosis. Am J Pathol 146: 16–19
11. Kerr JFR (1965) A histochemical study of hypertrophy and ischemic injury of rat liver with special references to changes in lysosomes. J Pathol Bacteriol 90: 419–435
12. Kerr JFR, Winterford CM, Harmon, BV (1994) Apoptosis: its significance in cancer and cancer therapy. Cancer 73: 2013–2026

13. Yamada T, Ohyama H, Kinjo, Y, Watanabe M (1981) Evidence for the internucleosomal breakage of chromatin in rat thymocytes irradiated in vitro. Radiat Res 85: 544–553
14. Litten M (1880) Untersuchungen uber der hemorrhagischen Infarct und uber die Einwirkung arterieller Anaemie awf das Lebende Gewebe. Z Klin Med 1: 131–227
15. Majno G, Joris I (1995) Apoptosis, oncosis and necrosis: an overview of cell death. Am J Pathol 146: 3–15
16. Masters JN, Finch CE, Sopolsky RM (1989) Glucocorticoid endangerment of hipppocampal neuron does not involve deoxyribomucleic acid cleavage. Endocrinology 124: 3083–3088
17. Nagasawa H, Kogure K (1989) Correlation between cerebral blood flow and histologic changes in a new rat model of middle cerebral artery occlusion. Stroke 120: 1037–1043
18. Siesjo B K, Katsura K, Zhao Q, Folbergrova J, Pahlmark K, Siesjo P, Smith M-L (1995) Mechanisms of secondary brain damage in global and focal ischemia: a speculative synthesis. J Neurotrauma 12: 943–956
19. Tomei LD, Shapiro JP, Cope FO (1993) Apoptosis in C3H/10T1/2 mouse embryonic cells: evidence for internucleosomomal DNA modification in the absence of double-strand cleavage. Proc Natl Acad Sci U S A 90: 853–857
20. Wijsman JH, Jonker RR, Keijer R et al. (1993) A new method to detect apoptosis in paraffin sections: in situ end-labelling of fragmentation DNA. J Histochem Cytochem 41: 7–12
21. Wyllie AH, Kerr JFR, Currie AR (1980) Cell death: the significance of apoptosis. Int Rev Cytol 68: 251–301

A Rat Model to Study Damage and Defense Mechanisms Under Penumbra Conditions

T. Seiwert, A. Heimann, and O. Kempski

Summary. The destiny of the ischemic penumbra – defined as a territory of critically reduced blood flow in the close neighborhood of an ischemic core – determines outcome from stroke. Currently, the pathophysiology of the penumbra is studied mainly in rat models with occlusion of the middle cerebral artery. Here, we propose another rat model with distinct advantages. It produces a large territory of critical flow reduction in the cortex of one hemisphere without the presence of an infarct core; this model is suited to study mediator mechanisms that may turn the penumbra into necrotic tissue. It is produced by occluding one carotid artery and, in addition, reducing arterial pressure to 50 mmHg using the hypobaric hypotension technique. Cortical flow is assessed by laser Doppler scanning. Induction of cortical spreading depression is used to evaluate whether spreading-depression-induced increases of cortical blood flow are absent as an indicator of penumbra conditions.

Introduction

The ischemic penumbra [1, 3] is gaining greater recognition as a critical determinant of outcome in stroke. There is now agreement that mediators activated or released from the ischemic core may negatively affect surrounding tissues with critically reduced flow. Peri-infarct depolarizations (PID) are discussed in this context [5]. Pathophysiological studies of the subject are hampered by the fact that, in rat models, the volume of the penumbra zone is rather small compared with the ischemic core. To evaluate potential mediators of secondary damage to the penumbra, models with a large penumbra would be desirable. Therefore, we have established a rat model with a large zone of critically reduced cortical blood flow and no ischemic core. Damage mechanisms may be evaluated by artificially applying mediators of secondary damage to the tissue suffering from penumbra-like conditions; defense mechanisms can be easily studied following defined penumbra episodes by employing immune histology or polymerase-chain-reaction (PCR) techniques.

Methods

Wistar rats [250–350 g body weight (bw)] were pretreated with 0.5 mg atropine, anesthetized with chloral hydrate (36 mg/100 g bw i.p.), and ventilated after intubation. Rectal temperature was controlled at 37 °C by means of a feedback-controlled homeothermic blanket (Harvard, Edenbridge GB). Blood gases were controlled after can-

Maturation Phenomenon in Cerebral Ischemia III
U. Ito et al. (Eds.)
© Springer-Verlag Berlin Heidelberg 1999

nulation of the right carotid artery (ABL 615 blood gas analyzer, Radiometer Copenhagen, Denmark). The head was fixed in a stereotactic frame (Stoelting, Wood Dale, Ill., USA) and the skull exposed by a 20-mm midline sagittal skin incision. Access to the brain surface was gained via a 6·3-mm cranial window over the right or left hemisphere (see protocol). During the craniotomy, the drill tip was cooled continuously with physiological saline to avoid thermal injury to the cortex. The dura was left intact (OP-microscope, Zeiss, Oberkochen, Germany). During the experiment, the skull was continuously rinsed with 37 °C physiological saline and skull temperature was measured in the temporal muscle.

Local cortical blood flow (lCBF) was measured using a laser flow blood-perfusion monitor (model BPM 403a, TSI, St. Paul, Minn., USA) with a 0.8-mm needle probe. lCBF is expressed as LD units, since the calibration of laser-Dopplers (LD) to absolute-flow units remains controversial. The LD system has a reproducibly low biological zero and, with the scanning technique, data from individual animals and locations may be compared [4, 6, 7, 8, 9]; this technique measures lCBF sequentially at 32(8·4) or 48(8·6) cortical locations, using a computer-controlled micromanipulator scanning. A fast analog-to-digital (A/D) conversion board with on-board signal processing capacity (DAP, Microstar Laboratories, Redmont, Wash., USA) allows data to be sampled in a running average of 8 s (i.e., approximately ten breathing cycles) for each point of measurement. Therefore, one scan takes 4–5 min.

Cortical direct current (DC)-potential was assessed between a Ag/AgCl-microelectrode inserted into the cortex and a reference electrode into the neck muscle using a DC amplifier (Gould, Cleveland, Ohio). Tissue alternating current (AC) impedance was measured between two cortical electrodes at 1 kHz (10 µV, HP4284 precision LCR meter). Spreading depression is elicited by microinjection of 150 mM KCl by glass micropipette.

Protocol

The right common carotid artery was permanently occluded. Hypobaric hypotension reduces cortical blood flow in the right hemisphere by lowering the systemic arterial pressure below the autoregulation threshold [2, 4]; the lower body portion of the animals is placed in a sealed chamber that is connected to an electronically controlled vacuum pump and the barometric pressure within the chamber is reduced to –30 cm H_2O, thereby causing a pooling of venous blood in the lower body of the rat. By doing so, arterial pressure can be fine-tuned to within 1–2 mmHg of a given level.

Using these methods, penumbra-like blood flow conditions are established in the right cerebral cortex. To study the effects of mean arterial blood pressure (MABP) reduction without carotid artery occlusion, the left cortex was studied. At the end of the experiment, the rats were returned to individual cages and allowed free access to water and food. Histological damage could be assessed later.

Results

On occlusion of the right common carotid artery, regional cerebral blood flow (rCBF) in the affected hemisphere was significantly reduced, without, however, dropping to critical levels, i.e., lCBF values below 15–20 LD units were observed in fewer than 10 % of locations which, in earlier studies, was found to be normal [4, 6, 9]. It was only after the systemic arterial pressure was additionally reduced (i.e., below the autoregulation threshold) to 50 mmHg, that rCBF decreased enough to establish penumbra-like conditions. Median flow was less than 45 % of normal, and more than 40 % of locations have a flow of less than 15 LD units. The final proof, however, that penumbra-like conditions are established is shown in Fig. 1; after microinjection of potassium chloride (KCl) into the contralateral (left) cortex, lCBF increased with kinetics typical of spreading depression (SD; Fig 1A). During penumbra-like conditions, however, there was no lCBF response (Fig. 1B), since the flow reserve of the tissue was exhausted. The model does not include the spontaneous development of an infarct core. Therefore, it is not surprising that PIDs did not occur during the 30-min period of penumbra-like CBF.

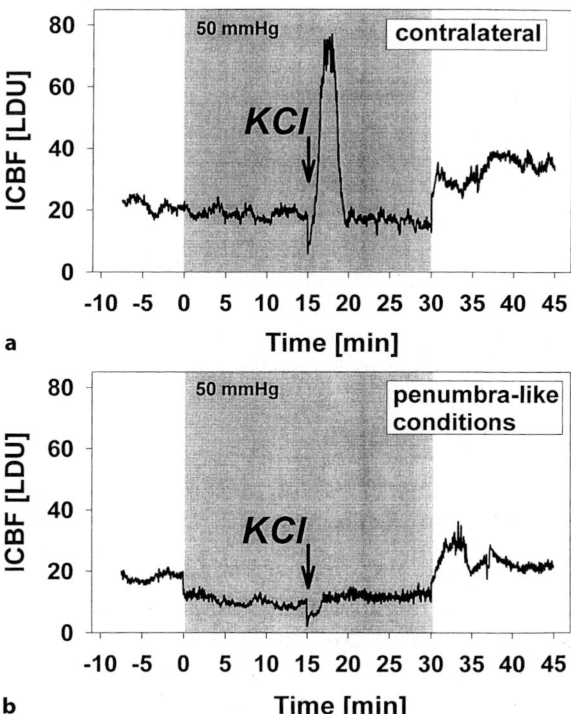

Fig. 1a, b. Effects of spreading depression from microinjection of KCl (*arrow*, time point of injection) on local cerebral blood flow detected 1.5 mm from the injection site in two typical experiments. **a** Contralateral (left) hemisphere; local laser-Doppler signal does not change during reduction of systemic arterial pressure to 50 mmHg. Upon induction of spreading depression after an initial flow decrease, there is a more than threefold flow increase which normalizes after 3–4 min. **b** Right hemisphere (right carotid artery occluded); laser-Doppler flow decreases after reduction of arterial pressure. Upon induction of spreading depression (*arrow*) there is a temporary decrease of flow but no increase at all, indicating the exhaustion of flow reserves as a characteristic of penumbra-like conditions

Discussion

The ischemic penumbra has been studied in rat, cat and monkey models with a temporary or permanent occlusion of the middle cerebral artery. In the rat, in particular, the resulting infarct is rather large compared with the penumbra volume. It is known that large portions of the penumbra are rather quickly, i.e., within hours, transformed into necrotic tissue [3]. The exact kinetics and dimensions of these changes are unknown, and the mechanisms involved in secondary tissue damage are still debated. To study mediator mechanisms, the model proposed herein appears suitable, given that no spontaneous infarct is found. Therefore, potential mediators of secondary damage may be applied, and the reactions used to rank the significance of the mediator mechanism tested.

In detail, the new model has distinct advantages and some drawbacks. Hypobaric hypotension has been shown to be an excellent method for reducing arterial blood pressure. Any desired pressure level below the physiological arterial blood pressure is adjustable by tuning the electronically controlled vacuum pump. To induce penumbra-like conditions, MABP is reduced to 50 mmHg, which is below the lower autoregulation threshold of $\sim$55 mmHg in Wistar rats [4]. As such, temporary local hypoperfusion is induced without heparinization or bleeding. The laser-Doppler scanning technique used in the present study allows for verification of the regional occurrence of low-flow conditions. Low-flow areas are defined as locations with a laser Doppler flow below 15 LD units, which are never observed under baseline conditions and are found following unilateral carotid artery occlusion in fewer than 10 % of cases (see above). We have to assume, however, that penumbra-like conditions develop at higher flow levels. The exact threshold can be assessed by reducing arterial blood pressure to predefined levels, measuring rCBF with the scanning technique, and assessing the flow reserve under these conditions either by inducing SD (cf. Fig. 1) or using CO_2 stimulation. Such studies are under way.

Certainly, this model allows for conclusions to be drawn following the application of mediators that worsen the penumbra and that may be responsible for the transition of the penumbra to necrotic tissue. Therapeutic principles can only be studied after additional induction of such a mediator mechanism. An example is the effect of SD, which is currently studied using this model. If SD is really a risk factor, histological outcome should worsen if enough SD waves were applied. The model may therefore allow for the evaluation of the amount of time required for SDs to kill penumbra tissue.

A contribution of SD to secondary brain damage suggested not only by previous studies [5], but also by initial data obtained with the new model (unpublished data). The major differences between the new penumbra model and that which surrounds an arterial infarct concern the temporal and spatial dimensions of the decay of penumbra tissue. The absence of an ischemic core may become a critical element if potential mediators are either rapidly eliminated by surrounding healthy tissue or require high concentrations that are only liberated from large necrotic tissue sections. In fact, this is the major advantage of the new model, since the only mediators that can exert such an effect are those that are either released or activated as a consequence of the low-flow conditions in the penumbra-like tissue or are exogenously applied by the investigator. Therefore, the model allows to screen for mediator mechanisms and their interactions with one another.

In conclusion, a model with penumbra-like conditions is proposed, which may help to study pathophysiological mechanisms contributing to the secondary decay of the penumbra. Current research is focussed on evaluating the effect of SD, and on the temporal window required to kill tissue under penumbra conditions.

References

1. Astrup J, Siesjö, BK, Symon L (1981) Thresholds in cerebral ischemia – the ischemic penumbra. Stroke 12: 723–725
2. Dirnagl U, Thoren P, Villringer A, Sixt G, Them A, Einhäupl KM (1993) Global forebrain ischemia in the rat: controlled reduction of cerebral blood flow by hypobaric hypotension and two-vessel occlusion. Neurol Res 15: 128–130
3. Ginsberg MD (1997) Injury mechanisms in the ischemic penumbra – approaches to neuroprotection in acute ischemic stroke. Cerbrovasc Dis 7[Suppl 2]:7–12
4. Heimann A, Kroppenstedt S, Ulrich P, Kempski OS (1994) Cerebral blood flow autoregulation during hypobaric hypotension assessed by laser Doppler scanning. J Cereb Blood Flow Metab 14: 1100–1105
5. Hossmann K-A (1996) Periinfarct depolarizations. Cerebrovasc Brain Metabol Reviews 8: 195–208
6. Kempski O, Heimann A, Strecker U (1995) On the number of measurements necessary to assess regional cerebral blood flow by local laser Doppler recordings: a simulation study with data from 45 rabbits. Int J Microcirc 15: 37–42
7. Nakase H, Heimann A, Kempski O (1996) Alterations of regional cerebral blood flow and oxygen saturation in a rat sinus–vein thrombosis model. Stroke 27: 720–728
8. Nakase H, Heimann A, Kempski O (1996) Local cerebral blood flow in a rat cortical vein occlusion model. J Cereb Blood Flow Metab 16: 720–728
9. Nakase H, Kempski O, Heimann A, Takeshima T, Tintera J (1997) Microcirculation after cerebral venous occlusions as assessed by laser Doppler scanning. J Neurosurg 87: 307–314

Instrumental Diagnosis and Treatment of Acute Ischemic Stroke: The Clinician's Perspective

C. Fieschi, C. Argentino, A. Falcou, M. Fiorelli, M. L. Sacchetti, G. Sette, and D. Toni

Introduction

It is difficult to estimate the impact of experimental work on mechanisms of induction and protection of cellular damage in the "real world" of neurological diseases. This is particularly difficult for ischemic stroke, although clinicians are now actively collaborating with basic scientists and technologists in order to implement effective therapeutic strategies for stroke victims. Important tasks for the clinician include: (1) the identification of the most appropriate diagnostic techniques, (2) the set up of organized stroke care, and (3) the design and realization of rigorous clinical trials. In the following pages, we review the current options for instrumental diagnosis and treatment of acute ischemic stroke.

Instrumental Diagnostic Techniques

Differential Diagnosis

Stroke is a clinical syndrome, the vascular origin of which can be presumed at the bedside, but needs instrumental confirmation. This is especially true for patients under the age of 50 years and for those whose clinical history is unclear. The questions clinicians ask during instrumental investigations are summarized in Table 1. Although challenged by magnetic resonance imaging (MRI), the computed tomography (CT) scan remains, for the time being, the mainstay of the diagnosis of acute ischemic stroke. Conventional spin-echo MRI has little more to offer than CT in acute stroke [10, 25], with the possible exception of clinical pictures suggesting brainstem/cerebellar lesions, and the rare cases of cerebral venous thrombosis. Superiority of CT over

Table 1. What clinicians ask in an instrumental work-up for patients with presumed acute ischemic stroke

Differential diagnosis	Investigation
Hemorrhage	CT
Identification and quantitation of hypoperfusion	SPECT, PWI–DWI
Identification of arterial occlusion	X-ray angiography, ultrasound, MRA, angio-CT
Evaluation of residual tissue viability	PWI–DWI?

SPECT, single-photon emission computed tomography; *PWI*, perfusion-weighted imaging; *DWI*, diffusion-weighted imaging; *MRA*, magnetic resonance imaging; *CT*, computed tomography

Maturation Phenomenon in Cerebral Ischemia III
U. Ito et al. (Eds.)
© Springer-Verlag Berlin Heidelberg 1999

MRI is due to its better accuracy in detecting fresh hemorrhage and skull fractures, but also to its wide availability and low costs. Recent reports challenge the view that MRI does not accurately differentiate acute hematoma from infarction, and propose that MRI should become the first-line imaging technique for patients with acute stroke [28].

Identification and Quantitation of Hypoperfusion

Single-photon emission tomography (SPET) is the only non-experimental technique that can assess regional perfusion in acute stroke patients. SPET hypoperfusional patterns in acute ischemic stroke appear to be relevant to functional prognosis [14] as well as to patient selection for thrombolytic therapy [39]. Diffusion-weighted MRI (DWI) is based on the translational diffusion of water in the tissues. Changes in the apparent coefficient of diffusion of water after an ischemic insult can be detected rapidly and non-invasively, thus allowing the topographical definition of the ischemic area in the brain parenchyma within minutes from onset. Perfusion-weighted MRI (PWI) allows the evaluation of the microcirculation of the brain using intravenously (i.v.) administered paramagnetic contrast agents. DWI and PWI can be rapidly carried out in acute stroke patients. Both DWI and PWI abnormalities have shown a strong correlation with the severity of the neurological deficit in acute stroke patients [38, 42]. DWI and PWI have many drawbacks that continue to prevent their utilization in the clinical routine: (1) the large magnetic field gradient needed for echo planar imaging, (2) the ultrafast technique on which most current DWI–PWI protocols are based cannot be implemented on low-field tomographs, (3) the reconstruction of perfusion images is time consuming and hardly feasible in an emergency setting, and (4) the clinical usefulness of DWI and PWI still needs to be compared with that of routinely used techniques such as CT [29].

Identification of Arterial Occlusion

The advent of new non-invasive techniques has limited the use of conventional angiography, although this remains the gold-standard imaging modality of the cerebral vessels. Due to the high rate of complications and high skill required from the operator [17], X-ray angiography cannot represent a first-line diagnostic procedure in the emergency setting for such a frequent disease as acute ischemic stroke. Currently, the role of angiography in the acute phase seems limited to the detection of occlusive disease of the carotid or basilar artery, especially in view of invasive therapeutic interventions.

Duplex sonography of the neck is a quick, simple, inexpensive, non-invasive technique, which is capable of detecting, with sufficient accuracy, an occlusive disease of the extracranial inferior cerebellar artery (ICA) in stroke patients [3]. Color-coded Doppler is a recent innovation, which has increased the reliability of Duplex sonography in the estimation of the severity of the stenosis. Ultrasound examination of the neck can be easily carried out in the acute phase of stroke, allowing, in a few minutes, the detection of a significant stenosis of the ICA at its origin [16]. The more distal segments of the extracranial ICA and the siphon cannot be properly investigated using this technique. However, the insonation of the supraorbital artery can reveal an inversion of the flow, which is indirect evidence of a distal stenosis or occlusion.

Transcranial Doppler sonography (TCD) can provide information on the state of the intracranial circulation, especially the middle cerebral artery (MCA) stem [16]. Compared with angiography as gold standard, TCD reliably depicts the modifications of flow occurring in acute ischemic stroke [44], including the recanalization of a previously occluded MCA [45]. However, this technique is not free of disadvantages. TCD cannot be performed in the 5–10 % of stroke patients with temporal bones too thick to be crossed by the ultrasound beam. In addition, the examination requires a considerable degree of cooperation from the patient, since an unforeseeable amount of time is needed for the identification of the various intracranial vessels. Contrast-enhanced insonation could circumvent the problem of absent cranial window and improve the sensitivity of the technique [27].

Early after onset, plain CT may also demonstrate a focal hyperdensity along the course of the MCA, a finding that has been interpreted as an indication of embolic occlusion [4]. Rarely, other intracerebral arteries may exhibit a similar abnormality. Dynamic CT conjugates a higher speed of acquisition than conventional tomographs with the possibility of reconstructing images in various planes [20] This technique allows the combined evaluation of the parenchyma and, after contrast injection, of the vessels, but its usefulness in acute stroke has never been evaluated. Preliminary data suggest its value in case of a stroke secondary to a suspected dissection of the extracranial ICA [22], and for selecting patients for thrombolysis [43]. MR angiography (MRA) visualizes large-caliber vessels well, therefore, allowing the diagnosis of occlusive disease of the ICA, or of the vertebral and basilar arteries. Dissections, coilings, kinkings and dolichoectasias are abnormalities of the large vessels, which underlie a minority of ischemic strokes and can similarly be diagnosed using MRA. Long acquisition times and susceptibility to movement artefacts may limit the applicability of this technique in the acute phase. However, rapid technological advances will likely obviate to these shortcomings in the near future [11].

Assessment of Tissue Viability

Shortly after the onset of an acute ischemic stroke, the area of cerebral parenchyma distal to the arterial occlusion, which underlies the clinical picture, gradually evolves towards necrosis. Theoretically, until necrosis occurs, the tissue is salvageable. The portion of tissue with reduced or abolished function due to ischemia, but which is still recoverable, has been called penumbra. Left to its spontaneous evolution, penumbral tissue can either recover spontaneously or deteriorate and die [12]. The identification of viable cerebral tissue has obvious therapeutic implications. This is especially true after the advent of thrombolysis, a potentially beneficial approach, but also harmful in other conditions. Local cerebral metabolic rates for oxygen and glucose ($CMRO_2$ and CMR_{Glu}, respectively) are the best indicators of viability. Unfortunately, the assessment of these two parameters requires positron emission tomography (PET), which is not available in the clinical practice. To what extent tissue viability can be inferred from levels of cerebral blood flow (CBF) is a matter of debate. Neurological function is directly dependent on adequate CBF levels. A correlation between decreasing levels of CBF and increasing neurological impairment after occlusion of the MCA was demonstrated in the experimental animal [19]. Studies in the acute phase of human ischemic stroke consistently show that severity and extent of hypoperfusion are associated with the severity of initial neurological deficit and final prognosis [1, 14, 23, 38]. However, things become much more complicated when it comes to defining CBF thresholds for tissue viability. A recent PET study of cerebral perfusion within 2 h of ischemic stroke onset demonstrated that CBF levels well below the classical thresholds for irreversibility may still be followed by recovery, following timely pharmacological reperfusion [15].

It is unclear how much information on tissue viability can be inferred from CT. Older concepts, that CT scan is negative within the first 24 h after the onset of an ischemic stroke, have been superseded by the recognition that early signs of focal ischemic damage can be identified as early as 1 h after onset. At least half of the patients with presumed carotid stroke submitted to CT within 5 h of onset exhibit a tenuous hypodensity and/or a focal swelling corresponding to the infarction in maturation [40, 41]. The spontaneous evolution of these abnormalities may be infarction. However, there are at least two published cases of reversal of focal hypodensity after thrombolysis [13, 34], suggesting that early CT signs of focal ischemic damage do not necessarily represent a point of no return. It has been claimed that DWI–WI can help delineate the irretrievably damaged tissue. The areas characterized by abnormal perfusion and normal diffusion might correspond to the ischemic penumbra and, therefore, represent the target for tissue-saving therapy [2].

Treatment

The care of stroke patients in specialized units has repeatedly and convincingly shown to result in a better outcome, compared with hospitalization in general wards. After the first claims from single centers [18, 31], meta-analyses conducted on multicenter cohorts of several thousands of patients [21, 32] have confirmed that mortality, dependency and need for institutional care are all reduced by organized stroke care. The results were adjusted for age, sex, stroke severity and variations in stroke-unit organizations. A very important concomitant finding was that, on average, stroke-unit care reduced the length of hospital stay. Several explanations for these findings have been put forward, the most realistic being that specialized care reduces the frequency and the severity of the complications that arise during the course of stroke [33]; that specific rehabilitation programs contribute to this improved outcome is a reasonable, but unproven hypothesis. The need for an optimization of stroke care from a general point of view stems evidently from these observations.

Therapeutic Trials

Therapeutic experimentation in stroke patients dates back several decades. Starting in the 1960s and 1970s, the systematic failure of clinical trials can be accounted for by numerous methodological pitfalls. Lack of CT confirmation of the clinical diagnosis of ischemic stroke and samples of insufficient size were the most common errors made. Many molecules have been dismissed after negative trials in the past years, but often methodological pitfalls alone could explain their failure.

From the pathophysiological standpoint, our knowledge of the basic aspects of ischemia are increasingly elucidated. Inspired by the new discoveries in terms of basic mechanisms and motivated by the economical implications behind stroke therapy, pharmaceutical companies are synthesizing and proposing for experimentation a great number of new compounds. Thus far, virtually all trials of cytoprotectants have failed to show significant benefits in an intention-to-treat analysis [35]. However, there are some encouraging results of potential efficacy in post-hoc defined subgroups for nimodipine [24], piracetam [6], citicoline [5] and lubeluzole [7]. Due to their mechanisms of action, which aim at circumscribing the consequences of the ischemic damage rather than removing its causes, it is unlikely that cytoprotectants will provide striking benefits to stroke patients. The net usefulness of cytoprotectants will, therefore, be strictly dependent on their safety profile.

"Cocktails" of cytoprotective agents could, theoretically, antagonize the ischemic damage, acting synergistically at many crucial points of the biochemical cascade, thus leading from ischemia to infarction. Another association therapy of theoretical appeal is that between cytoprotectants and thrombolytics. Of all the trials of thrombolytic agents performed so far, only that of the NINDS study group has proven that i. v. thrombolysis can improve the functional outcome without increasing mortality [36]. Patients in this trial were treated within 0.9 mg/kg (i. v.) recombinant tissue plasminogen activator (rt-PA) within 3 h of onset. European Cooperative Acute Stroke Study (ECASS 1) [9], a European trial of 1.1 mg/kg i. v. rt-PA administered within 6 h of onset, also showed an improvement of functional outcome associated with rt-PA. However, mortality was higher among treated patients, therefore, a new trial (ECASS II) with the same rt-PA dose used in NINDS was deemed necessary to evaluate the efficacy and safety of this drug in the 6-h time frame. The results of ECASS II are to be published soon. Three trials of relatively large size were carried out using streptokinase. All were interrupted because of an excess of deaths in the treated arm [8, 26, 37].

Although rt-PA may be considered the first drug to demonstrate its efficacy in acute ischemic stroke after a rigorously conducted clinical trial, it still has several crucial drawbacks. First, the results of the NINDS trial have not yet been replicated. Second, the number of patients, who are potential candidates for thrombolytic therapy with the current selection criteria, do not exceed 5 % of all patients hospitalized with an acute ischemic stroke. It is, therefore, highly unlikely that thrombolysis will become the treatment of choice for a significant proportion of stroke patients over the next few years. What seems likely is that the appropriate combination of drugs will soon be identified that can increase the proportion of treatable patients and minimize the damage caused by thrombolytic agents [30]. On the basis of the experience accumulated so far, trials in acute stroke must come of age. The foreseeable developments of therapeutic experimentation in acute ischemic stroke are summarized in Table 2.

Table 2. Foreseeable developments of therapeutic experimentation in acute ischemic stroke

- Larger trials, i.e., myocardial infarction style
- More accurate patient selection
- More drugs tested in the same trial
- New (more sensitive) end-points
- Elimination of placebo arm
- Closer implication of basic scientists in clinical trial design
- Sponsorship by non-profit institutions

References

1. Baird AE, Austin MC, McKay WJ, Donnan GA (1996) Changes in cerebral tissue perfusion during the first 48 h of ischaemic stroke: relation to clinical outcome. J Neurol Neurosurg Psychiatry 61: 26–29
2. Baird AE, Benfield A, Schlaug G, Siewert B, Lovblad KO, Edelman RR, Warach S (1997) Enlargement of human cerebral ischemic lesion volumes measured by diffusion-weighted magnetic resonance imaging. Ann Neurol 41: 581–589
3. Barnes RW, Nix L, Rittgers SE (1981) Audible interpretation of carotid doppler signals. Arch Surg 116: 1185–1189
4. Bastianello S, Pierallini A, Colonnese C, et al. (1991) Hyperdense middle cerebral artery sign. Comparison with angiography in the acute phase of ischemic supratentorial infarction. Neuroradiology 33: 207–211
5. Clark WM, Warach SJ, Pettigrew LC, Gammans RE, Sabounjian L (1997) A randomized dose-response trial of citicoline in acute ischemic stroke patients. Citicoline Stroke Study Group. Neurology 49: 671–678
6. De Deyn PP, Reuck JD, Deberdt W, Vlietinck R, Orgogozo JM (1997) Treatment of acute ischaemic stroke with piracetam. Members of the Piracetam in Acute Stroke Study (PASS) Group. Stroke 28: 2347–2352
7. Diener HC (1998) Multinational randomised controlled trial of lubeluzole in acute ischaemic stroke. European and Australian Lubeluzole Ischaemic Stroke Study Group. Cerebrovasc Dis 8: 172–181
8. Donnan GA, Davis SM, Chambers BR, Gates PC, Hankey GJ, McNeil JJ, Rosen D, Stewart-Wynne EG, Tuck RR (1996) Streptokinase for acute ischemic stroke with relationship to time of administration: Australian Streptokinase (ASK) Trial Study Group. JAMA 276: 961–966
9. European Cooperative Acute Stroke Study (ECASS) (1995) Intravenous thrombolysis with recombinant tissue plasminogen activator for acute ischaemic stroke. JAMA 274: 1017–1025
10. Fiorelli M, Sacchetti ML, Toni D, et al. (1993) Feasibility and usefulness of conventional spin-echo MR imaging in hyperacute ischemic stroke: a comparison with CT scan. Circ Metabol Cerveau 10: 5–10
11. Fisher M, Sotak CH, Minematsu K, Li L (1992) New magnetic resonance techniques for evaluating cerebrovascular disease. Ann Neurol 32: 115–122
12. Furlan M, Marchal G, Viader F, Derlon JM, Baron JC (1996) Spontaneous neurological recovery after stroke and the fate of the ischemic penumbra. Ann Neurol 40: 216–226
13. Gholkar A, Davis M, Barer D, Mendelow AD (1998) Early computed-tomography abnormalities in acute stroke. Lancet 351: 679
14. Giubilei F, Lenzi GL, Di Piero V, Pozzilli C, Pantano P, Bastianello S, Argentino C, Fieschi C (1990) Predictive value of brain perfusion single-photon emission computed tomography in acute ischemic stroke. Stroke 21: 895–900
15. Heiss WD, Grond M, Thiel A, von Stockhausen HM, Rudolf J (1997) Ischaemic brain tissue salvaged from infarction with alteplase. Lancet 349: 1599–1600
16. Hennerici M, Mohr JP, Rautenberg W, Steinke W (1992) Ultrasound imaging and doppler sonography in the diagnoses of cerebrovascular diseases. In: Barnett HJM, Mohr JP, Stein BM, Yatsu FM (eds) Stroke: pathophysiology, diagnosis and management, 2nd edn. Churchill Livingstone, New York pp 241–268
17. Hessel SJ, Adams DF, Abrams HL (1981) Complications of angiography. Radiology 138: 273–281
18. Indredavik B, Bakke F, Solberg R, Rokseth R, Haaheim LL, Holme I (1991) Benefit of a stroke unit: a randomized controlled trial. Stroke 22: 1026–1031
19. Jones TH, Morawetz RB, Crowell RM, Marcoux FW, FitzGibbon SJ, DeGirolami U, Ojemann RG (1981) Thresholds of focal cerebral ischemia in awake monkeys. J Neurosurg 54: 773–782

20. Kalender WA, Polacin A (1991) Physical performance characteristics of spiral CT scanning. Med Phys 18: 910–915
21. Langhorne P, Williams BO, Gilchrist W, Howie K (1993) Do stroke units save lives? Lancet 342: 395–398
22. Leclerc X, Godefroy O, Salhi A, Lucas C, Leys D, Pruvo JP (1996) Helical CT for the diagnosis of extracranial internal carotid artery dissection. Stroke 27: 461–466
23. Marchal G, Serrati C, Rioux P, Petit-Taboué MC, Viader F, de la Sayette V, Le Doze F, Lochon P, Derlon JM, Orgogozo JM, et al. (1993) PET imaging of cerebral perfusion and oxygen consumption in acute ischaemic stroke: relation to outcome. Lancet 341: 925–927
24. Mohr JP, Orgogozo JM, Harrison MJG, Hennerici M, Wahlgren NG Gelmers JH, Martinez-Vila E, Dycka J, Tettenborn D (1994) Meta-analysis of oral nimodipine trials in acute ischemic stroke. Cerebrovasc Dis 4: 177–210
25. Mohr JP, Biller J, Hilal SK, et al. (1995) Magnetic resonance versus computed tomographic imaging in acute stroke. Stroke 26: 807–812
26. Multicentre Acute Stroke Trial-Italy (MAST-I) Group (1995) Randomised controlled trial of streptokinase, aspirin, and combination of both in treatment of acute ischaemic stroke. Lancet 346: 1509–1514
27. Otis S, Rush M, Boyajian R (1995) Contrast-enhanced transcranial imaging: results of an American phase-two study. Stroke 26: 203–209
28. Patel MR, Edelman RR, Warach S (1996) Detection of hyperacute primary intraparenchymal hemorrhage by magnetic resonance imaging. Stroke 27: 2321–2324
29. Powers WJ, Zivin J (1998) Magnetic resonance imaging in acute stroke: not ready for prime time. Neurology 50: 842–843
30. Sacchetti ML, Toni D, Fiorelli M, Argentino C, Fieschi C (1997) The concept of combination therapy in acute ischemic stroke. Neurology 49[Suppl 4]:S70–S74
31. Strand T, Asplund K, Eriksson S, Hegg E, Lithner F, Wester PO (1985) A non intensive stroke unit reduces functional disability and the need for long term hospitalization. Stroke 16: 29–34
32. Stroke Unit Trialists' Collaboration (1997) Collaborative systematic review of the randomised trials of organised inpatient (stroke unit) care after stroke. BMJ 314: 1151–1159
33. Stroke Unit Trialists' Collaboration (1997) How do stroke units improve patient outcomes? A collaborative systematic review of the randomized trials. Stroke 28: 2139–2144
34. Tarr R, Taylor CL, Selman WR, Lewin JS, Landis D (1996). Good clinical outcome in a patient with a large CT scan hypodensity treated with intra-arterial urokinase after an embolic stroke. Neurology 47: 1076–1078
35. The European Ad Hoc Consensus Group (1998) Neuroprotection as initial therapy in acute stroke. Cerebrovasc Dis 8: 59–72
36. The NINDS rt-PA Stroke Study Group (1995) Tissue plasminogen activator for acute ischemic stroke. N Engl J Med 333: 1581–1587
37. The Multicenter Acute Stroke Trial-Europe Study Group (1996) Thrombolytic therapy with streptokinase in acute ischemic stroke. N Engl J Med 335: 145–150
38. Tong DC, Yenari MA, Albers GW, O'Brien M, Marks MP, Moseley ME (1998) Correlation of perfusion- and diffusion-weighted MRI with NIHSS score in acute (<6.5 hour) ischemic stroke. Neurology 50: 864–870
39. Ueda T, Hatakeyama T, Kumon Y, Sakaki S, Uraoka T (1994) Evaluation of risk of hemorrhagic transformation in local intra-arterial thrombolysis in acute ischemic stroke by initial SPECT. Stroke 25: 298–[Font:ZapfDingbats]z[ZapfDingbatsEnde]30312
40. von Kummer R, Bozzao L, Manelfe C (1995) Early CT diagnosis of hemispheric brain infarction. Springer, Berlin Heidelberg New York
41. von Kummer R, Weber J (1997) Brain and vascular imaging in acute ischemic stroke: the potential of computed tomography. Neurology 49[Suppl 4]:S52–S55
42. Warach S, Dashe JF, Edelman RR (1996) Clinical outcome in ischemic stroke predicted by early diffusion-weighted and perfusion magnetic resonance imaging: a preliminary analysis. J Cereb Blood Flow Metab 16: 53–59
43. Wildermuth S, Knauth M, Brandt T, Winter R, Sartor K, Hacke W (1998) Role of CT angiography in patient selection for thrombolytic therapy in acute hemispheric stroke. Stroke 29: 935–938
44. Zanette EM, Fieschi C, Bozzao L, et al. (1989) Comparison of cerebral angiography and transcranial doppler in acute stroke. Stroke 20: 899–903
45. Zanette EM, Roberti C, Mancini G, et al. (1995) Spontaneous middle cerebral artery reperfusion in ischemic stroke. Stroke 26: 430–433

V Special Lecture

Mechanisms of Regulation of Cerebral Blood Flow

L. Sokoloff

Summary. The physiological mechanisms that regulate cerebral blood flow (CBF) have long been studied, but are still not fully defined. Neurogenic mechanisms probably exist, but their role is still undefined. Chemical mechanisms are widely believed to mediate a "coupling" between cerebral energy metabolism and CBF to assure adequate supply of substrates to meet the brain's energy demands. We have used two experimental models of cerebral glucose deprivation, i.e., insulin-induced hypoglycemia and glycolytic blockade by loading doses of 2-deoxyglucose, to examine mechanisms underlying the associated large increases in CBF, despite lowered energy metabolism in these conditions. Mechanisms excluded thus far are: (1) changes in blood pH and pCO_2, (2) direct insulin action, (3) increased lactate and decreased K+ levels in plasma induced by insulin, and (4) nitric oxide production. Both caffeine, an adenosine receptor antagonist, and glibenclamide, which blocks ATP-sensitive K^+ channels, reduce until abolition the increases in CBF in these conditions in a dose-dependent manner. Adenosine receptors, which mediate vasodilation, and ATP-sensitive K^+ (K_{ATP}) channels, which, when open, promote smooth-muscle relaxation, exist in vascular smooth muscle. We have measured and found, during glucose deprivation, marked rises in brain levels of adenosine and its degradation products, inosine and hypoxanthine, indicating increased adenosine release. There is evidence in a variety of tissues that adenosine-receptor activation stimulates cyclic adenosine monophosphate (cAMP) formation, which activates protein kinase A, an enzyme that phosphorylates proteins. There is also evidence that the activity of the K_{ATP} channels can be altered by such phosphorylation. These results suggest the following sequence: (1) when the ATP/ADP balance is shifted toward ADP by stimulation of Na^+/K^+-ATPase activity, e.g., during functional activation, or by reduced ATP generation, e.g., during glucose or oxygen deprivation, some of the ADP is converted to AMP by adenylic kinase; (2) AMP is dephosphorylated by 5'-nucleotidase to produce adenosine; (3) adenosine activates adenosine receptors in vascular smooth muscle to produce cAMP, and (4) cAMP-dependent protein kinase A phosphorylates the K^+ channels, which then open, allowing K^+ efflux, membrane hyperpolarization, smooth-muscle relaxation and vasodilatation. Increasing adenosine diphosphate (ADP) and inorganic phosphate concentrations is known to stimulate glycolytic and oxidative metabolism. The shift in the ATP/ADP balance toward ADP accompanying functional activation would then not only lead to increased CBF, but also to increased energy metabolism, thus, resulting in their being related, not by a direct coupling mechanism, but as separate, yet correlated, consequences of one prior event.

Maturation Phenomenon in Cerebral Ischemia III
U. Ito et al. (Eds.)
© Springer-Verlag Berlin Heidelberg 1999

Introduction

Regulation of cerebral blood flow (CBF) has been a subject of continual investigation for more than a century. In 1890, Roy and Sherrington [50] proposed that CBF is determined mainly by the balance between mean arterial blood pressure (MABP) and cerebral vascular resistance (CVR). They provided evidence that CVR could be intrinsically regulated by chemical factors, in particular, chemical products of tissue-energy metabolism. Although they did not measure energy metabolism, they further hypothesized that functional activation stimulated metabolic activity to produce these products, thus providing the brain with an "intrinsic mechanism, by which its vascular supply can be varied locally in correspondence with local variations of functional activity".

Roy and Sherrington [50] actually appeared to favor the view that the intrinsic regulation was merely fine tuning, that the influence of MABP predominated, and that CBF tended to follow the MABP passively. This view was most likely based on observations in deeply anesthetized animals, in which autoregulatory mechanisms had been suppressed. It was later realized that CBF is normally maintained relatively constant over a wide range of MABP by intrinsic modulation of cerebral vascular tone and that it passively follows MABP only when the limits of the autoregulatory range are exceeded [34]. The exact mechanisms by which CVR is regulated are yet to be defined. Many have been considered, investigated and found to have some of the necessary properties, but not one has yet proved adequate to account, by itself, for all the observed phenomena. Some of the many factors proved, suspected or speculated to be involved in some way in the regulation of CVR and CBF are illustrated in Fig. 1.

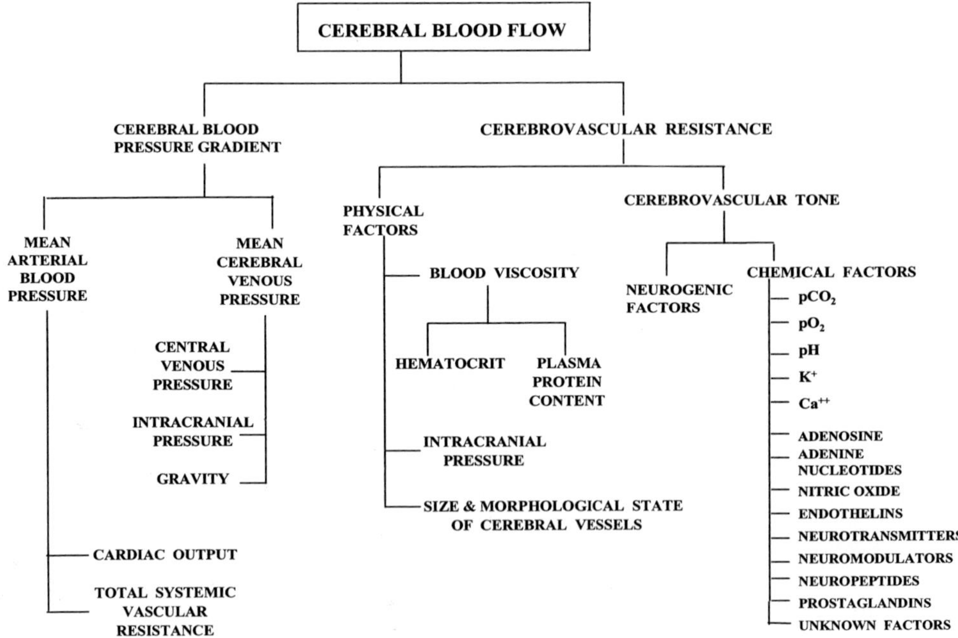

Fig. 1. Schema of the multiple factors regulating cerebral blood flow (CBF)

Neurogenic Mechanisms

It is beyond the scope of this report to review and evaluate the almost innumerable studies on the role of neurogenic and related factors in the control of CVR and CBF. This subject has been comprehensively covered by Edvinsson et al. [16]. There is abundant anatomical evidence of the existence of nerve supplies to the dural, pial and intracerebral vessels. Myelinated and unmyelinated fibers and perivascular nerves of adrenergic, cholinergic and peptidergic origin have been demonstrated on intracerebral arterioles down to 15–20 μm in diameter. Many of the associated neurotransmitters, neuropeptides and their receptors, as well as enzymes for the synthesis and degradation of the neurotransmitters and/or neuromodulators, have been found on or in close proximity to the cerebral vessels. Some of these pathways appear to have vasomotor effects on the pial and superficial vessels of the brain. For example, stimulation of cervical sympathetic nerves constricts pial arteries, but the decreases in diameter of the pial arteries are small, compared with the effects on extra-cerebral vessels. Also, a parasympathetic cerebral vasodilator pathway via the facial and greater superficial petrosal nerves and the internal carotid plexus has been described, which, when stimulated, dilates pial arteries over the ipsilateral parietal cortex [10].

The functional significance of such neurogenic influences on diameters of pial and superficial cerebral vessels to the physiological regulation of blood flow in the tissues of the brain is uncertain. Such effects might not apply to the small parenchymal resistance vessels, which contribute most to the CVR and regulation of blood flow. The evidence that neurogenic factors play a major role in the regulation of cerebral vascular tone and blood flow is unconvincing. For example, procaine block of the stellate ganglion, performed bilaterally in normotensive and hypertensive human patients [21] and unilaterally in patients with cerebral vascular disease [34], does not alter CVR or blood flow. Shenkin et al. [58] did find reduced CVR after bilateral stellate ganglionectomy, but this result was most likely due to the development of anemia in the interval between the control and postoperative measurements. There is, therefore, no support for an important tonic role for the cervical sympathetics in the regulation of cerebral vascular tone and blood flow. Neither is there any cogent evidence of a tonic neurogenic vasodilator tone. Furthermore, cerebral-vasomotor mechanisms do not appear to be integrated into extrinsic general circulatory reflexes of the baroreceptor type.

There have been reports of intrinsic neural pathways within the brain, which affect parenchymal resistance vessels and increase blood flow in specific regions of the brain. For example, electrical stimulation of the fastigial nucleus in the cerebellum results in increased blood flow in most of the cerebral cortex in laboratory animals [37, 48]. This effect of fastigial nucleus stimulation on local CBF was recently shown, however, to be associated with increases in metabolism in the same brain structures [64], raising doubts that the effects on blood flow were due to a neurogenic vasomotor mechanism. Indeed, a number of so-called neurogenic vasodilator effects on CBF elicited by stimulation of regions of the brain have been found to be associated with metabolic activation, and the relevance of such reported effects, which are still under consideration, is questionable until further examined.

There is evidence for a role of the sympathetics, that is not directly on regulation of the tone of the cerebral resistance vessels (e.g., arterioles) or blood flow, but rather on larger arteries preceding the resistance vessels. Its effect appears to be to adjust the blood-pressure range over which autoregulation is effective. Harper et al. [22] found that cervical sympathetic stimulation shifts the autoregulatory range to a higher level, thus maintaining a constant CBF and protecting the brain from too high a level of blood pressure at the arteriolar ends of the capillaries, despite an elevated arterial blood pressure. Ablation of the cervical sympathetics has opposite effects, thus extending the protection against low arterial blood pressures.

Chemical Factors

It is generally believed that regulation of cerebral vascular tone is achieved mainly by chemical factors. There are many chemical substances that have effects on the tone of the cerebral vessels and have been, and often still are, candidates for the role of main mediator of regulation of cerebral vascular tone and blood flow. These are listed in Fig. 1. Most prominent among them are the respiratory gases. It has been repeatedly demonstrated in animals and man that elevated arterial and/or tissue pCO_2 dilates cerebral vessels and increases CBF, and that reverse changes in CO_2 tensions have the opposite effects [31, 34, 59]. Less pronounced, but still quite effective, are the influences of alterations in arterial and/or tissue pO_2; reduced pO_2 dilates cerebral vessels and increases CBF, while raised pO_2 has the opposite effect [31, 34, 59]. Blood and tissue pH also influence cerebral vascular tone. Acids dilate and bases constrict cerebral vessels [34, 59]. Indeed, some of the effects of CO_2 may be mediated by its effects on pH. For example, with chronic exposure to high CO_2 levels, CBF is at first elevated, but then adapts and returns toward normal, despite continued high pCO_2, when compensation for the respiratory acidosis occurs and CSF pH returns to normal. Adaptation to low arterial pCO_2 also occurs. During the respiratory alkalosis and low arterial pCO_2 caused by hyperventilation at high altitudes, CBF is initially reduced, but returns to near normal when compensation occurs and CSF pH returns to normal, despite the continued low arterial pCO_2. The vasodilator effects of CO_2 cannot, however, be entirely due to the lowering of the pH that it produces, because opposite effects, i.e., vasoconstriction with low pH and vasodilatation with elevated pH, have also been observed [55, 59].

Because elevated pCO_2 and reduced pO_2 and pH (changes to be expected in tissues when their rate of energy metabolism is increased) cause cerebral vasodilation, whereas changes in gas tensions and pH in the opposite direction (to be expected from decreased metabolism) cause cerebral vasoconstriction, it has been widely assumed that, as proposed by Roy and Sherrington [50], local CBF and metabolic rate are tightly coupled through the regulation of cerebral vascular tone by products of tissue-energy metabolism.

Local energy metabolism in neural tissues has been shown to vary with functional activity [60], but it has been difficult to prove that products of energy metabolism are the sole mediators of the adjustment of CBF to functional activity. This is because many other chemical factors, not directly related to energy metabolism, but possibly to functional activity, have been found to influence the cerebral circulation and have not been excluded. Some of them are listed in Fig. 1. For example, K^+, which has vasodilator effects, is released from neuronal elements in the generation of action potentials, and extracellular K^+ concentration may rise during excitation. Ca^{2+} exchange between extracellular and intracellular compartments is involved in most of the processes associated with excitation and neural activity, and Ca^{2+} uptake into vascular smooth muscle is involved in its contractility. Nitric oxide is a potent vasodilator, which is produced by two different isoforms of the nitric oxide synthase, one in vascular endothelium and the other in some neurons; the activity of both is activated by Ca^{2+}/calmodulin. Adenosine and adenine derivatives have vasodilator effects and are released from functionally activated cerebral tissues [46]. Prostaglandins have been reported to have influence on the cerebral circulation [45]. Many other naturally occurring chemical substances exert effects on cerebral vascular tone. It may well be that the search for a single chemical factor that regulates the CBF to meet the metabolic demands of the tissue is fruitless; the regulation may be achieved not by one, but rather by combinations of many or all of them [33].

Effects of Restriction of Cerebral Glucose Utilization on CBF

In order to investigate further possible mechanisms that might be involved in the regulation of CBF, we chose a model in which energy metabolism and CBF are dissociated. Restriction of the brain's glucose utilization, either by limiting its glucose supply, as, for example, in insulin-induced hypoglycemia, or by pharmacological block-

Table 1. Effects of insulin in euglycemic conditions, insulin-induced hypoglycemia, and pharmacological doses of 2-deoxyglucose (2-DG) on blood constituents. Values are mean ± SD calculated from the numbers in parentheses. Insulin-treated rats were administered 10 U/kg of insulin, and plasma glucose level was maintained englycemic by administration of a 10 % glucose solution

Physiological variables	Saline treated	Insulin treated		Deoxyglucose treated
		Hypoglycemia	Euglycemia	
	($n=7$)	($n=11$)	($n=7$)	($n=6$)
Mean arterial blood pressure (mmHg)	119±7	118±7	118±9	122±10
Arterial pO_2 (mmHg)	88±7	88±4	95±3[c]	92±8
Arterial pCO_2 (mmHg)	37±1	39±1	38±2	42±1[b, d]
Arterial pH	742±0.02	7.37±0.03[b]	7.38±0.04[b, d]	7.36±0.02[b, c]
Arterial blood HCO_3 concentration (mM)	24±1	23±2[a]	22±2[b]	24±1[a]
Arterial plasma glucose concentration (mM)	7.4±0.8[a]	2.3±0.1[b]	7.3±1.5	13.3±3[b, c]
Arterial plasma insulin concentration (mM)	0.6±0.1	-	>9.3	0.8±0.6 ($n=3$)
Arterial plasma K^+ concentration (mM)	4.2±0.3	3.2±0.4[b]	3.2±0.4[b, d]	3.6±0.8
Arterial plasma lactate concentration (mM)	0.9±0.1	1.3±0.3[a]	1.4±0.3[a, d]	1.1±0.2
Plasma epinephrine (ng/ml)	0.5±0.11	7.45±0.33	-	3.32±0.45[a]

[a]$P<0.05$ [b]$P<0.01$, compared with values before treatment in the same animal (paired t test)
[c]$P<0.05$ [d]$P<0.01$, compared with saline-treated group (grouped t test)

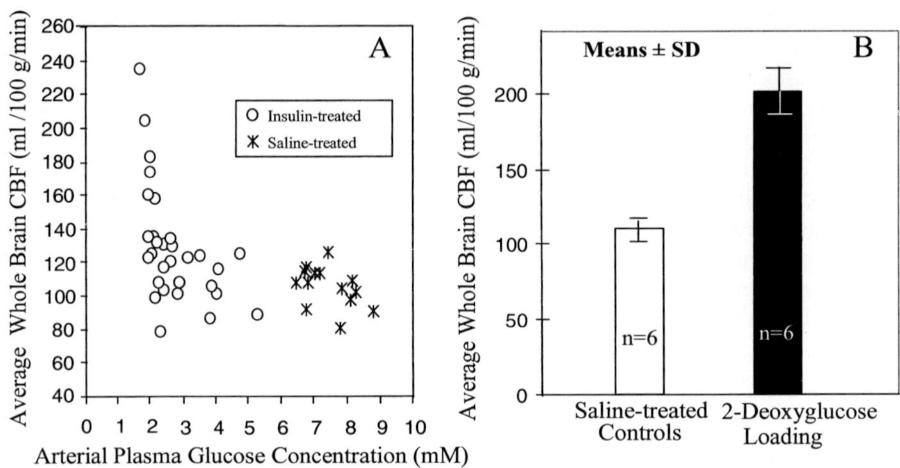

Fig. 2. A Global cerebral blood flow (CBF) as a function of arterial plasma glucose level in conscious rats, in which hypoglycemia was induced by insulin (0.125–15 U/kg intravenously) and in saline-treated control rats. **B** Effects of pharmacological doses (200 mg/kg intravenously) of 2-deoxyglucose (2-DG) on global CBF in conscious rats. From Horinaka et al. [25]

ade of glycolysis with loading doses of 2-deoxyglucose (2-DG) results in marked increases in CBF [1, 7, 8, 14, 23, 25, 26, 43]. Because cerebral energy metabolism is inhibited in these conditions, increased production of vasodilator products of metabolism cannot explain the enhancement of CBF. The effect of the hypoglycemia on CBF is not graded; CBF, measured quantitatively in unanesthetized rats with the $[^{14}C]$iodoantipyrine ($[^{14}C]$IAP) method [53], does not change with falling arterial plasma-glucose level until arterial plasma-glucose levels reach 2–3 mM (Fig. 2A); at this level, the rats are still conscious and free of seizure activity. Several systemic factors, e.g., MABP, arterial pCO_2, pO_2, pH, and hematocrit, etc., which could influence CBF have been excluded [25] (Table 1).

Lack of Direct Effect of Insulin on CBF

The possibility that the increase in CBF was not due to hypoglycemia, per se, but rather to a direct action of insulin on the cerebral circulation, was also excluded. Equivalent administration of insulin combined with glucose to maintain euglycemic conditions had no significant effects on CBF (Fig. 3A). Furthermore, when cerebral glycolysis is blocked by pharmacological doses of 2-DG, the enhancement of CBF is even greater than that elicited by insulin administration (Fig. 2B).

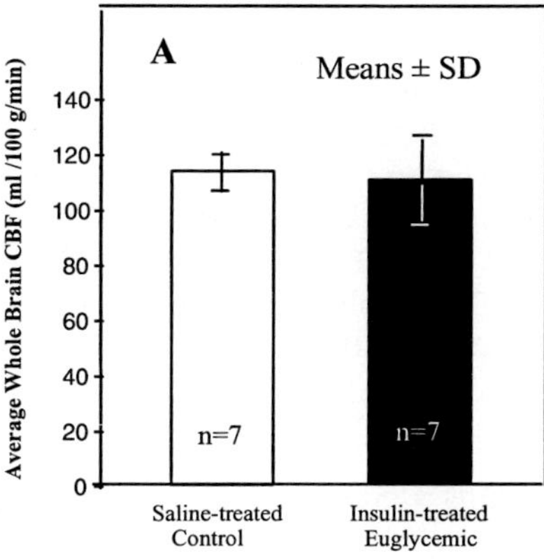
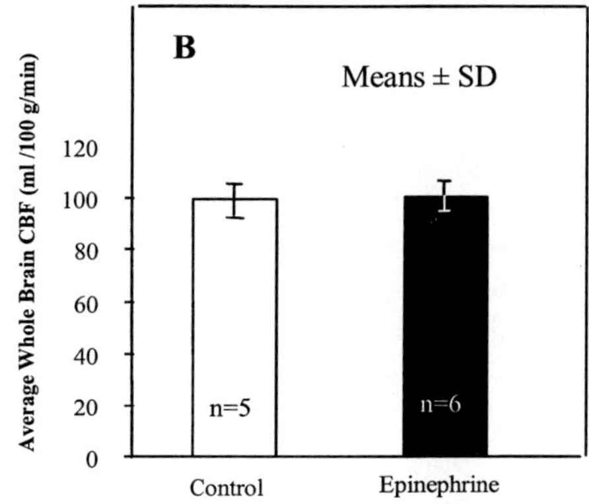

Fig. 3A, B. Effects of insulin under euglycemic conditions (A) and epinephrine (B) on global cerebral blood flow (CBF). A, Insulin (10 U/kg) and glucose (2.5 ml/10 % glucose in water) were injected intravenously. Additional glucose was injected as needed. From Horinaka et al. [25]. B Effects of continuous intravenous infusion of epinephrine (2.3–2.6 µg/kg/min) at sufficient rate to raise arterial plasma levels 10- to 20-fold, as much or greater than observed during glucoprivation. From Horinaka et al. [24]

Lack of Influence of Insulin-Induced Changes in Plasma Lactate and K$^+$ Concentrations on CBF

Insulin promotes uptake of glucose and K$^+$ into skeletal muscle where the glucose is metabolized to lactate for excretion into the blood. These effects were manifested in rats with insulin-induced hypoglycemia by a significant rise in lactate and decrease in K$^+$ levels in the plasma (Table 1). These changes in plasma constituents did not, however, cause the increases in CBF, because the same plasma changes were seen in the insulin-treated euglycemic animals with no changes in CBF (Table 1) (Fig. 3A). Furthermore, loading doses of 2-DG produced even more profound increases in CBF without any effects on plasma lactate and K$^+$ concentrations (Table 1) (Fig. 2B).

Lack Of Effects of Epinephrine on CBF

Hypoglycemia is one of Cannon's stresses known to stimulate the sympathetic nervous system. Indeed, both insulin-induced hypoglycemia and 2-DG loading resulted in marked increases in arterial plasma-epinephrine levels from control levels of about 0.5 ng/ml to 7.5 ng/ml and 3.3 ng/ml, respectively [24]. To determine whether these rises in plasma-epinephrine levels contributed to the increases in CBF during cerebral glucose deprivation, epinephrine was continuously infused intravenously at rates that raised arterial plasma-epinephrine levels 10- to 20-fold, at least as much and even more than those occurring during glucose deprivation. There were absolutely no effects whatsoever on either global CBF (Fig. 3B) or on local CBF and glucose utilization in any of 25 cerebral structures examined [24]. These results clearly excluded rises in plasma-epinephrine levels as responsible for the increased CBF during cerebral glucose deprivation.

Effects of Inhibition of Nitric Oxide Synthase Activity

Acute intravenous administration of 30 mg/kg of N^G-nitro-L-arginine methyl ester (L-NAME) raised MABP ($P<0.0002$) and lowered CBF ($P<0.0001$), indicating that the drug had effectively inhibited some nitric oxide synthase activity and that nitric oxide normally exerted tonic influence on systemic and cerebral vascular beds. Despite its effects on MABP and baseline CBF, acute L-NAME administration did not significantly reduce the percentage increases in CBF, evolted by insulin-induced hypoglycemia or pharmacological doses of 2-DG [25] (Fig. 4).

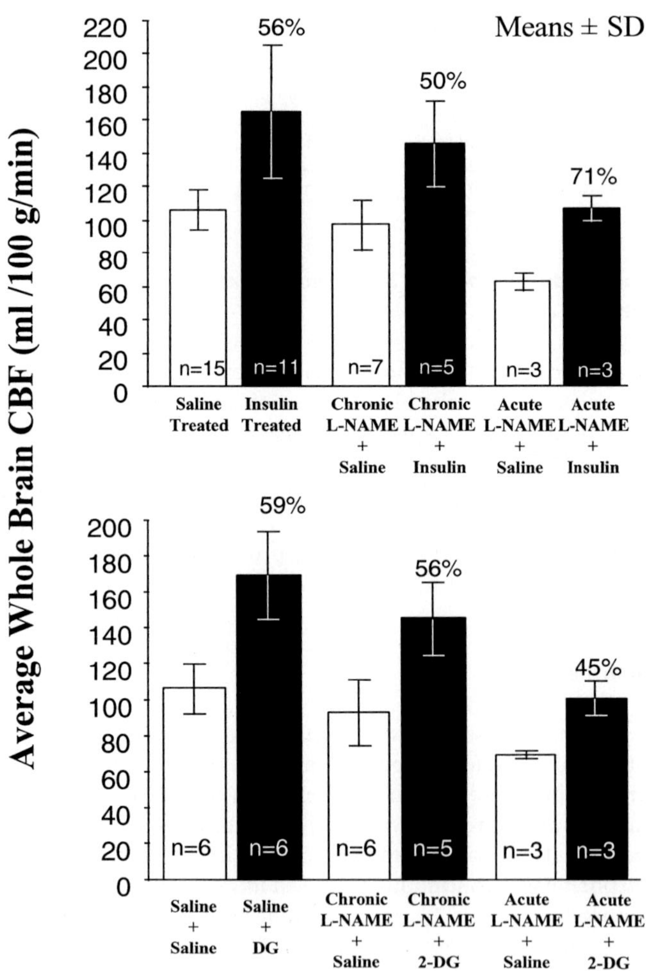

Fig. 4. Effects of acute [single intravenous dose of 30 mg/kg of N^G-nitro-L-arginine methyl ester (L-NAME)] and chronic (50 mg/kg L-NAME intraperitoneally twice daily for 4 days) inhibition of nitric oxide synthase activities on cerebral blood flow (CBF) responses to insulin-induced hypoglycemia (*upper*) or pharmacological doses of 2-deoxyglucose (2-DG) (*lower*). From Horinaka et al. [25]

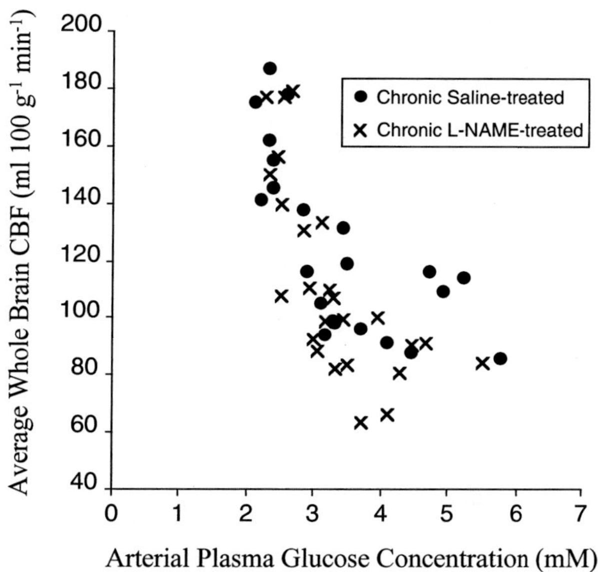

Fig. 5. Influence of arterial plasma glucose concentration on global cerebral blood flow (CBF) in insulin-treated (0.25–20 U/kg) rats after intraperitoneal injections of either saline or N^G-nitro-L-arginine methyl ester (L-NAME) (50/mg/kg) twice daily for 4 days. From Horinaka et al. [25]

Although the increases in MABP and decreases in CBF produced by acute intravenous injections of L-NAME indicated that at least endothelial nitric synthase activity was inhibited, it was conceivable that neuronal nitric oxide synthase within the brain was unaffected because of limited transport of L-NAME across the blood–brain barrier. Chronic pretreatment with L-NAME by intraperitoneal injections of 50 mg/kg twice daily for 4 days has been shown to inhibit 85–95 % of total brain nitric-oxide-synthase activity [2, 15], suggesting that both the neuronal and endothelial nitric-oxide-synthase activities were inhibited. When we employed this dosage regimen, MABP rose to levels similar to those following acute L-NAME administration ($P<0.001$), and in normoglycemic rats with arterial plasma glucose levels in the 3-mM to 6-mM range, CBF tended to be reduced below the levels in the saline-treated control rats (Fig. 5). When arterial plasma glucose levels were reduced to 2–3 mM, however, CBF rose in the L-NAME-treated rats just as precipitously as it did in the saline-treated rats (Fig. 5). Also, the percentage increases in CBF due to hypoglycemia or 2-DG loading were unaffected by the chronic L-NAME-treatment (Fig. 4). Therefore, nitric oxide does not appear to play a role in the enhancement of CBF by cerebral glucose deprivation.

Evidence for Role of Adenosine in Mechanism of Enhancement of CBF by Cerebral Glucose Deprivation

Another possible candidate to be considered was adenosine, which is known to have vasodilator effects in various tissues, including brain [6, 33]. Because it has many properties to be expected of a physiological regulator of cerebral vascular tone, it has been proposed as a mediator of metabolic regulation of CBF [52, 69]. For example,

Table 2. Effects of insulin-induced hypoglycemia and pharmacological doses of 2-deoxyglucose (2-DG) on adenosine, inosine and hypoxanthine levels in conscious rat brain. Values are expressed as mean ± SD of the number of animals in parentheses

Compound	Saline-treated normo-glycemic controls (*n*=8)	Insulin-induced hypoglycemia (*n*=9)	2-DG loading (*n*=9)
Adenosine (nmol/g brain)	0.70±0.14	2.79±1.62**	5.81±3.90**
Inosine (nmol/g brain)	0.39±0.38	1.41±1.26*	16.54±13.25**
Hypoxanthine (nmol/g brain)	9.65±5.86	23.09±14.79*	132.94±53.27***

2-DG 2-deoxyglucose
*$P<0.05$, **$P<0.01$, ***$P<0.001$ compared with normoglycemic saline-treated controls (grouped *t*-test). Data from Horinaka et al. [26]

adenosine levels in brain tissue rise during cerebral ischemia [6, 44, 66], hypotension [67], hypoxia [68], seizures [56], and during chemical or electrical stimulation [57]; these are all conditions in which cerebral-resistance vessels are dilated. It is noteworthy that the increases in CBF in hypoglycemia appear or become prominent when arterial plasma-glucose concentrations fall to about 2–3 mM [25], the level at which the brain's ability to metabolize glucose and to phosphorylate adenosine diphosphate (ADP) to adenosine triphosphate (ATP) levels is impaired [19, 63]. Conditions that tend to raise ADP levels favor formation of adenosine (see Discussion). It, therefore, seemed advisable to examine the possibility of a role for adenosine in the increases in CBF during cerebral glucose deprivation.

First, we measured the effects of insulin-induced hypoglycemia and 2-DG loading on the levels of adenosine and its metabolic-degradation products, inosine and hypoxanthine, in rat brains that had been rapidly frozen in vivo by the freeze-blowing technique of Veech et al. [65]. The results confirmed that, in both conditions, adenosine release is markedly enhanced in the brain, particularly with the loading doses of 2-DG, which led to average 8-fold, 41-fold, and 13-fold increases for adenosine, inosine and hypoxanthine, respectively (Table 2). We, therefore, examined the effects of caffeine, a nonselective adenosine receptor antagonist, on the CBF response to insulin-induced hypoglycemia in unanesthetized rats. Acute intravenous injections of caffeine (10 mg/kg and 20 mg/kg) produced dose-dependent reductions in the percentage increases in CBF in hypoglycemia, to the point of complete abolition of the response (Fig. 6, upper panel). This result clearly implicates adenosine in the mechanism of the response.

Evidence for Role of Inwardly Rectifying ATP-Sensitive K⁺ Channels in the Mechanism of Enhancement of CBF in Hypoglycemia

Whatever the mediator of the increased CBF in glucose deprivation may be, adenosine or some other agent, it must ultimately invoke additional mechanisms that will lead to relaxation of cerebral-vascular smooth muscle. K⁺ channels may well be involved in this process. ATP-sensitive K⁺ (K_{ATP}) channels, first described in cardiac muscle [42], have also been found in skeletal muscle [61], β cells of the pancreas [4, 12], neurons [5] and vascular smooth muscle [39, 62]. These channels are regulated

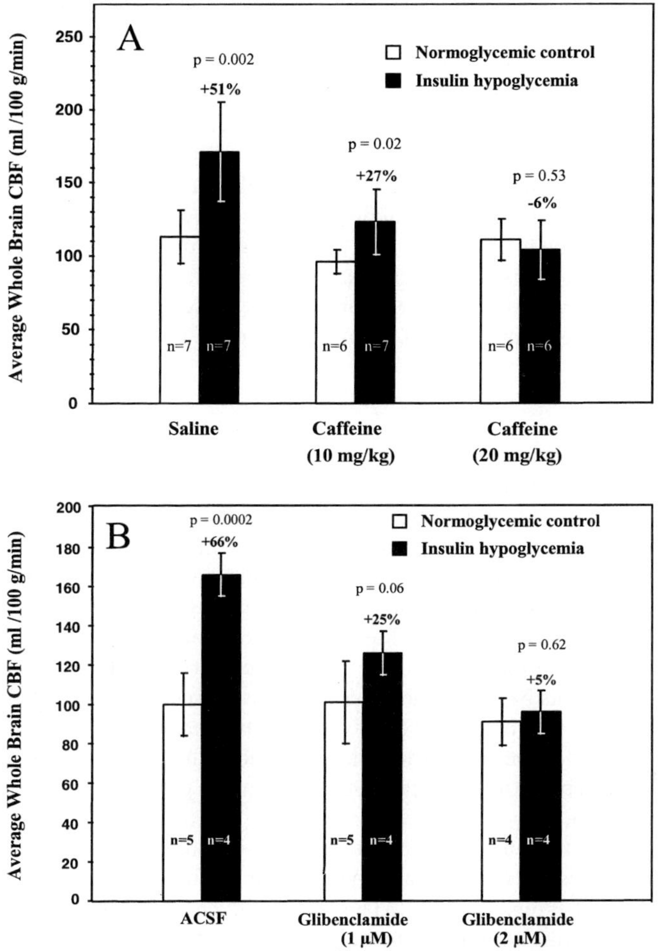

Fig. 6A, B. Effects of blockade of adenosine receptors by caffeine or of ATP-sensitive K^+ channels by glibenclamide on the cerebral blood flow (CBF) response to insulin-induced hypoglycemia. A Effects of intravenous caffeine administration in doses indicated. B Effects of continuous 30-min intracisternal infusions of 1 μM and 2 μM glibenclamide, dissolved in artificial cerebrospinal fluid (ACSF) on the CBF response to insulin-induced hypoglycemia. From Horinaka et al. [26]

by intracellular ATP and open when intracellular ATP levels fall. When open, K^+ efflux occurs, and the smooth-muscle-cell membrane is hyperpolarized, voltage-gated Ca^{2+} channels are closed, the smooth muscle is relaxed and, in the case of blood vessels, dilatation occurs [40, 41]. These channels appear to be involved in cerebral arterial dilatation, which can be induced by treatment with K_{ATP} channel openers [18]. Decreased glucose concentration has been shown to open K_{ATP} channels in pancreatic β cells and neurons in the brain [17]. K_{ATP} channels are also modulated by various normal endogenous substances. For example, the vasodilators, CGRP and adenosine, have been shown to activate K_{ATP} channels in smooth muscle of systemic arteries and gallbladder [13, 40, 47, 72]. Presumably, adenosine and K_{ATP} channels could be acting independently, sequentially or in concert to increase CBF during glucose deprivation.

To investigate the possibility that K_{ATP} channels might be involved in the increases in CBF in cerebral glucose deprivation, we examined the effects of the K_{ATP} channel blocker, glibenclamide, on the CBF response to insulin-induced hypoglycemia in unanesthetized rats [26]. Because glibenclamide does not readily cross the blood-brain barrier, it was administered by continuous intracisternal infusion in concentrations of 1 µM and 2 µM in artificial cerebrospinal fluid (ACSF) for 30 min prior to and for 1 min during the measurement of CBF by the $[^{14}C]IAP$ method. Glibenclamide produced dose-dependent reductions in the percentage increases in CBF in hypoglycemia to the point of complete abolition of the response (Fig. 6, lower panel), suggesting that K_{ATP} channels are, indeed, involved in the mechanisms of the effect.

Discussion

These studies provide cogent evidence that adenosine plays an important role in the regulation of CBF. Insulin-induced hypoglycemia or blockade of cerebral glucose utilization by pharmacological doses of 2-DG result in marked enhancements of CBF, which are not due to insulin, per se, or its effects on blood constituents, elevated blood epinephrine levels or nitric oxide. The glucose deprivation leads to large increases in levels of adenosine and its metabolites in the brain, indicating increased adenosine formation. There is abundant evidence in the literature (see above) that adenosine has vasodilator actions by interactions with adenosine receptors on vascular smooth muscle. Caffeine, a relatively nonselective antagonist of adenosine receptors, inhibits in a dose-dependent manner and, ultimately, abolishes the increase in CBF due to cerebral glucose deprivation, indicating that adenosine plays a crucial role in the mechanism of the effect.

How does an interaction of adenosine with its receptors result in relaxation of smooth muscle in cerebral resistance vessels and vasodilation? Other results of these studies implicate inwardly rectifying channels, ATP-sensitive K^+ channels, which have been demonstrated in vascular smooth muscle, including that of cerebral vessels. When opened, these channels allow K^+ efflux from the cells, resulting in hyperpolarization and closure of voltage-gated Ca^{2+} channels, relaxation of the smooth muscle, and vasodilation. The evidence implicating these channels is the finding that glibenclamide, a specific inhibitor of these channels, can inhibit in a dose-dependent manner, to the point of extinction, the increases in CBF due to cerebral glucose deprivation. It is relevant that glibenclamide also blocks the 2-DG-induced hyperpolarization and dilatation in rat coronary arteries [11]. Adenosine and its receptors as well as K_{ATP} channels in vascular smooth muscle appear, therefore, to be fundamentally involved in the regulation of CBF during cerebral glucose deprivation, and possibly in many other conditions, such as hypoxia, in whichcaffeine has also been found to block the usual increases in CBF [28].

If the blockades of the CBF response to cerebral glucose deprivation by caffeine and glibenclamide are due to their presumed probable actions, i.e., caffeine antagonism of adenosine at adenosine receptors and glibenclamide inhibition of K_{ATP} channels in vascular smooth muscle, then they suggest the following unifying hypothesis about a mechanism that includes both adenosine and K_{ATP} channels and is common

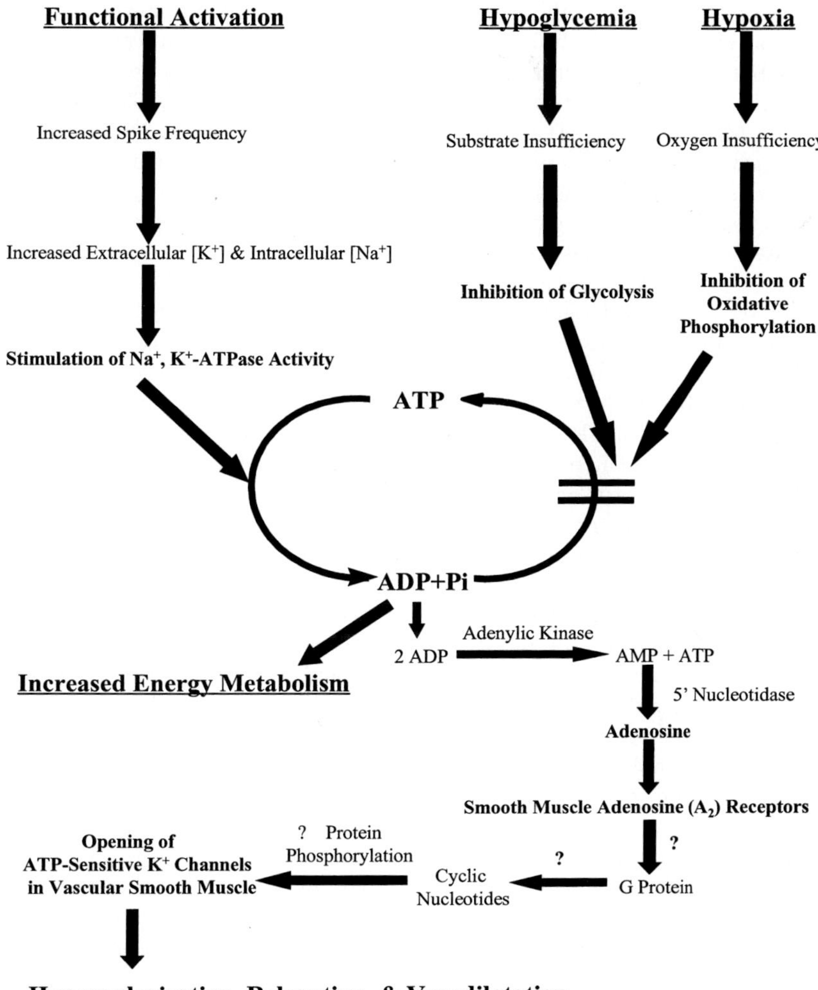

Fig. 7. Diagram of proposed sequence of events involved in the regulation of cerebral blood flow (CBF) in response to deficient substrate supply and/or activated neural activity (see Discussion). The question marks placed at several sites in the schema do not imply that such factors have not yet been found; they have been found to operate in some tissues, but have not yet been proved to be involved in the regulation of the cerebral circulation. Modified from Horinaka et al. [26]

to both the adjustment of CBF to the increased energy demand associated with functional activation and to inadequate substrate supply (Fig. 7). Functional activation in neural tissues is essentially synonymous with increased neuronal spike activity, and local glucose utilization is increased in direct proportion to the increase in local spike frequency [29]. The stimulation of glucose utilization is due to the activation of Na⁺/K⁺-ATPase activity to restore ionic gradients across the cell membranes, which have been partially degraded by the spike activity [35].

ATPase activation increases the ADP/ATP ratio and the ADP and inorganic phosphate (Pi) concentrations, which in turn stimulate glycolysis, electron transport, and energy metabolism. Electrical stimulation of brain tissue in vitro has been shown to result in the release of adenosine and its metabolites from the tissue [46]. Glucose deprivation [9, 25, 26], hypoxia [31, 51] and bicuculline-induced seizures [36, 70] are all conditions in which both CBF and brain adenosine levels have been shown to be elevated. In addition, there are conditions, such as hypotension [66] and ischemia [67], in which, for obvious reasons, CBF does not increase, but in which brain adenosine levels rise and cerebral vessels dilate. In all these conditions the ADP/ATP ratio and ADP levels tend to increase, due to either over-utilization or under production of ATP. Higher ADP levels lead to increased adenosine monophosphate (AMP) by action of the ubiquitous enzyme, adenylic kinase, thus providing substrate for the ecto-enzyme, 5'-nucleotidase, to produce adenosine. Adenosine action at smooth-muscle A_2 receptors produces cyclic AMP (cAMP), which has been shown to increase in brain tissue during electrical stimulation [30]. cAMP activates protein kinase A, which can phosphorylate the K_{ATP} channels in vascular smooth muscle. The phosphorylated channels may tend to open, resulting in increased K^+ efflux, hyperpolarization of cell membranes, decreased influx of Ca^{2+} through voltage-gated Ca^{2+} channels, relaxation of the vascular smooth muscle and vasodilation. Phosphorylation of K_{ATP} channels by cAMP-dependent protein kinase activity has been reported in vascular and other tissues [3, 20, 32, 49, 71]. This cascade is initiated by increased ADP levels, which leads to increased metabolism and/or formation and release of adenosine by brain tissue, followed by adenosine's action on caffeine-sensitive adenosine receptors on smooth muscle cells, and culminating in opening of the glibenclamide-sensitive K^+ channels. This sequence is diagrammed in Fig. 7.

This hypothesis does not include an obligatory relationship, e.g., "tight coupling", between energy metabolism and CBF. One is not a direct consequence of the other. Both are derived from the same initial chemical change, a shift in the balance from ATP to ADP, but they then evolve by separate, independent mechanisms (Fig. 7). Because the shift from ATP to ADP can stimulate both energy metabolism and adenosine formation and increased CBF, there may appear to be a so-called "coupling" of the two, but it is more a correlation than a true "coupling". Metabolism and CBF may, and often do, vary independently as, for example, in the moderate hypoglycemia used in the present studies [25, 26, 63].

Some reservations must be considered before this hypothesis can be accepted. First, it assumes that the observed effects of caffeine and glibenclamide are due to their specific actions on adenosine receptors and K_{ATP} channels in vascular smooth muscle. Caffeine also has other actions; for example, it acts on adenosine receptors in neurons, has localized effects on glucose utilization in the brain [38] and inhibits cyclic nucleotide phosphodiesterases, which degrade cyclic AMP and cyclic GMP. It may have a direct effect on K_{ATP} channels, bypassing the adenosine receptors; it has been reported to raise intracellular Ca^{2+} concentration in pancreatic β cells by directly inhibiting the K_{ATP} channels, resulting in depolarization-induced opening of L-type voltage-dependent Ca^{2+} channels [27]. Investigations on the effects of more-specific adenosine-receptor antagonists on the increases in CBF induced by cerebral-glucose deprivation as well as studies on the effects of inhibitors of adenosine receptors and K_{ATP} channels on the increases in CBF associated with functional activation are needed. Such studies are currently in progress.

References

1. Abdul-Rahman A, Agardh CD, Siesjö BK (1980) Local cerebral blood flow in the rat during severe hypoglycemia and in the recovery period following glucose injection. Acta Physiol Scand 109: 307–314
2. Adachi K, Takahashi S, Melzer P, Campos KL, Nelson T, Kennedy C, Sokoloff L (1994) Increases in local cerebral blood flow associated with somatosensory activation are not mediated by nitric oxide. Am J Physiol 267:H2155–H2162
3. Ashcroft SJH (1994) Protein phosphorylation and beta-cell function. Diabetologia 37[Suppl 2]:S21–S29
4. Ashcroft FM, Harrison DE, Ashcroft SJH (1984) Glucose induces closure of single potassium channels in isolated rat pancreatic β-cells. Nature 312: 446–448
5. Ashford ML, Sturgess NC, Trout NJ, Gardner NJ, Hales CN (1988) Adenosine-5'-triphosphate-sensitive ion channels in neonatal rat cultured neurones. Pflügers Arch 412: 297–304
6. Berne RM, Rubio R, Curnish RR (1974) Release of adenosine from ischemic brain: effect on cerebral vascular resistance and incorporation into cerebral adenine nucleotide. Circ Res 35: 262–271
7. Breier A, Crane AM, Kennedy C, Sokoloff L (1993) The effects of pharmacologic doses of 2-deoxy-D-glucose on local cerebral blood flow in the awake, unrestrained rat. Brain Res 618: 277–282
8. Bryan RM, Hollinger BR, Keefer KA, Rage RB (1987) Regional cerebral and neural lobe blood flow during insulin-induced hypoglycemia in unanesthetized rats. J Cereb Blood Flow Metab 7: 96–102
9. Chapman AG, Westerberg E, Siesjö BK (1981) The metabolism of purine and pyrimidine nucleotides in rat cortex during insulin-induced hypoglycemia and recovery. J Neurochem 36: 179–189
10. Chorobski J, Penfield W (1932) Cerebral vasodilator nerves and their pathway from the medulla oblongata. Arch Neurol Psychiatr Chicago 28: 1257–1289
11. Conway MA, Nelson MT, Brayden JE (1994) 2-Deoxyglucose-induced vasodilation and hyperpolarization in rat coraonary artery are reversed by glibenclamide. Am J Physiol 266:H1322–H1326
12. Cook DL, Hales CN (1984) Intracellular ATP directly blocks K^+ channels in pancreatic β-cells. Nature 311: 271–273
13. Dart C, Standen NB (1993) Adenosine-activated potassium current in smooth muscle cells isolated from the pig coronary artery. J Physiol (Lond) 471: 767–786
14. Della Porta P, Maiolo AT, Negri VU, Rossella E (1964) Cerebral blood flow and metabolism in the therapeutic insulin coma. Metabolism 13: 131–140
15. Dwyer MA, Bredt DS, Snyder SH (1991) Nitric oxide synthase: irreversible inhibition by L-N^G-nitroarginine in brain in vitro and in vivo. Biochem Biophys Res Commun 176: 1136–1141
16. Edvinsson L, MacKenzie ET, McCulloch J (1993) Cerebral blood flow and metabolism. Raven, New York, pp 57–91 and pp 183–312
17. Edwards G, Weston AH (1993) The pharmacology of ATP-sensitive potassium channels. Annu Rev Pharmacol Toxicol 33: 597–637
18. Faraci FM, Heistad DD (1993) Role of ATP-sensitive potassium channels in the basilar artery. Am J Physiol 264:H8–H13
19. Ghajar JBG, Plum F, Duffy TE (1982) Cerebral oxidative metabolism and blood flow during acute hypoglycemia and recovery in unanesthetized rats. J Neurochem 38: 397–409
20. Hamada Y, Nakaya Y, Hamada S, Kamada M, Aono T (1994) Activation of K^+ channels by ritodrine hydrochloride in uterine smooth muscle cells from pregnant women. Eur J Pharmacol 288: 45–51
21. Harmel MH, Hafkenschiel JH, Austin GM, Crumpton CW, Kety SS (1949) The effect of bilateral stellate ganglion block on the cerebral circulation in normotensive and hypertensive patients. J Clin Invest 28: 415–418
22. Harper AM, Deshmukh VD, Fitch W, Graham DI, MacKenzie, ET (1977) Effect of cervical sympathetic stimulation and ablation on CBF in normotensive, hypotensive and hypertensive primates. In: Owman C, Edvinsson L (eds) Neurogenic control of the brain circulation. Wenner-Gren Center International Symposium Series, Vol. 30, Pergamon, Oxford, pp 357–368
23. Hollinger BR, Bryan RM (1987) b-Receptor-mediated increase in cerebral blood during hypoglycemia. Am J Physiol 253:H949–H955
24. Horinaka N, Artz N, Cook M, Holmes C, Goldstein DS, Kennedy C, Sokoloff L (1997) Effects of elevated plasma epinephrine on glucose utilization and blood flow in conscious rat brain. Am J Physiol 272:H1666–H1671
25. Horinaka N, Artz N, Jehle J, Takahashi S, Kennedy C, Sokoloff L (1997) Examination of potential mechanisms in the enhancement of cerebral blood flow by hypoglycemia and pharmacological doses of deoxyglucose. J Cereb Blood Flow Metab 17: 54–63
26. Horinaka N, Kuang T-Y, Pak H, Wang B, Jehle J, Kennedy C, Sokoloff L (1997) Blockade of cerebral blood flow response to insulin-induced hypoglycemia by caffeine and glibenclamide in conscious rats. J Cereb Blood Flow Metab 17: 1309–1318

27. Islam S, Larsson O, Nilsson T, Berggren P-O (1995) Effects of caffeine on cytoplasmic free Ca^{2+} concentration in pancreatic β-cells are mediated by interaction with ATP-sensitive K^+ channels and L-type voltage-gated Ca^{2+} channels but not the ryanodine receptor. Biochem J 306: 679–686
28. Isozumi K, Fukuuchi Y, Takeda, H, Itoh Y (1994) Mechanisms of CBF augmentation during hypoxia in cats: probable participation of prostacyclin, nitric oxide, and adenosine. Keio J Med 43: 31–36
29. Kadekaro M, Crane AM, Sokoloff L (1985) Differential effects of electrical stimulation of sciatic nerve on metabolic activity in spinal cord and dorsal root ganglion in the rat. Proc Natl Acad Sci U S A 82: 6010–6013
30. Kakiuchi S, Rall TW, McIlwain H (1969) The effect of electrical stimulation upon the accumulation of adenosine 3', 5'-phosphate in isolated cerebral tissue. J Neurochem 16: 485–491
31. Kety SS, Schmidt CF (1948) The effects of altered arterial tensions of carbon dioxide and oxygen on cerebral blood flow and cerebral oxygen consumption of normal young men. J Clin Invest 27: 484–492
32. Kleppisch T, Nelson MT (1995) Adenosine activates ATP-sensitive potassium channels in myocytes via A_2 receptors and cAMP-dependent protein kinase. Proc Natl Acad Sci USA 92: 12441–12445
33. Kuschinsky W, Wahl M (1978) Local chemical and neurogenic regulation of cerebrovascular resistance. Physiol Rev 58: 656–689
34. Lassen NA (1959) Cerebral blood flow and oxygen consumption in man. Physiol Rev 39: 183–238
35. Mata M, Fink D J, Gainer H, Smith CB, Davidsen L, Savaki H, Schwartz WJ, Sokoloff L (1980) Activity-dependent energy metabolism in rat posterior pituitary primarily reflects sodium pump activity. J Neurochem 34: 213–215
36. Meldrum BS, Nilsson B (1976) Cerebral blood flow and metabolic rate early and late in prolonged epileptic seizures induced by bicuculline. Brain 99: 523–542
37. Nakai M, Iadecola C, Reis DJ (1982) Global cerebral vasodilation by stimulation of rat fastigial cerebellar nucleus. Am J Physiol 243:H226–H235
38. Nehlig A, Lucignani G, Kadekaro M, Porrino LJ, Sokoloff L (1984) Effects of acute administration of caffeine on local cerebral glucose utilization in the rat. Eur J Pharmacol 101: 91–100
39. Nelson MT (1993) Ca^{2+}-activated potassium chanels and ATP-sensitive potassium channels as modulators of vascular tone. Trends Cardiovasc Med 3: 54–60
40. Nelson MT, Huang Y, Brayden JE, Heschler JK, Standen NB (1990) Arterial dilations in response to calcitonin gene-related peptide involve activation of K^+ channels. Nature 344: 770–773
41. Nelson MT, Patlak JB, Worley JF, Standen NB (1990) Calcium channels, potassium channels, and voltage-dependence of arterial smooth muscle tone. Am J Physiol 259:C3–C18
42. Noma A (1983) ATP-regulated K^+ channels in cardiac muscle. Nature 305: 147–148
43. Norberg K, Siesjö BK (1976) Oxidative metabolism of the cerebral cortex of the rat in severe insulin-induced hypoglycemia. J Neurochem 26: 345–352
44. Nordstrom C-H, Rehncrona S, Siesjö BK, Westerberg E (1977) Adenosine in rat cerebral cortex: its determination, normal values, and correlation to AMP during shortlasting ischemia. Acta Physiol Scand 101: 63–71
45. Pickard JD (1981) Role of prostaglandins and arachidonic acid derivatives in the coupling of cerebral blood flow to cerebral metabolism. J Cereb Blood Flow Metab 1: 361–384
46. Pull I, MCIlwain H (1972) Adenine derivatives as neurohumoral agents in the brain. The quantities liberated on excitation of superfused cerebral tissues. Biochem J 130: 975–981
47. Quayle JM, Standen NB (1994) K_{ATP} channels in vascular smooth muscle. Cardiovasc Res 28: 797–807
48. Reis DJ, Iadecola C (1986) Regulation by the brain of its blood flow and metabolism: role of intrinsic neuronal networks and circulating catecholamines. In: Owman C, Hardebo JE (eds) Neural regulation of brain circulation. Elsevier, Amsterdam, pp 125–145
49. Roch B, Baro I, Hongre AS, Escande D (1995) ATP-sensitive K^+ channels regulated by intracellular CA^{2+} and phosphorylation in normal (T84) and cystic fibrosis (CFPAC-1) epithelial cells. Pflügers Arch 429: 355–363
50. Roy CS, Sherrington CS (1890) On the regulation of the blood supply of the brain. J Physiol (Lond) 11: 85–108
51. Rubio R, Berne RM, Bockman EL, Curnish RR (1975) Relationship between adenosine concentration and oxygen supply in rat brain. Am J Physiol 228: 1896–1902
52. Rubio R, Berne RM, Winn HR (1978) Production, metabolism and possible functions of adenosine in brain tissue in situ. In: Purves M, Elliott K (eds) Cerebral vascular smooth muscle and its control. Ciba Foundation Symposium 56, Elsevier/Excerpta Medica/North Holland, Amsterdam, pp 355–378
53. Sakurada O, Kennedy C, Jehle J, Brown JD, Carbin GL, Sokoloff L (1978) Measurement of local cerebral blood flow with iodo[^{14}C]antipyrine. Am J Physiol 234:H59–H66

54. Scheinberg P (1950) Cerebral blood flow in vascular disease of the brain, with observations on the effect of stellate ganglion block. Am J Med Sci 8: 139–147
55. Schieve JF, Wilson WP (1953) The changes in cerebral vascular resistance of man in experimental alkolosis and acidosis. J Clin Invest 32: 33–38
56. Schrader J, Wahl M, Kuschinsky W, Kreutzberg W (1980) Increase of adenosine content in cerebral cortex of the cat during bicuculline-induced seizure. Pflügers Arch 387: 245–251
57. Sciotti VM, Park TS, Berne RM, Van Wylen DGL (1993) Changes in extracellular adenosine during chemical or electrical brain stimulation. Brain Res 613: 16–20
58. Shenkin HA, Cabieses F, Van den Noordt G (1951) The effect of bilateral stellectomy upon the cerebral circulation of man. J Clin Invest 30: 90–93
59. Sokoloff L (1959) The action of drugs on the cerebral circulation. Pharmacol Rev 11: 1–85
60. Sokoloff L (1981) Localization of functional activity in the central nervous system by measurement of glucose utilization with radioactive deoxyglucose. J Cereb Blood Flow Metab 1: 7–36
61. Spruce AE, Standen NB, Stanfield PR (1985) Voltage-dependent ATP-sensitive potassium channels of skeletal muscle membrane. Nature 316: 736–738
62. Standen NB, Quayle JM, Davies NW, Brayden JE, Huang Y, Nelson MT (1989) Hyperpolarizing vasodilators activate ATP-sensitive K^+ channels in arterial smooth muscle. Science 245: 177–180
63. Suda S, Shinohara M, Miyaoka M, Lucignani G, Kennedy C, Sokoloff L (1990) The lumped constant of the deoxyglucose method in hypoglycemia: effects of moderate hypoglycemia on local cerebral glucose utilization in the rat. J Cereb Blood Flow Metab 10: 499–509
64. Takahashi S, Crane AM, Jehle J, Cook M, Kennedy C, Sokoloff L (1995) Role of the cerebellar fastigial nucleus in the physiological regulation of cerebral blood flow. J Cereb Blood Flow Metab 15: 128–142
65. Veech RL, Harris RL, Veloso D, Veech EH (1973) Freeze-blowing: a new technique for the study of brain in vivo. J Neurochem 20: 183–188
66. Winn HR, Rubio R, Berne RM (1979) Brain adenosine production in the rat during 60 seconds of ischemia. Circ Res 45: 485–492
67. Winn HR, Welsh JE, Rubio R, Berne RM (1980) Brain adenosine production in rat during sustained alteration in systemic blood pressure. Am J Physiol 239:H636–H641
68. Winn HR, Rubio R, Berne RM (1981) Brain adenosine concentration during hypoxia in rats. Am J Physiol 241:H235–H242
69. Winn HR, Rubio R, Berne RM (1981) The role of adenosine in the regulation of cerebral blood flow in brain. J Cereb Blood Flow Metab 1: 239–244
70. Winn HR, Welsh J, Rubio R, Berne RM (1981) Changes in brain adenosine during bicuculline-induced seizures in rats: effects of hypoxia and altered systemic blood pressure. Circ Res 47: 481–491
71. Xu ZC, Yang Y, Hebert SC (1996) Phosphorylation of the ATP-sensitive, inwardly rectifying K^+ channel, ROMK, by cyclic AMP-dependent protein kinase. J Biol Chem 271: 9313–9319
72. Zhang L, Bonev AD, Mawe GM, Nelson MT (1994) Protein kinase A mediates activation of ATP-sensitive K^+ currents by CGRP in gallbladder smooth muscle. Am J Physiol 267:G494–G499

VI Poster Presentations (Abstracts)

The Protective Effect of DY9760e, a Novel Calmodulin Antagonist, on Rat Permanent Middle Cerebral Artery Occlusion

K. Takagi, A. Tamura, H. Nakayama, K. Narita, M. Aoki,
T. Sato, and Y. Shirasaki

Background and Purpose. A newly synthesized calmodulin antagonist, DY9760e (3-[2-[4-(3-chloro-2-methylphenyl)-1-piperazinyl]ethyl]-5,6-dimethoxy-1(-imidazolyl-methyl)-1H-indazole dihydrochloride 3.5 hydrate), has been shown to possess a cytoprotective effect against cytotoxicity induced by Ca^{2+} overload [1]. Since Ca^{2+} overload is suspected to be one of the major causes of ischemic neuronal cell damage [2], we examined the effect of this drug on infarct volume in the rat permanent focal ischemia model.

Method. Eighteen spontaneously hypertensive rats were used (DY9760e: $n=8$, vehicle: $n=10$). The left middle cerebral artery was permanently occluded. DY9760e (0.5 mg/kg/hr) or vehicle was continuously administered intravenously for 6 h starting just after the ischemic insult. The rectal body temperature was kept at 37.5±0.5 °C. The animals were sacrificed 24 h after ischemia. Cerebral infarct volume was evaluated by 2,3,5-triphenyltetrazolium chloride stain.

Results. Mean arterial blood pressure was not affected by the treatment at this dose. In the vehicle and DY9760e groups, mean infarct volumes were 192.8±7.8 mm^3 and 150.3±9.2 mm^3 (mean±SE), respectively. Significant differences were recognized ($P<0.05$).

Conclusions. Intravenous administration of DY9760e, a novel calmodulin antagonist, showed a protective effect in the permanent focal ischemia model when treatment was begun just after the onset of ischemia. The effect of delayed post-ischemic treatment is now under way.

References

1. Sugimura M, Sato T, Nakayama W, Morishima Y, Fukunaga K, Omitsu M, Miyamoto E, Shirasaki Y (1997) DY-9760e, a novel calmodulin antagonist with cytoprotective action. Eur J Pharmacol 336: 99–106
2. Siesjö BK, Bengtsson F (1989) Calcium fluxes, calcium antagonists, and calcium-related pathology in brain ischemia, hypoglycemia, and spreading depression: a unifying hypothesis. J Cereb Blood Flow Metab 9: 127–140

Maturation Phenomenon in Cerebral Ischemia III
U. Ito et al. (Eds.)
© Springer-Verlag Berlin Heidelberg 1999

Amelioration of Brain Damage Following Transient Focal Ischemia in Rats by ONO-2506: Relevance of Its Modulating Action on Astroglial Functions

N. Tateishi, Y. Kagamiishi, T. Shimoda, K. Shintaku,
S. Satoh, and K. Kondo

Introduction. Accumulating evidence indicates that overexpression of S-100 protein, an astrocyte-derived protein, is detrimental to neuronal cells, resulting in various pathological conditions. Since ONO-2506 was shown to have a modulating action on the increase of S-100β content in cultured astrocytes, its time-dependent effects on the neurological deficits, brain water content, infarct volume, immunoreactivities of S-100 protein, and expression of inducible NO synthase messenger ribonucleic acid (iNOS mRNA) following transient focal ischemia in rats, were examined. We report here that ONO-2506 significantly ameliorates brain damage following transient focal ischemia, presumably through its inhibitory action on the overexpression of S-100 protein and iNOS mRNA.

Methods. Male Wistar rats anesthetized with diethylether were subjected to ischemia by insertion of a silicone-coated nylon suture (4–0) from the right internal carotid artery to the middle cerebral artery (MCA). Only those rats that exhibited focal neurological deficits (evaluated by the postural degree of rotation while being dangled by the tail, and by the decrease in traction force of the left hind leg) were used. One hour after MCA occlusion, the suture was pulled out for recirculation. In the first experiments, designed to determine the astroglial activation, rats were anesthetized with pentobarbital at the appropriate time after the transient ischemia, and perfusion fixation of brain was performed with 10% neutral-buffered formalin solution. Brain sections (7 µm) stained with hematoxylin and eosin were used for determination of the infarct area. The astroglial activation was evaluated by immunoreactive staining for S-100 protein and glial fibrillary acidic protein (GFAP). The expression of iNOS mRNA was examined using the reverse-transcription polymerase-chain-reaction method. In the second experiments, designed to determine the efficacy of ONO-2506 (1, 3, and 10 mg/kg, intravenously administered at 6, 24, and 48 h after recirculation), the infarct area and water content were examined at 72 h after recirculation.

Results and Conclusion. In the first experiments, the neurological deficits were steadily depressed throughout the observation period. The infarct volumes at 24, 48, 72, 120 and 168 h after recirculation were 13.7±3.6, 58.2±13.6, 102.3±9.2, 120.1±22.3 and 95.3±16.0 mm^3, in descending order. At each time point, GFAP immunoreactivity was observed around the infarct area. However, S-100 protein immunoreactivity was recognized as early as 6–9 h within the ischemic area, which was thought to correspond the ischemic core. Later, S-100 protein immunoreactivity became recognizable, not within but outside the periphery of the degenerative area, adjacent to the GFAP immunoreactivity area. At 24 h after recirculation, iNOS mRNA was induced in the

Maturation Phenomenon in Cerebral Ischemia III
U. Ito et al. (Eds.)
© Springer-Verlag Berlin Heidelberg 1999

ischemic area that was stained for S-100 protein. The overexpression of both S-100 protein and iNOS mRNA following recirculation was significantly suppressed in the ONO-2506 treated group compared with vehicle group. The neurological deficits, infarction area, and brain water content at 72 h were markedly ameliorated by ONO-2506.

The above results suggest that astroglial activation, which may be designated as "pre-mitotic S-100 peak (PSP)", precedes the neurodegeneration following transient focal ischemia, and should be distinguished from the so-called gliosis observed in the post-neurodegeneration and GFAP-dependent astroglial proliferation. It is surmised that the marked ameliorative effect of ONO-2506 on the brain damage is due to its suppressive action on the PSP.

The Effect of ONO-2506 on Permanent Focal Ischemia in Rats

T. Asano, T. Matsui, E. Mori, A. Tamura, N. Tateishi, Y. Kagamiishi, S. Satoh, and K. Kondo

Introduction. A novel synthetic agent, ONO-2506, which inhibits the production of S-100 protein by cultured astrocytes, was shown to ameliorate the brain damage following transient focal ischemia in rats. In the present study, we aimed to further examine its effects in the permanent middle cerebral artery occlusion (MCAO) model in rats.

Methods. Under halothane anesthesia, a total of 76 male Sprague-Dawley rats were subjected to MCAO according to modified Tamura's method. In the first experiment, rats were randomly divided into the following three groups: vehicle ($n=10$), ONO-2506 3 mg/day ($n=10$), and ONO-2506 10 mg/day ($n=10$). Drug administration (i. v., bolus) was started immediately after MCAO. The neurological status and body temperature were examined once per day, just prior to the daily drug administration. Perfusion fixation of the brain was carried out using 10 % formalin 72 h after MCAO. In the second experiment, rats were divided into two groups which received either vehicle ($n=24$) or ONO-2506 10 mg/day ($n=22$). Except for the fact that perfusion fixation of the brain was carried out 168 h after MCAO, they underwent the same procedures as in the first. Hematoxylin and eosin and terminal dUTP nick-end labeling (TUNEL) stains were used for histological evaluation of the brain damage. The infarct volume of each rat was calculated as the sum of necrotic areas in ten serial sections (1 mm apart) stained with hematoxylin and eosin.

Conclusion. As compared to the vehicle-treated group, the neurological deficits in the drug-treated groups were significantly ameliorated throughout the observation period. Whereas the infarct volume was not significantly different between the experimental groups at 72 h, the number of TUNEL-positive nuclei in the affected hemisphere was highly significantly increased in the ONO 2506-treated group. At 168 h, the total infarct volume was further increased in the vehicle group (70–92 mm^3), but not in the ONO-2506 group (64–58 mm^3). Hence, the difference became highly significant between the two groups. The above results indicate the progression of "maturation phenomena" beyond 72 h after permanent MCAO, thereby implicating the existence of the "secondary therapeutic time window" for permanent focal cerebral ischemia. The brain-protective effects of ONO-2506 and its mechanism of action in relation to astrocytic S100 protein certainly deserve further investigation.

Maturation Phenomenon in Cerebral Ischemia III
U. Ito et al. (Eds.)
© Springer-Verlag Berlin Heidelberg 1999

Preconditioning with 5 Min Forebrain Ischemia Ameliorated Mortality and Brain Edema Caused by 15 Min Forebrain Ischemia in the Gerbil

T. Mima, M. Fukuoka, and K. Mori

Introduction. Recent evidence that apoptosis, a programmed cell death, is at least partially involved in delayed neuronal death prompted us to hypothesize that selective and vulnerable death in the hippocampal CA1 sector acts like a "fuse system" in an electrical circuit to save the whole brain and the life system from further ischemic insults. To test this hypothesis, we used the ischemia model of the gerbil subjected to a 15-min occlusion of bilateral carotid arteries. The gerbils subjected to 15 min forebrain ischemia die slowly, until finally about 60 % of the animals die during a 14-day observation period. We examined whether or not preconditioning with 5 min forebrain ischemia, which almost always causes selective death of the hippocampal CA1 sector, ameliorates the mortality and brain edema caused by 15 min forebrain ischemia.

Materials and Methods. Male Mongolian gerbils, 60–70 g, were used. Under 2 % halothane anesthesia, bilateral common carotid arteries were occluded with Zen clips. Rectal temperature was maintained at 37.0–38.0 °C during ischemia and up to 1 h after reperfusion. A total of 101 gerbils were divided into two groups. Gerbils were given either a single insult of 15-min forebrain ischemia ($n=61$) or a double ischemic insult, i.e., 5-min forebrain ischemia followed by 15-min forebrain ischemia after a 10-day interval ($n=40$).

Results. During the 14-day observation, 59 % (36/61) of the gerbils died in the 15-min group; in contrast, as few as 35 % (14/40) of the gerbils died in the 5- to 15-min group ($P<0.05$, Mantel-Cox in Kaplan Meier method). Body-weight loss in the survivors at 14 days after the last ischemic insult was also significantly less in the 5- to 15-min group than in the 15-min group ($P<0.005$). The water content in each group was highest at 2 h, then subsided gradually. The water content in the 5- to 15-min group was significantly attenuated at all the time points compared with that in the 15-min group: 2 h ($P<0.0001$), 2 days ($P<0.01$), and 7 days ($P<0.0001$) after the last ischemic insult.

Conclusion. The beneficial effect of preconditioning with 5 min forebrain ischemia on mortality and body-weight loss was at least partially supported by the evidence that brain edema was significantly attenuated after 15 min forebrain ischemia. At present, however, it is not yet clear whether selective death of the hippocampal CA1 sector acted as a "fuse system", as we hypothesized, or other mechanisms induced by preconditioning with 5 min forebrain ischemia influenced the results.

Maturation Phenomenon in Cerebral Ischemia III
U. Ito et al. (Eds.)
© Springer-Verlag Berlin Heidelberg 1999

References

1. Kirino T, Sano K (1984) Selective vulnerability in the gerbil hippocampus following transient ischemia. Acta Neuropathol (Berl) 62: 201–208
2. Stummer W, Weber K, Tranmer B, Baethmann A, Kempski O (1994) Reduced mortality and brain damage after locomotor activity in gerbil forebrain ischemia. Stroke 25: 1862–1869
3. Fukuoka M, Mima T, Mori K (1997) Jpn J Stroke 19: 145–152

Alteration of Control Mechanisms of Endoplasmic Reticulum Calcium Pools in Focal Cerebral Ischemia

T. Dembo, K. Fukuuchi, K. Tanaka, T. Shirai, E. Nagata, D. Ito, S. Suzuki, and A. Futatsugi

Introduction. We previously reported that specific inositol 1,4,5-trisphosphate (IP_3) receptor binding was decreased only in the hippocampus CA1 following 2- or 4-h severe hemispheric ischemia of the gerbil brain [1, 2]. However, specific ryanodine receptor binding was already decreased in the hippocampus CA1 at 15 min of severe hemispheric ischemia in the gerbil brain [3]. In the present study, we performed autoradiographic analysis of $^{45}Ca^{2+}$ uptake into the endoplasmic reticulum (ER), Ca^{2+} release response via the IP_3 receptor (IP_3-induced Ca^{2+} release, or IICR) or the ryanodine receptor (Ca^{2+}-induced Ca^{2+} release, or CICR), binding capacity of IP_3 receptor and local cerebral blood flow (lCBF) in the rat brain subjected to 3- or 5-h occlusion of the right middle cerebral artery.

Materials and Methods. Eleven male Sprague-Dawley rats weighing 280–330 g were used. The right middle cerebral artery was permanently occluded via a transvascular approach using a nylon 3–0 or 2–0 suture, whose tip was coated with poly-L-lysine. The ^{14}C-iodoantipyrine method was employed to measure lCBF at the end of 3- or 5-h ischemia [4]. Sequential coronal brain sections were obtained on a cryostat. The sections for the measurement of IP_3 receptor binding were incubated with ^3H-IP_3 for 10 min. The remaining brain sections were preincubated in permeabilization buffer containing digitonin and incubated in the buffer containing $^{45}Ca^{2+}$ and adenosine triphosphate (ATP) for 1 h for the measurement of $^{45}Ca^{2+}$ uptake [5, 6]. IICR was examined by incubating the sections with $^{45}Ca^{2+}$ and IP_3, whereas CICR was examined by incubating the sections with $^{45}Ca^{2+}$ and caffeine [5, 6]. The obtained autoradiograms were analyzed using the image processor to quantify $^{45}Ca^{2+}$ uptake, IP_3 receptor binding and lCBF in the same regions of interest.

Results and Conclusion. Arterial blood gases, pH and mean arterial blood pressure were within the normal range. The obtained results were compared between the regions with $lCBF \leq 20$ ml/100 g/min (ischemic area and those with $lCBF \geq 90$ ml/100 g/min (non-ischemic area). Ca^{2+}-release response was evaluated by the ratio of $^{45}Ca^{2+}$ uptake obtained by incubating with only $^{45}Ca^{2+}$ to that obtained using $^{45}Ca^{2+}$ plus IP_3 or caffeine. Significant reduction in $^{45}Ca^{2+}$ uptake was noted only in the ischemic areas of the caudate putamen in the 3-h ischemia group. In contrast, Ca^{2+} uptake was significantly reduced in each ischemic area in the 5-h ischemia group. The binding capacity of IP_3 receptor was maintained at the normal level in each ischemia group. However, IICR was suppressed in the ischemic area of the caudate putamen in both ischemia groups. CICR remained normal in each structure of both ischemia groups. These data suggest that (1) the Ca^{2+}-uptake mechanism of ER in the caudate

Maturation Phenomenon in Cerebral Ischemia III
U. Ito et al. (Eds.)
© Springer-Verlag Berlin Heidelberg 1999

putamen may be significantly impaired even in the presence of ATP after 3 h severe ischemia, (2) impairment of Ca^{2+}-ATPase on ER may become apparent in the cerebral cortex following 3–5 h of ischemia, (3) the functional pathway between the activation of IP_3 receptor by IP_3 and IP_3-induced Ca^{2+} release from ER may be disrupted in the ischemic caudate putamen at 3 h of ischemia, and (4) intracellular Ca^{2+}-control mechanisms may be more vulnerable to ischemia in the caudate putamen than in the cerebral cortex in the present ischemia model, in which the former region belongs to the ischemic core.

References

1. Nagata E, Tanaka K, Gomi S, Mihara B, Shirai T, Nogawa S, Nozaki H, Mikoshiba K, Fukuuchi Y (1994) Alteration of inositol 1,4,5-trisphosphate receptor after six-hour hemispheric ischemia in the gerbil brain. Neuroscience 61: 983–990
2. Nagata E (1995) The autonomic nervous system 34: 119–126
3. Nozaki H, Tanaka K, Nagata E, Kondo T, Koyama S, Dembo T, Fukuuchi Y (1997) Rapid reduction in ryanodine binding of hippocampus CA1 in cerebral ischemia. Keio J Med 46: 85–89
4. Sakurada O, Kennedy C, Jehle J (1978) Measurement of local cerebral blood flow with iodo [14C] antipyrine. Am J Physiol 234:H59–H66
5. Verma A, Ross CA, Verma D (1990) Rat brain endoplasmic reticulum calcium pools are anatomically and functionally segregated. Cell Regul 1: 781–790
6. Verma A, Hirsch DJ, Snyder SH (1992) Calcium pools mobilized by calcium or inositol 1,4,5-trisphosphate are differentially localized in rat heart and brain. Mol Biol Cell 3: 621–631

Global Ischemia Induces Downregulation of GluR2 mRNA and Increases AMPA Receptor-Mediated Ca^{2+} Influx in Hippocampal CA1 Neurons

J. A. GORTER, E. M. ARONICA, T. OPITZ, M. V. L. BENNETT, J. A. CONNOR, and R. S. ZUKIN

Introduction. Transient, severe forebrain or global ischemia leads to delayed cell death of pyramidal neurons in the hippocampal CA1. The precise molecular mechanisms underlying neuronal cell death after ischemia are as yet unknown. Ca^{2+}-permeable GluR2 lacking alpha-amino-3-hydroxy-5-methyl-4-isoxazoleproprionate (AMPA) receptors are implicated in the pathogenesis of ischemia-induced degeneration. Global ischemia leads to reduced expression of GluR2 mRNA in vulnerable CA1 neurons prior to the delayed cell death. After ischemia, AMPA-receptor-mediated excitatory postsynaptic currents at the CA1/Schaffer collateral synapse are enhanced and increased in sensitivity to channel blockers selective for Ca^{2+}-permeable AMPA receptors. Moreover, 2,3-dihydroxy-6-nitro-7-sulfamoyl-benzo(F)-quinoxaline (NBQX), an AMPA antagonist, protects CA1 neurons against ischemia-induced damage, even when administered 16–24 h after ischemia. These observations suggest that "switching off" GluR2 expression in CA1 after an ischemic insult is translated into formation of new AMPA receptors lacking the GluR2 subunit. This change in receptor composition increases AMPA-receptor-mediated Ca^{2+} entry in response to endogenous glutamate and enhances glutamate pathogenicity in this region (the GluR2 hypothesis). The present study was performed to test whether GluR2 downregulation leads to AMPA-receptor-gated Ca^{2+} entry into CA1 neurons.

Materials and Methods. Forebrain ischemia in the gerbil was induced by temporary bilateral occlusion of the carotid arteries. Control gerbils were sham-operated. Neuronal damage was monitored by histological examination of toluidine-blue-stained brain sections at the level of the hippocampus. Glutamate receptor mRNA expression was assessed by in situ hybridization with [^{35}S] UTP-labeled RNA probes specific for GluR1, GluR2 and NR1. Slides were exposed to film (72 h) or, for higher resolution, dipped in photographic emulsion. For quantification, autoradiograms were analyzed with an image analysis system (NIH-IMAGE program). AMPA-receptor-mediated Ca^{2+} influx was assessed by intracellular recording and optical ratio imaging of individual fura-2-injected CA1 neurons in transverse slices of dorsal hippocampus from control and ischemic gerbils.

Results and Conclusions. In situ hybridization revealed that expression of RNA encoding GluR2 was markedly and specifically reduced in gerbil CA1 pyramidal neurons following global ischemia, but preceding the onset of neuron degeneration, to 85±2 %, 48±6 %, and 17±10 % of control at 24, 48 and 72 h, respectively. Expression of GluR1 and *N*-methyl-D-aspartate receptor subunit 1 was unchanged at 24 h and exhibited only modest decreases to 87±5 % and 93±5 % of control at 48 h in CA1. The

Maturation Phenomenon in Cerebral Ischemia III
U. Ito et al. (Eds.)
© Springer-Verlag Berlin Heidelberg 1999

ratio of GluR2 to GluR1 mRNA expression in a given region may be a predictor of the fraction of Ca^{2+} permeable receptors; this ratio declined steadily to 33 % of control by 72 h. Receptor expression showed little or no change in other subfields of the hippocampus. No changes in expression of glutamate receptor mRNAs were noted in other brain areas. To determine whether the change in GluR2 expression is functionally significant, we examined the AMPA receptor-mediated rise in cytoplasmic free Ca^{2+} in individual CA1 pyramidal neurons. At 72 h after ischemia, CA1 neurons that retained the ability to fire action potentials exhibited a greatly enhanced AMPA-elicited rise in intracellular free Ca^{2+}. Basal intracellular free-Ca^{2+} concentration in these neurons was unchanged. These findings provide evidence for Ca^{2+} entry directly through AMPA receptors in pyramidal neurons destined to die. Moreover, Ca^{2+} influx through AMPA receptors lacking the GluR2 subunit may be an important factor contributing to delayed neurodegeneration following global ischemia.

SPD 502 (NS 1209), a New Selective AMPA Antagonist, Reduces the Infarct Size in Rats Following Permanent Occlusion of the Middle Cerebral Artery

T. N. SAGER, A. MØLLER, F. WÄTJEN, O. B. PAULSON, and J. DREJER

Introduction. Alpha-amino-3-hydroxy-5-methyl-4-isoxazoleproprionate (AMPA)-antagonists (i.e., 2,3-dihydroxy-6-nitro-7-sulfamoyl-benzo(F)quinoxaline [NBQX] and 6-(1-imidazolyl)-7-nitroquinoxaline-2,3(1H,4H)-dione [YM900]) have shown protective effects in different animal models of focal and global cerebral ischemia. We have developed a new highly selective and water-soluble AMPA antagonist (SPD 502). The compound is well-tolerated in rodents producing no liver or kidney pathology after doses up to 120 mg/kg. The aim of the present study was to evaluate whether SPD 502 was also neuroprotective in a focal cerebral ischemia model.

Materials and Methods. Male spontaneous hypertensive rats (SHR), weighing 270–353 g were anaesthetized in 1.5–2.5 % halothane (30 % O_2 and 70 % N_2O) and the middle cerebral artery (MCA) was exposed through a craniotomy made at the base of the skull. Bipolar diathermy was used to permanently occlude the MCA between the inferior cerebral vein and the optic tract. SPD 502 was administered 2 h post-occlusion via a bolus dose (8 mg/kg bolus) followed by a 24-h infusion (4 mg/kg/h) through an indwelling jugular-vein cannula. The temperature was registered every fifth minute by means of a transmitter placed in the peritoneum, and heating lamps were activated if the temperature dropped below 36 °C. The infarct volumes were determined 2 days and 4 days after MCA occlusion by magnetic resonance (MR) imaging (diffusion- and T2-weighted images) on a 4.7 T SISCO MR scanner. Following the last MR scanning (day 4), the rats were decapitated and the brains frozen on dry ice for histological evaluation of the infarcts using hematoxylin and eosin staining. The total volume of the cerebral infarct was estimated using the Cavalieri volume estimator. Data were analyzed using Student's *t*-test.

Results and Conclusion. A total of 40 rats were operated. Fourteen animals were excluded from the study due to either striatal infarction or hemorrhagia; this was done prior to decoding the experiment. The resulting 26 animals consisted of 14 animals in the control group and 12 animals in the treated group. No difference in body temperature was seen between the two groups receiving SPD 502 treatment. In all three types of volume-measurements, SPD 502 induced a significant $\approx$20 % reduction of the infarct volume (Table 1).

Several first-generation competitive AMPA antagonists, including NBQX and YM900, have shown robust neuroprotective activity in models of global and focal cerebral ischemia. However, due to very poor water solubility, rapid kidney elimination and consequent kidney precipitation/necrosis at doses at or lower than neuroprotective doses, these first-generation AMPA antagonists have not been developed

Maturation Phenomenon in Cerebral Ischemia III
U. Ito et al. (Eds.)
© Springer-Verlag Berlin Heidelberg 1999

Table 1. Infarct volumes at different times after middle cerebral artery occlusion evaluated by magnetic resonance imaging and by hematoxylin and eosin staining. Values are mean ± SEM

	Control (mm^3)	SPD 502 (mm^3)	Reduction (%)	2P
Diffusion-weighted image (2d)	244±9.8	194±17.9	20.6	0.02
T2-weighted image (4d)	220±10.4	181±12.9	17.6	0.03
Hematoxylin and eosin (4d)	148±6.2	122±9.2	19.6	0.01

d = days

clinically. SPD 502 has an in vitro profile similar to NBQX and YM900 but, in contrast to these compounds, SPD 502 is highly water soluble (>100 mg/ml over a wide pH range) and has shown a long-lasting block of AMPA responses in vivo after a single intravenous dose. SPD 502 has also been found to be highly neuroprotective in a global cerebral ischemia model. The demonstration, in the present study, of a significant 20% reduction in infarct volumes by SPD 502, when administered 2 h post-occlusion in rats exposed to permanent MCAO, strongly suggests that SPD 502 should be evaluated clinically as treatment for acute neurodegenerative conditions such as stroke.

Neuroprotective Effects of Magnesium and Tirilazad in Rats Subjected to Transient Focal Cerebral Ischemia

R. Schmid-Elsaesser, E. Hungerhuber, S. Zausinger, A. Baethmann, and H.-J. Reulen

Introduction. Neuronal death after cerebral ischemia is mediated by a massive release of excitatory amino acids and generation of free radicals. Calcium influx into cells is considered to be a crucial step of the deleterious cascade triggered by ischemia. Magnesium competes with calcium to reduce calcium entry into cells, blocks voltage-sensitive and N-methyl-D-aspartate-activated ion channels, and inhibits the release of excitatory amino acids. The 21-amino steroid tirilazad is a well-known antioxidant. We speculated that combined administration of these clinically available drugs might be superior to current monotherapy.

Methods. Forty male Sprague-Dawley rats were intubated and ventilated with 0.8–1 % halothane in a mixture of 70 % N_2O and 30 % O_2. The animals were subjected to middle cerebral artery occlusion (MCAO) for 90 min by a silicone-coated 4–0 nylon monofilament. The temporalis muscle and rectal temperature were maintained at 37 °C. Physiological variables were monitored and kept within normal limits. The local cerebral blood flow (LCBF) was bilaterally recorded by means of continuous laser-Doppler flowmetry in cerebral cortex supplied by the MCA throughout ischemia and 1 h of reperfusion. The rats were randomly assigned to one of four treatment arms ($n=10$ each) that received an isovolumetric dose of (1) vehicle, (2) $MgCl_2$, (3) tirilazad, or (4) $MgCl_2$+tirilazad. $MgCl_2$ (2×1mmol/kg i. v.) and tirilazad (2×3mg/kg i. v.) were administered 15 min before ischemia and at reperfusion. Neurological deficits were quantified by daily neurological examinations. Infarct volume was histologically assessed in hematoxylin and esoin-stained coronal sections after 7 days. Statistical comparisons were made using the Kruskal-Wallis analysis of variance by rank, followed by comparison of all groups versus the control group using Dunnett's method. Differences were considered to be significant at $P<0.05$.

Results. Laser-Doppler flow measurements showed no significant difference in LCBF between the treatment groups and the control group. MCAO resulted in a reduction of blood flow to 20 % of baseline in the ipsilateral cortex supplied by the MCA. Post-ischemic hyperemia was observed for the first 15–20 min after reperfusion, followed by a gradual decrease in blood flow to about 70 % of baseline. Delayed hypoperfusion persisted until the end of the recording period. LCBF in the contralateral hemisphere remained unchanged throughout the experiment. Animals that received $MgCl_2$ or tirilazad monotherapy showed significantly ($P<0.05$) less neurological deficits than controls only on postoperative days 3 and 4, whereas treatment with both drugs significantly ($P<0.05$) improved neurological function from postoperative days 2–7. The infarct volume was 65.8 ± 21.2 mm^3 in controls, 49.3 ± 18.4 mm^{3}i n animals that

Maturation Phenomenon in Cerebral Ischemia III
U. Ito et al. (Eds.)
© Springer-Verlag Berlin Heidelberg 1999

received MgCl$_2$, 34.5±17.1 mm^3 in animals that received tirilazad, and 27.1±7.9 mm^3 in animals that received both drugs (mean±SD). Tirilazad and combination therapy significantly ($P<0.05$) reduced infarct volume compared with controls by 48 % and 59 %, respectively. The limitation of infarction by 24 % in rats treated with MgCl$_2$ alone did not reach a statistically significant level.

Conclusion. Combined antagonism of excitatory amino acids and free radicals enhances neuroprotective efficacy compared with monotherapy in transient focal cerebral ischemia. The results suggest that these drugs act without directly influencing CBF. In contrast to many experimental agents, magnesium and tirilazad offer the advantage that they are licensed for clinical use. It is conceivable that this drug combination could be of great benefit when given before temporary artery occlusion in cerebrovascular surgery.

Acknowledgement. Supported by DFG Schm 1067/2–1.

Do Natural Antioxidants Protect Neurons from Oxidative Stress Due to Their Anti-Radical Activity?

A. Boldyrev, P. Johnson, Y. Wei, Y. Tan, and D. Carpenter

Introduction. Carnosine, melatonin and taurine are compounds possessing antioxidant properties and protecting cells against oxidative stress. We have compared protection of rat neurons by carnosine, melatonin and taurine against free radicals generated by kainic acid, N-methyl-D-aspartate (NMDA), 3-(2-hydroxy-1-methyl-2-nitrosohydrazino)-N-methyl-1-propanamine (NOC-7) or 3-morpholinosydnonimine hydrochloride (SIN-1). Kainic acid and NMDA stimulate free-radical formation within the cells by activation of glutamate receptors, while NOC-7 and SIN-1 spontaneously generate nitric oxide and peroxinitrite, respectively, in aqueous solution.

Materials and Methods. Generation of reactive oxygen species (ROS) induced by the above compounds in neurons previously loaded with the ROS-trap, 2,7-dichloro-dihydro-fluorescein diacetate (DCF-DA), was measured by flow cytometry; the quantity of dead cells was estimated with propidium iodide. The protecting effects of the compounds used were tested after 1 h of preloading of neurons with each compound in physiological concentrations.

Results and Conclusion. Exposure of the cerebellum granule cells to 500 μM kainate, 500 μM NMDA, 100 μM NOC-7 or 100 μM SIN-1 results in an increase in intracellular fluorescence and partial death of neurons. Kainate or NMDA stimulates fluorescence by 50 %, the other two compounds by 200–400 %. In agreement with this observation, there is a decrease in viability of the neurons, from a few percent in the case of kainic acid or NMDA to 50 % in the case of NOC-7. Stimulation of ROS formation by kainate or NMDA is calcium dependent (it can be prevented by substitution of calcium ions in the medium by 1 mM EGTA). Contrary to these data, removal of calcium ions from the incubation medium did not affect ROS generation by SIN-1 or NOC-7. Carnosine was found to be the only compound able to suppress fluorescence induced by both stimulation of glutamate receptors and by SIN-1 and NOC-7 action, and to decrease neuronal death. Other compounds were partially effective: taurine protected cells against death induced by kainic acid (with no effect on the fluorescence) and melatonin increased viability in the presence of kainic acid or SIN-1, with no decrease in DCF-DA fluorescence (actually, in the presence of SIN-1, melatonin slightly stimulated the ROS level). We conclude that ROS generation is not the only reason for cell death induced by oxidative stress in tissues.

Maturation Phenomenon in Cerebral Ischemia III
U. Ito et al. (Eds.)
© Springer-Verlag Berlin Heidelberg 1999

Carnosine Protects Neurons from Excitoxic Effects of NMDA and Kainate

A. Boldyrev, D. Carpenter, Z. Kovalenko, N. Kuleva,
D. Lawrence, and R. Song

Introduction. Among different signals inducing apoptopic cell transformation, the most prominent are reactive oxygen species (ROS), overproduction of which usually accompanies oxidative stress in the cell. Long-lasting activation of glutamate receptors in neurons results in excitotoxic cell death (either apoptopic or necrotic), accompanied by an increased generation of ROS. In order to discover natural defense mechanisms against this kind of excitotoxicity, we focused our attention on the neuropeptide carnosine, which had been shown to be a hydrophilic antioxidant in both in vivo and in vitro experiments.

Materials and Methods. In the experiments, 12-day-old Wistar rats were used to prepare cerebellum granule cells, whose levels of ROS generation, necrotic and apoptopic transformation were then measured by flow cytometry with 2,7-dichlorofluorescein diacetate (DCF-DA), propidium iodide (PI) and annexin V, respectively. In order to stimulate ROS generation, the cells were exposed to 50–500 M NMDA or kainate for 10 min. Two sets of neurons were compared: those not treated and those pre-treated with carnosine or its acetylated derivative (10 mM each) 1 h prior to measurements.

Results and Conclusion. Exposure of DCF-DA-loaded cells to NMDA or kainic acid resulted in the increase of DCF-DA fluorescence, reflecting the level of intracellular ROS generation. However, in the case of neurons pre-loaded with carnosine or acetylcarnosine, their fluorescent response was several times lower. Carnosine was shown to suppress the response of cerebellum granule cells to excitotoxic ligands in both concentration-dependent and time-dependent manners, the $K_{0.5}$ value being about 0.75 mM. This effect could be related to the radical-scavenging ability of carnosine. Moreover, we had observed significant carnosine protection of neurons; excitotoxic death measured with PI or with annexin V demonstrated that the anti-radical effect is accompanied by prevention of both apoptopic and necrotic cell death.

Although acetylcarnosine was shown to be as effective as carnosine in suppression of DCF-DA-induced fluorescence, it did not prevent cell death. At the same time, acetylcarnosine did not protect cell histones against glycation. The conclusion is that the anti-glycating effect is an important condition of effective protection of neurons against excitotoxic death.

Acknowledgments. This work was supported by the Fullbright Foundation (21224, 1996–97, USA) and the Russian Foundation for Basic Research (96-04-49078).

Maturation Phenomenon in Cerebral Ischemia III
U. Ito et al. (Eds.)
© Springer-Verlag Berlin Heidelberg 1999

Aspects of Tolerance and Apoptosis: Cell and Molecular Biological Studies

V. COLANGELO, W. C. GORDON, W. J. LUKIW, P. K. MUKHERJEE, I. KLATZO, and N. BAZAN

Introduction. We have studied cell survival, intracellular signal transduction and gene expression responses in gerbils subjected to transient bilateral carotid artery occlusion at variable time intervals. We have tested the hypothesis that induction of tolerance has a biphasic character and is associated with attenuation of the signal leading to the upregulation of inducible cyclooxygenase isoform 2 (COX-2).

Methods. Gerbils were subjected to bilateral carotid artery occlusion and divided into the following groups: sham operated, 6 min of ischemia alone and 2 min of ischemia followed by either 15 min, 60 min or 3–4 days of circulation, and then by 6 min of ischemia . Three days later, some animals were sacrificed and cresyl violet and fluorescein isothiocyanate/deoxyuridine triphosphate terminal deoxynucleotidyl transferase-mediated dUTP nick-end labeling analyses were performed. Mitogen-activated protein (MAP) kinases were also assayed, and a reverse-transcription polymerase chain reaction (RT-PCR) was performed for several genes.

Results and Conclusion. We have found that 2 min of sublethal ischemia followed by 15 min and 3 days of recirculation and then 6 min of ischemia attenuates ischemia-induced activation of stress-sensitive MAP kinases and COX-2 expression. This correlates with decreased apoptosis in the CA1 sector and thalamus.

Acknowledgement. Study was funded by NIH NS 23002.

Maturation Phenomenon in Cerebral Ischemia III
U. Ito et al. (Eds.)
© Springer-Verlag Berlin Heidelberg 1999

VII Round Table Discussion

Round Table Summary

The round table discussion started with a brief history of the conceptual development of the maturation phenomenon and its experimental support provided by Professor Igor Klatzo. Professor Bazan then gave his impressions. He stated that it is enlightening to picture cell-signaling transduction as leading to different phases in cell death, activation, propagation, execution and final process. He felt that there is more to be learned about the messengers and receptor-mediated mechanisms that trigger the transcription and activation of genes encoding neurotrophic factors. Another area of interest to Professor Bazan involved the identification of mediators which allow communication between glial and neuronal cells. Some of these messengers are inflammatory mediators and the list would also include glutamate and several other diffusable messengers. It is becoming apparent that the inflammatory response has a neuronal component such that neuronal inflammatory signaling occurs in addition to the well-recognized contribution of microvasculature and inflammatory cells to inflammation. Professor Bazan also suggested that the way signaling dysfunction affects the fate of neurons will probably be a widely studied question. Mitochondria are very important in the final stages of cell death and should be addressed along with synaptic signaling dysfunction and uncoupling of oxidative phosphorylation.

Professor Siesjö noted that mitochondria have a high-capacity uniporter system that makes use of the electrochemical gradient for taking up calcium. Their capacity to extrude calcium is far more limited and involves a calcium-sodium exchange followed by normalization of the sodium by a further sodium ion exchange. Nearly 20 years ago a high-conductance calcium channel was described in mitochondria, the permeability transition pore. It was inhibited by cyclosporin A. The pore is voltage-sensitive and Ca^{2+}-activated and is modulated by many factors. Opening of the pore can be transient and reversible but if it is opened for a long time, free radicals form and mitochondria become irreversibly damaged. Redox changes appear to be important in that oxidants tend to open and reductants tend to close the pore. Professor Siesjö further noted that it has been recently shown that pore opening is regulated by gene expression, particularly by Bcl-2 and Bcl-xL, which are anti-apoptotic and make it more difficult to open the pore. BAX, which is a pro-apoptotic protein, promotes opening of the pore. It has been shown that cytochrome c, which is bound to the outer part of the inner mitochondrial membrane, is released when the permeability transition pore forms and activates caspase 3, leading to apoptosis. Apoptosis then can be triggered by mitochondria, in particular by mitochondrial depolarization.

Professor Choi addressed apoptosis vs necrosis and stated that the distinction between apoptotic and necrotic death is very important because they are counteracted by different maneuvers. For instance, caspase inhibition is likely to be good for

Maturation Phenomenon in Cerebral Ischemia III
U. Ito et al. (Eds.)
© Springer-Verlag Berlin Heidelberg 1999

stopping apoptosis and glutamate receptor blockers are indicated if a cell is dying because of excitotoxicity. In addition, Professor Choi suggested that factors operating in the ischemic brain actually might affect apoptotic and necrotic cell death in opposite directions. For instance, growth factors tend to prevent programmed cell death, but have in many cases a remarkably potentiating effect on excitotoxic cell death. Calcium is another example. Excessively high levels of intracellular calcium are associated with necrosis, but raising intracellular calcium toward an optimal point can actually attenuate programmed cell death. Although the distinction between apoptosis and necrosis is critically dependent on morphology at present, ultimately there needs to be a molecular definition of apoptosis. Failure to redefine the term restricts our use of it to very clear extreme examples. Professor Hossmann maintained that separation of ischemic cell death mechanisms does not just involve a distinction between apoptosis and necrosis. Different types of ischemia lead to different forms of injury. An oxidative stress response can lead to mitochondrial damage and opening of mitochondrial transition pores and a signal cascade of events leading to apoptosis. This is most evident in brief global ischemia models and transient focal ischemia models with selective vulnerability. Mechanisms are probably different in prolonged reduction of cerebral blood flow in the penumbra of a focal ischemic lesion. Cardiac arrest may also have a different pathophysiology, and these varying mechanisms may respond to different kinds of drugs. Professor Hossmann also felt that Professor Spatz's demonstration that hippocampal delayed selective neuronal injury can be prevented by an ETA antagonist (which reduces hemodynamic compromise) expands our concept of the mechanisms involved in delayed neuronal death following brief global ischemia. He also proposed that although the signal cascade in models of transient focal ischemia and selective vulnerability following global ischemia is very interesting, it may have little clinical relevance. These studies may be out of focus with respect to stroke or irreversible brain death after cardiac arrest.

Professor Baethamm then asked what is the point of no return in ischemic brain damage. He emphasized the need for a quantitative endpoint. Professor Klatzo stated that we are dealing with a threshold phenomenon. In CA1 neurons which stain for apoptosis, signs of necrosis can also be identified. Professor Choi agreed that there can be mixed complexes between necrotic and apoptotic pathways. A cell can be predestined to undergo programmed cell death but encounter conditions that divert it to a necrotic pathway. Even if apoptosis is blocked, such a cell would not survive. He observed that at the cell biological level, the treatment windows are expanding as we gain more knowledge about the internal pathways of cell death. Professor Ito asserted that from a clinical point of view, ischemic injury is not a complex of different processes, but is instead a continuum. Beyond a threshold there is a continuum that leads from selective neuronal necrosis to infarction. During selective neuronal necrosis, revascularization is possible and effective for some patients even up to 12 h after the ictus, but after this time infarction evolves. Professor Ito maintained that it is important to find a way to prolong the phase of selective neuronal necrosis without evolving infarction in order to extend the period during which patients can be revascularized to prevent infarction. Professor Bazan also agreed that the definition of the point of no return is a very important issue. He stated that there are a series of physiological components in the brain that are critical for plasticity and repair on the one hand and for damage on the other. The point of no return may be reached when a series of messengers and genes that are physiological go beyond a certain threshold. It may be possible to explore this further by studying the dual-type mediators that are especially prominent in neurons. Professor Bazan also thought that people can be somewhat obsessive about trying to distinguish between apoptosis and necrosis. TUNEL staining demonstrates DNA damage and it does not matter whether the cell is going to die by apoptosis or necrosis. What is clear is that DNA has been damaged and it would be important to learn more about DNA repair mechanisms. Professor Bazan also observed that several enzyme exist within the brain that are known to repair damaged proteins and do not require proteolysis and re-synthesis of the protein. There is, for example, a reductase that is very efficient in reducing disulfide groups and preventing the active sites of proteins from being denatured so that proteins can survive oxidative stress. Professor Bazan also mentioned that it is important to develop an understanding of the compartmentalization within neurons rather than to consider the interior of the cell a uniform microenvironment. Professor Siesjö asserted that in necrosis, breakage of the cell membrane or the mitochondrial membrane is the point of no return and that this has been a long-standing view. Under circumstances in which the cellular membranes are intact, the point of no return is determined by DNA damage that cannot be repaired.

According to Professor John, there is a tendency to look at individual cell types in the brain as if they were separate and unrelated rather than considering neurons, glia and other brain cells as constituting a very interactive system. In addition, connections between cells and the extracellular matrix and the intracellular matrix can be involved in signaling and can play a critical role in determining the survival and communication between cells. Professor John further suggested that discussion of whether a cell is necrotic or apoptotic doesn't really address the question of functional activity and recovery of the brain. It is more important to look at the gestalt, the system that involves interaction between all of the cells and the extracellular space. Furthermore, it is important to distinguish between protection and rescue. One can protect tissue from ischemia only when the ischemia can be anticipated, such as after cardiac bypass, but normally it is necessary to rescue tissue from unanticipated ischemia. During rescue it would be very helpful to have a surrogate marker to guide therapy and provide an endpoint for how much of a therapeutic agent to give and how long it must be given. Professor Krieglstein observed that there had been considerable discussion about the mechanisms of neural degeneration and that endogenous neuroprotection should also be discussed. Short ischemic periods may be neuroprotective and offer the possibility that endogenous neuroprotective mechanisms could be adapted for therapy. Activation of astrocytes, for example, might be beneficial. Professor Hossmann then affirmed that when DNA damage cannot be repaired the cell is going to die. It would be important to know how late the function of the cell can be restored after blood flow has stopped or, in other words, how long cells can be exposed to ischemia and still be rescued. Tissue can have identifiable markers of damage such as very low pH or very high lactate and still be rescued. One relevant question is how long thrombolysis can be delayed. Professor Bazan suggested that there are DNA repair enzymes that can reverse some of the changes and these questions will be addressed to some degree by papers that are in press at present. Professor Choi indicated that although it is valuable to identify system failure such as breakdown of DNA, it is still important to identify the overall envelope process. In this regard he disagreed with Professor Hossmann's perspective. Professor Hossmann responded that he agreed with that point and he stated that we are looking for a quantitative measure to indicate whether tissue is dead or not. On another subject he wondered why we have not yet started to test hypothermia in clinical trials for stroke and cardiac arrest. Hypothermia can be induced in humans and it is effective in models. Professor Kearney then mentioned that tPA does not work very well at temperatures as little as 2–3 °C below normal. Professor Ito agreed that dropping temperature is very dangerous because coagulopathy and other derangements of metabolic homeostasis can occur. He thought ischemia should be treated at normal temperature as early as possible. He further suggested it might be possible to raise the threshold for developing infarction to higher levels by pharmacologic means. Professor Klatzo agreed that cells in the penumbra survive the ischemic insult but ventured that some of the neurons that survive may not the normal. They appear hypertrophic. He had seen cells of this sort in a cardiac arrest model in rats in which there was selective damage in the reticular nucleus of the thalamus. In the roughly 20 % surviving cells in this area, the processes can be seen to hypertrophy. Professor Klatzo also mentioned that inhibition of protein synthesis is probably important and it seems to precede morphological cell death. He wondered whether DNA damage or protein synthesis inhibition is the initiating factor for cell death. Professor Hossmann stated that inhibition of protein synthesis is a very good predictor of impending cell death. All types of ischemic injury are closely associated with inhibition of global protein synthesis. The question is whether it is a causal factor or not. Inhibition of protein synthesis can be reversed and does not always lead to cell death.

A point raised by Professor Bazan was that the study of induction of tolerance may reveal endogenous mechanisms of resistance to ischemia and this is an important area for future meetings to discuss. Studies of tolerance tend to be in young animals which would probably model stroke in teenagers, and this is a deficiency because most strokes occur in people who are 50 years old or older. Professor Johanson agreed with the latter point and observed that aged brain has a different response in terms of inflammatory mechanisms than the brain of younger individuals, particularly with respect to microglial activation. Professor LaManna mentioned that his group had performed cardiac arrest followed by resuscitation in 24- to 26-month-old rats and young rats. Sixty percent of the old rats and 90 % of the young rats could be resuscitated.

Attention was then directed to pathologic events in the presynaptic terminal by Professor LaManna. He mentioned that there are three to four mitochondria in each terminal that can become damaged and impair function during ischemia. Professor Bazan also felt that damage to terminal mitochondria might be an important target in ischemic damage and cited work by Professor Kogure's group on this problem. The concept that terminal mitochondria are a target in ischemia was further described by Professor Siesjö, who quoted work by Abe. The terminal mitochondria need to be transported back to the cell body in order to synthesize some essential proteins, particularly for complex IV.

During ischemia there is a breakdown of the cytoskeleton and damage to motor proteins such as kynesin such that the mitochondria cannot be transported in retrograde fashion. This was regarded as a very stimulating hypothesis of mitochondrial damage in ischemia. Professor Kuroiwa agreed that energy failure is the point of no return, but he did not think it would occur 4–5 h after recirculation. He also indicated that the paper by Abe dealt with neurons and the findings probably could not be applied to glia. Professor Siesjö responded that the mitochondrial dysfunction hypothesis involved delayed loss of energetic state in neurons primarily. There is a gradual calcium accumulation that may stop the function of mitochondria, damage them, and lead to a secondary deterioration of the energy state.

The current state of neuroprotection was summarized briefly by Professor Krieglstein. He observed that a variety of drugs such as calcium antagonists, NMDA antagonists, and free radical scavengers have been found to be effective in experimental animal models of ischemia, but have not provided a clinical breakthrough. This increases the attractiveness of an endogenous process that could be activated and protects cells. Professor Klatzo expanded the idea of endogenous protection by suggesting that there can be transneuronal induction of tolerance. His group has observed that ipsilateral MCA occlusion for a brief period or spreading depression can induce neuroprotection in the hippocampus of the contralateral hemisphere and this probably involves transneuronal signaling.

Professor Spatz raised the point that animal models do not generally take into account the fact that patients who develop stroke have changes in their vascular trees such as atherosclerosis. Another point is that progressive damage in ischemia is multifactorial and should be probably be treated by a combination of drugs that lead to vascular, glial and neuronal responses. The need for surrogate measures to predict outcome after interventions to treat stroke was highlighted by Professor Kearney. Clinicians need outcomes other than the pathologic determination of infarct volume that is so characteristic of experimental animal models of ischemia. It may not be possible in the end to compare therapeutic windows determined in rodents with those in humans because of the wide variability in the presentation of human stroke. Professor Buchan concluded that as the lessons from animal models are incorporated into clinical trials and control of temperature and dose of agent are optimized and patients are treated in an early phase, the results will be favorable, as demonstrated by the tPA trial. We now can resupply oxygen and glucose to the ischemic injury zone and this may increase the incidence of the maturation phenomenon, which will have to be managed with experimental drugs.

December, 1998   J. M. HALLENBECK
                                                                           F. ORZI
                                                                           U. ITO

Subject Index

Numbers indicate starting pages of where each subject included.

Springer
and the
environment

At Springer we firmly believe that an international science publisher has a special obligation to the environment, and our corporate policies consistently reflect this conviction.

We also expect our business partners – paper mills, printers, packaging manufacturers, etc. – to commit themselves to using materials and production processes that do not harm the environment. The paper in this book is made from low- or no-chlorine pulp and is acid free, in conformance with international standards for paper permanency.

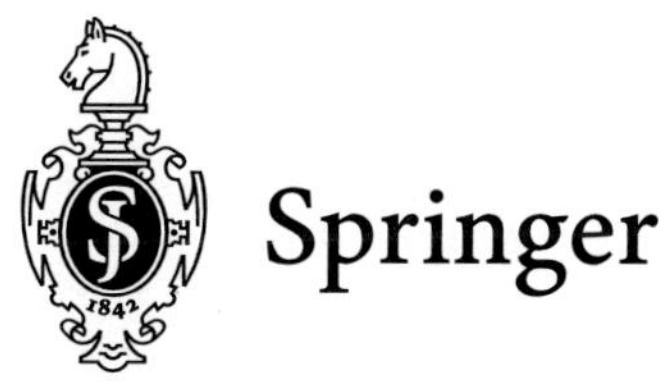

Computer to plate: Mercedes Druck, Berlin
Binding: Buchbinderei Lüderitz & Bauer, Berlin